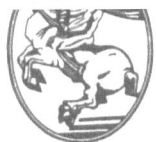

Topics in Infectious Diseases
Vol. 1

Drug Receptor Interactions in Antimicrobial Chemotherapy

Symposium, Vienna, September 4-6, 1974

Edited by
J. Drews and F. E. Hahn

Springer-Verlag
Wien   New York
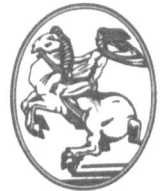

Drug Receptor Interactions
in Antimicrobial Chemotherapy

Sandoz-Symposium, Vienna, September 4—6, 1974

With 130 figures

Prof. Dr. Jürgen Drews
Sandoz Forschungsinstitut Gesellschaft m. b. H.
Vienna, Austria

Prof. Fred E. Hahn, Ph. D.
Walter Reed Army Medical Center
Washington, D.C., U.S.A.

ISBN-13:978-3-7091-8407-3   e-ISBN-13:978-3-7091-8405-9
DOI: 10.1007/978-3-7091-8405-9

Introduction

The concept of chemotherapy as originated by Paul Ehrlich is based
on the premise that antiparasitic drugs must have two properties:
they must first bind to specific structures of the parasite which
Ehrlich called chemoreceptors. Subsequent to their attachment to the
chemoreceptor and by virtue of this binding they must possess the
capacity to kill the parasite. Since the host which is to be cured
of an invading parasite also contains a large number of chemoreceptors,
that have the potential to bind toxic compounds, the task of the chemo-
therapist is to identify chemoreceptors of the parasite which are not
represented in the host and to design drugs which bind selectively to
them. In this context, Ehrlich called for "the complete and exhaustive
knowledge of all the different chemoreceptors of a certain parasite"
as a "*sine qua non* for success in chemotherapy".

Paradoxically and in spite of the fact that chemotherapy has become a
very advanced and successful therapeutic discipline, few of its tri-
umphs have been achieved by following Ehrlich's original precepts. On
the contrary, in the overwhelming majority of cases, effective drugs
have been discovered without any knowledge of their chemoreceptors,
and these drugs themselves have conversely been used as tools to study
the nature of the chemoreceptors involved. In other words: chemotherapy, notably antibacterial chemotherapy, has been successful without
ever living up to the fundamental standards put forward by Paul Ehrlich.

Two reasons should lead us to reassess the basic postulates of chemotherapy: the first one can be deduced from the present state of antimicrobial chemotherapy itself. Clearly, the rate of progress in this
area as judged by the number of genuinely novel drugs becoming available to the physician each year has slowed down. The rediscovery
problem in the search for new antibiotics and the paucity of known
biochemical differences between parasites and hosts which might be
exploited for the design of antimetabolites are contributory factors
to the decreasing rate of discovery of new chemotherapeutic drugs.
Moreover, the current situation is characterized by the appearance
of new problems such as multiple drug resistance of bacteria and the
increasing frequency of infections with gram-negative pathogens and
fungi as well as by the persistence of old problems best exemplified
by our distressing inability to make progress in the area of antiviral
chemotherapy.

The second, and more positive reason is that since the days of Paul
Ehrlich tremendous advances have been made in the fields of physical
chemistry, biochemistry, biophysics, genetics and molecular biology.
Studies on the molecular structure of drug-receptors and on the interaction of such receptors with antimicrobial compounds should, therefore, have a distinctly better chance of success today than they had

sixty years ago when their necessity was first recognized. While during the first decades following Ehrlich's death (1915) chemotherapy research was constrained to use empirical search and development procedures, we feel that with the current state of the art the field can no longer afford the luxury of unguided empiricism; the time has arrived to apply the knowledge of principles and mechanisms of drug action which has been gained during three decades of intensive research to premediated efforts to develop novel chemotherapeutic agents.

It is for these reasons that the Sandoz Research Institute decided to ask a number of scientists well known for their work in areas such as structure-activity relationships, structure and function of plasmid DNA, bacterial protein biosynthesis and bacterial enzymes to reassess their own work in the context of its possible applicability to the search for new antimicrobial drugs or to the improvement of already existing compounds. In selecting the general topics for our symposium on drug-receptor interactions in antimicrobial chemotherapy we were led by the intention to include only such areas of research which had already contributed to the generation of novel chemotherapeutic agents or in which relevant practical contributions towards this goal could be expected in the forseeable future. We believe that the general subjects, microbial enzymes as drug-receptors, ribosomes as drug-receptors, DNA as drug-receptors and, last but not least, a general consideration of the receptor hypothesis, satisfy these criteria.

The proceedings of this symposium are not meant to compete with more systematic texts on molecular aspects of chemotherapy or pharmacology. The exciting responses of basic scientists to the challenges and problems of drug therapy and drug development were revealed during this symposium. We hope that some of this excitement will be conveyed to the readers of this volume.

J. Drews   F.E. Hahn
Vienna   Washington

February 1975

Contents

I. Receptor Hypothesis

Structure-Activity Rules and the Receptor Hypothesis
Fred E. Hahn

I. INTRODUCTION

Chemotherapy as a science began with the postulation of the receptor hypothesis by Paul Ehrlich. His famous doctrine, corpora non agunt nisi fixata, substances do not act unless they are bound, should perhaps today be rephrased to say, corpora agunt quia fixata, substances do act because they are bound. Through much of his scientific life, Ehrlich propounded his embattled side chain theory in order to explain the interaction of chemotherapeutic drugs with bioreceptors which were still hypothetical. Ehrlich's early observations of vital staining offered the first visible evidence of selective binding of chemicals to bioreceptors, and his demonstration, in 1891 (Guttmann and Ehrlich, 1891), of the therapeutic value of methylene blue in the treatment of vivax malaria was directly based upon the selective staining properties of this dye for malarial parasites.

Today, the receptor hypothesis has an established place in the molecular pharmacology of antimicrobial drugs. The identification of receptors to which drugs bind is an integral part of any research effort toward the explanation of mechanisms of action of drugs at the molecular level. With the introduction of antimetabolite hypothesis (Fildes, 1940) as well as with the recognition of double-helical DNA as one structurally well-known drug receptor (Lerman, 1963; Hahn, rev. 1971), knowledge of receptors also has become important to drug design. Furthermore, the analysis of structure-activity relationships must differentiate between structural contributions to permeability and electronic and steric contributions to primary drug action. These last two parameters are directly related to drug binding to complementary receptor sites.

II. DERIVATION OF RECEPTOR BINDING FROM DOSAGE-RESPONSE CORRELATIONS

Let us assume that a drug A binds to a receptor P in a reversible manner, obeying the law of mass action. Then it follows that the product of the molar concentrations of the receptor (P) and of the drug (X_A) divided by the molar concentration of the receptor-drug complex (PX_A) equals an equilibrium constant K_A, as shown in equation (I).

$$\frac{(P)\,(X_A)}{(PX_A)} = K_A \qquad\qquad (I)$$

If we now consider (P_T) the total receptor concentration and (PX_A) the concentration of receptor to which the drug A is bound, it follows that the difference $(P_T - PX_A)$ represents the concentration of free receptor. Substituting this into equation (I) one obtains equation (II).

$$\frac{(P_T - PX_A)\,(X_A)}{(PX_A)} = K_A \qquad\qquad (II)$$

which can be rearranged into equation (III)

$$\frac{(PX_A)}{(P_T)} = \frac{(X_A)}{K_A + (X_A)} \qquad\qquad (III)$$

When the concentration (PX_A) of the receptor-drug complex is isolated one obtains equation (IV)

$$(PX_A) = \frac{(P_T)\,(X_A)}{K_A + (X_A)} \qquad\qquad (IV)$$

This is the familiar Langmuir adsorption isotherm in which the concentration of the complex equals zero for drug concentration zero and approaches the total receptor concentration (P_T) when the drug concentration (X_A) becomes very large.

If one then makes the assumption that quantified biological responses to graded concentrations of a drug are proportional to the fractions of the receptor occupied by the drug, a plot of the dosage-response correlation should obey equation (IV).

For example, in 1956 we published precise dosage-response determinations of the decreases of growth rates of Escherichia coli by graded concentrations of chloramphenicol (Hopps, Wisseman, Hahn, Smadel and Ho, 1956). At that time, we only knew that the antibiotic was bacteriostatic, i.e. that its antibacterial action was reversible, and that chloramphenicol was a specific inhibitor of protein biosynthesis. But neither transfer RNA, nor ribosomes, nor messenger RNA, nor incorporation factors had been discovered, and the mechanism of protein biosynthesis was still a typical "black box problem" in which one can measure input and output but does not know the mechanics inside the box.

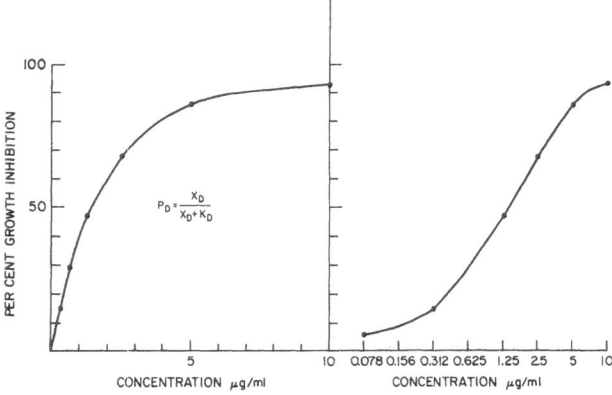

Fig. 1. Dosage-response correlation for inhibition of growth of Escherichia coli C2 by chloramphenicol.

Fig. 1 from these growth-inhibition experiments shows, at left, a dosage-response correlation for chloramphenicol; it has the shape of an hyperbolic adsorption isotherm. Usually one transforms such a curve by entering on the abscissa the logarithm of drug concentration. This is shown at right and results in a sigmoid curve with a linear portion which is grouped symmetrically around the fifty per cent inhibitory concentration.

A further transformation substitutes a probability term, the probit of the response, for the per cent response data. Instead of entering the per cent response on the ordinate, each percentage is converted to a normal equivalent deviation, i.e. to the corresponding multiple of the standard deviation. This cumulative Gaussian distribution assumes the form of a straight line throughout the entire dosage-response range. In order to avoid the use of negative numbers, the integer 5 is added to each normal equivalent deviation, i.e. the probit is this deviation plus 5.

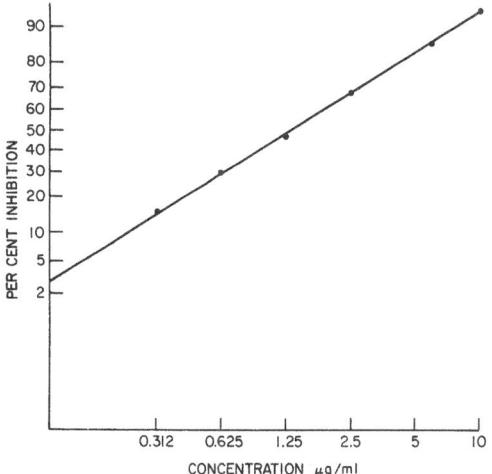

Fig. 2. Probit transformation of data from Fig. 1.

Fig. 2 shows a graphic probit transformation of the dosage-response data for chloramphenicol. The linearity of this plot proves that one is dealing, indeed, with a typical dosage-response correlation which obeys equation (IV) and permits one to fit the best line by the method of least squares and, thus, to obtain a precise measure of growth inhibition.

Let us now remember the basic assumption that the measured response is proportional to the extent of receptor occupancy by the drug. This can be tested by drawing the Hill plot, a double-logarithmic diagram in which each fractional response is entered as a function of the drug concentration. The Hill equation is a general form of equation (IV) of the adsorption isotherm. If one substitutes the response E for the concentration of bound drug (PX_A) and the maximally possible response E_{max} for the total receptor concentration (P_T) one obtains equation (V)

$$E = \frac{E_{max} \; X_A^{nh}}{K_A + X_A^{nh}} \qquad (V)$$

In this, the exponent nh is a constant, known as the Hill constant. It is apparent that for nh = 1, equation (V) reverts to the special form of the adsorption isotherm, equation (IV).

In order to draw the Hill plot, equation (V) is rearranged into equation (VI)

$$\log \frac{E}{E_{max} - E} = nh \log (X_A) + \log K_A \qquad (VI)$$

so that a linear regression of log $E/E-E_{max}$ on log (X_A) allows the slope, nh, to be determined. For nh = 1, the slope of the regression line is unity, meaning that the actual drug concentration (X_A) and not some function $(X_A)^{nh}$ of it is the determinant of the response.

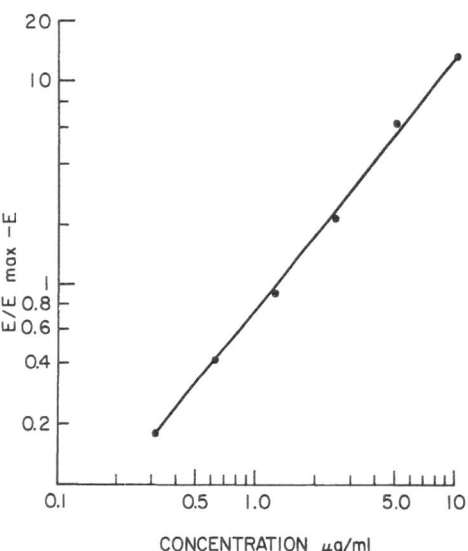

Fig. 3. Hill plot of data from Fig. 1.

Fig. 3 shows the Hill plot of the dosage-response data for chloramphenicol. The plot is, indeed, linear and has a slope of 1.16, i.e. close to unity. This means that the growth-inhibitory action of chloramphenicol is proportional to the occupancy of a receptor by one drug molecule and that one does not need to invoke allosteric effects or simultaneous binding of more than one drug molecule in order to explain the antibacterial action. Only much later was it found (Wolfe and Hahn, 1965) that, indeed, one molecule of chloramphenicol binds per 70s ribosome and also per isolated 50s ribosomal subunit (Nierhaus and Nierhaus, 1973).

I have deliberately gone through the handling of old data from a point in time at which neither the mechanism of protein biosynthesis nor the mechanism of action of chloramphenicol were known, in order to show that proof of the existence of a drug receptor and of microbiological effects resulting from receptor occupancy by a drug can be obtained from dosage-response data in abstraction, i.e. in the complete absence of biochemical information on the action of the drug or on the nature of its receptor. It is surprising that these procedures of data handling and the conclusions which can be drawn from their outcome have not seen much use in the study of antimicrobial drugs although they are well-established methods in pharmacology.

III. DNA AS A DRUG RECEPTOR

In considering the relationship of structure-activity rules to the receptor hypothesis, the most instructive drug receptor is double-helical DNA. Twenty five years ago, Albert and his associates (Albert, Rubbo and Burvill, 1949) established empirial rules for the structures of N-heterocyclic amines to possess antibacterial activity. Only after the macromolecular architecture of the double helix (Watson and Crick, 1953) became known, and the intercalation theory (rev. Lerman, 1964) was established, could one rationalize Albert's rules to be those for intercalation binding into the double helix. The first of these rules specifies that N-heterocyclic amines must possess a flat surface of minimally 28 $Å^2$. Planarity is one requirement for intercalation binding which must fit compounds into a slot not wider than 3.4 Å, and the total surface of an intercalant must be in a commensurate size relationship to the planar area of one base pair which approximates 40 $Å^2$. This appears to be necessary in order for van der Waals forces to hold an intercalated ring system in place.

The second rule of Albert specifies a requirement for amino groups to be ionized to more than 50 per cent at physiological pH levels. This is necessary for providing electrostatic attraction between these protonated centers and phosphoric acid groups in the sugar-phosphate backbones of the double helix. Since neither the double helix structure nor intercalation binding were known at the time of the postulation of these rules, no stereoelectronic requirements were specified, i.e. no thought was given to the optimal spatial separation of protonated centers.

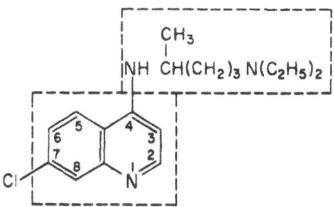

Fig. 4. Structure of antimalarial drug chloroquine.

This came into play from 1964 in our studies of the mechanism of action of the antimalarial drug chloroquine, Fig. 4. The two positive charges of the side chain are separated by a 4-carbon interval which provides the optimal distance to bridge the minor groove of DNA between phosphates of the two complementary strands. Fig. 5 shows the relative antimalarial activity of a series of chloroquine derivatives with variations in the interval between the two amino groups; this illustrates that a charge separation by a 4-carbon chain is, indeed, optimal (Hahn, O'Brien, Ciak, Allison and Olenick, 1966).

Knowledge of structure-activity rules for intercalation binding to DNA are developed to an extent that examination of structures of biologically active compounds can suggest that they bind to DNA in this manner and that even biological activity itself can be predicted as, for example, the ability of substances to eliminate bacterial plasmids (Hahn and Ciak, this volume).

Binding of drugs to DNA has been studied by a variety of biophysical methods. A given quantity of DNA can, for example, be titrated, usually spectrophotometrically, by graded concentrations of an intercalative drug. When the binding is reversible and obeys the law of mass action, the results

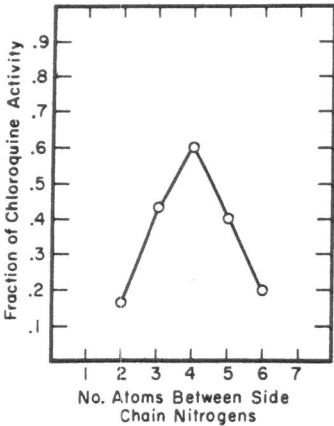

Fig. 5. Influence of charge separation in the side chain on antimalarial activity of chloroquine.

of such titration experiments can be expressed in a special form of the adsorption isotherm, known as the Scatchard plot. For this, we return to equation (II) which can be inverted into equation (VII).

$$\frac{(PX_A)}{(P_T - PX_A)(X_A)} = \frac{1}{K_A} \qquad (VII)$$

Expressing $\dfrac{1}{K_A}$ as an association constant k and isolating the term $\dfrac{PX_A}{X_A}$ i.e. the ratio of bound drug over free drug, one obtains

$$\frac{PX_A}{X_A} = kP_T - kPX_A \qquad (VIII)$$

For one binding process with one binding constant, the plot of the ratio of bound over free drug as a function of the amount of drug bound yields a straight line as, for example, in the binding of ethidium bromide to DNA at high inorganic ion concentrations. Usually, however, one obtains non-linear Scatchard plots.

Fig. 6 shows such a curve for the titration of calf-thymus DNA with quinacrine (Krey and Hahn, 1974). Extrapolation to the axes of the coordinate system yields for low concentrations of bound drug, i.e. for strong binding, a stoichiometry of one molecule of quinacrine per approximately four nucleotides with an apparent association constant of 1.2×10^6 M^{-1} and for a weaker process at high concentrations of bound drug a stoichiometry of one additional quinacrine molecule per 3 nucleotides with an apparent association constant of 4.6×10^4 M^{-1}. The stronger process is intercalation binding (Lerman, 1963) and the weaker process probably electrostatic binding to the outside of the helix.

A description of DNA binding in terms of only two classes of binding sites, however, is an evident oversimplification. Firstly, it assumes an independent site model in which partial occupancy of receptor sites does not change the binding properties of still vacant sites. Additionally, it is known for quinacrine and also for proflavine that not all intercalation spaces

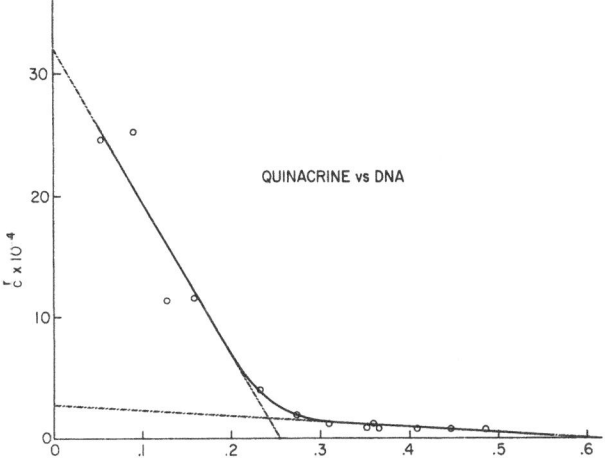

Fig. 6. Scatchard plot from spectrophotometric titration of quinacrine with
          calf-thymus DNA.

in DNA are equivalent. Both drugs have a greater affinity for binding regions
which consist of several AT-pairs (Thomas, Weill and Daune, 1969; Pachmann and
Rigler, 1972; Krey and Hahn, 1974).

     Even with such partially unresolved microheterogeneity of binding sites in
DNA, the consideration of the double helix as a drug receptor is revealing not
only because the structures of the receptor and of the drugs which interact
with it present a complementary and coherent relationship but also because the
biological function of DNA is understood. The polymer serves as a template for
its own semi-conservative replication as well as for the transcription of RNA.
The biochemical effect of DNA-binding drugs is one of template toxicity, i.e.
they inhibit DNA and RNA biosyntheses.

     Template toxicity for DNA is also exhibited by drugs which bind to DNA in
a non-intercalative manner for which the structural relationship to DNA is less
clear. The trypanocidal drug berenil (Newton and LePage, 1967; Newton, 1967)
and the antiviral antibiotics distamycin A and netropsin (rev. Hahn, 1974)
bind to DNA with preference for AT-pairs, and the mitomycins (Szybalski and
Iyer, 1967) which are converted by reduction into reactive metabolites of short
half-life form, in this condition, covalent bonds with DNA with preference for
GC-pairs.

IV. PROTEINS AS DRUG RECEPTORS

     Receptor sites for most chemotherapeutic drugs, however, are on proteins,
i.e. either on enzymes or on ribosomal proteins. Unlike for DNA, there exist
no general structure-activity rules for protein-binding drugs since proteins
do not possess a uniform macromolecular architecture in the sense that drug
molecules could address themselves to general protein features. Each drug-
receptor relationship becomes, therefore, a special case onto itself. Also,
while binding of drugs to DNA, despite variations in stoichiometry, always
involves a multiplicity of drug molecules, proteins usually contain only one
receptor site for a drug.

Relatively advanced knowledge of drug receptors of protein molecules exists in the area of antimetabolites, i.e. in those instances in which a drug is a structural analog and functional antagonist of, or substitute for, a natural enzyme substrate. Some inferences concerning the structure of the receptor site can be drawn from the substrate range of an enzyme, and among structure-activity rules will be those which are empirically employed in the design of antimetabolites. One can define three general principles of molecular modifications which convert metabolites into antimetabolites. The first of these is isosteric substitution, the second is introduction of sterically hindering substituents such as methyl, and the third principle is ring closure in aliphatic chains of which we will encounter one example in this lecture.

An antimetabolic drug which binds to the substrate receptor of an enzyme competes with the substrate for this site and, hence, exhibits functionally the phenomenon of competitive inhibition. For a theoretical consideration of this we return to equation (IV). If one postulates that the binding of a substrate S to the receptor P produces a proportional biochemical response E, usually a reaction velocity, and that the maximal response E_{max} is produced when the total receptor concentration P_T is occupied by the substrate, substitution of these terms into equation (IV) yields equation (IX).

$$E = \frac{E_{max} (X_S)}{K_S + (X_S)} \tag{IX}$$

This can be inverted into its reciprocal form (X).

$$\frac{1}{E} = \frac{K_S}{E_{max}} \cdot \frac{1}{(X_S)} + \frac{1}{E_{max}} \tag{X}$$

The equation is one of a straight line in which K_S/E_{max} is the slope and $1/E_{max}$ is the intercept when $1/E$ is plotted as a function of $1/(X_S)$. This yields the classical double-reciprocal plot.

For competitive antagonism, uncombined receptor (P) will be in simultaneous equilibria with the receptor-substrate complex (PX_S) and the receptor-drug complex (PX_A) with equilibrium constants K_S and K_A. For this situation mixed equations can be written which solve to yield (XI).

$$\frac{1}{E'} = \left(1 + \frac{(X_A)}{K_A}\right)\left(\frac{K_S}{E_{max}}\right)\left(\frac{1}{(X_S)}\right) + \frac{1}{E_{max}} \tag{XI}$$

In this equation for the inhibited response E', the y intercept $1/E_{max}$ is unchanged but the slope is increased by the factor $1 + \dfrac{(X_A)}{K_A}$.

Hence, whenever a double-reciprocal plot for the non-inhibited and inhibited reactions yields straight lines with different slopes but passing through the same y-intercept, this is considered experimental evidence for competitive inhibition.

Let us examine examples of this. The antibiotic D-cycloserine or oxamycin (Fig. 7) is a structural analog of D-alanine. We discovered (Ciak and Hahn, 1958) that cycloserine is bactericidal because it inhibits the biosynthesis of the cell-wall polymer and we predicted that this effect was a result of D-alanine antagonism. Since Jack Strominger was investigating the enzymology of cell-wall biosynthesis, I suggested to him to study the action of cycloserine.

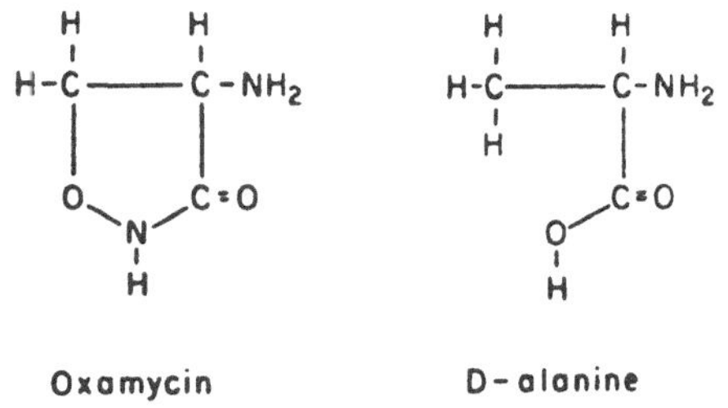

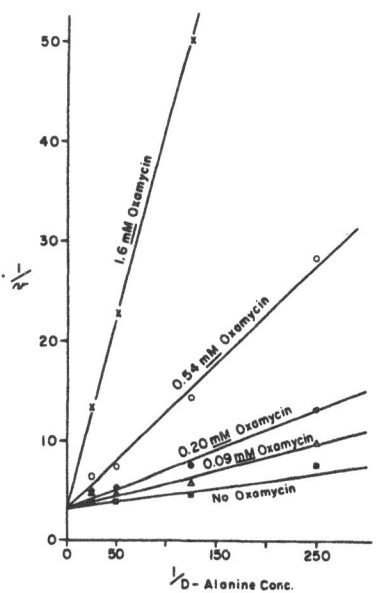

Oxamycin   D-alanine

Fig. 7.   Structures of oxamycin (cycloserine) and D-alanine.

        Fig. 8 shows Strominger's (1960) double-reciprocal plot for the effect
of cycloserine on alanine racemase, i.e. the enzyme which interconverts L-
and D-alanines.   This reaction is inhibited by cycloserine in competition with
D-alanine.   The next step in the pathway of peptidoglycan synthesis is the

Fig. 8.   Competitive inhibition of alanine racemase by oxamycin (cycloserine).

formation of D-alanyl-D-alanine. Fig. 9, again from Strominger (1960),
indicates that this reaction is also inhibited by cycloserine in competition
with D-alanine.   By substitution of his experimental data into the appropriate
equations, Strominger calculated that the binding of cycloserine to each of the
two enzymes is 100 times stronger than the binding of D-alanine.

        Beyond exemplifying competitive inhibitions of enzyme reactions by an
antimetabolite, the cycloserine case deserves additional comment. Inhibition of
sequential reaction steps in the same metabolic pathway produces potentiation
of the individual inhibitory actions. Cycloserine mimics, therefore, the
combined effects of two different drugs which act on different reaction steps
of the same pathway.   The greater affinity of cycloserine for the two enzymes as

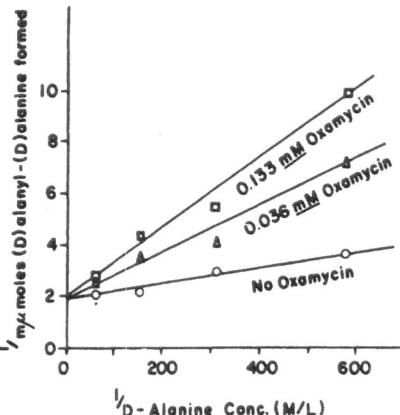

Fig. 9. Competitive inhibition of D-alanyl-D-alanine synthetase by oxamycin (cycloserine).

compared to that of the natural metabolite favors competition. Most anti-metabolites are poor drugs because they have no greater affinity for the respective enzyme than the natural enzyme substrate. In fact, one of the unsolved problems in the design of antimetabolites is to project compounds which are not merely antimetabolic on structural grounds but will bind to the enzyme more strongly than the natural substrate with which they must compete. In the case of cycloserine, this task has been solved by cyclization of the side chain of D-alanine which evidently stabilizes a structure which is preferred by the alanine receptor sites of enzymes.

A special case of antimetabolism is one in which an analog resembles the natural metabolite so closely that it is processed by the enzyme in lieu of its substrate. This is called fraudulent biosynthesis and leads to metabolic products of impaired or of no biochemical functionality. Among antimicrobial drugs, one example of this is the thymidine analog 5-iodo-2'-deoxyuridine, in which the methyl group of thymine is replaced by an iodine atom. This drug is used in the treatment of eye infections with herpes virus and has been shown to be vicariously incorporated into viral DNA (Prusoff, Bakhle and McCrae, 1963). Another example is puromycin which is processed by the ribosomal enzyme, peptidyl transferase and serves as a generalized acceptor of the peptidyl residue in peptide bond synthesis. Peptide elongation breaks off at this point because peptidyl puromycin does not remain bound to the ribosome (Nathans, 1964).

With this we have arrived at a consideration of ribosomal proteins as drug receptors. Aminoglycosides, tetracyclines, chloramphenicol, macrolides and many other antibiotic inhibitors of protein synthesis bind to ribosomes. However, neither the structures nor the functions of ribosomal proteins are sufficiently known for a definitive analysis of drug-receptor interactions. In no instance has an isolated protein of ribosomal origin been shown to have independent biochemical activity or to bind a drug.

V. MEMBRANES AS DRUG RECEPTORS

When it finally comes to chemotherapeutic drugs whose receptors are in membranes, we are in a still more difficult position since the biochemical inventory of membrane constituents is not yet developed to the completeness to which we know the constituents of ribosomes. Bacitracin, tyrocidins, gramicidins and polyene antibiotics act on microbial membranes and increase their permeability, and for polymyxin, membrane binding in vivo of a fluorescent derivative of the antibiotic has been demonstrated by fluorescence microscopy (Newton, 1955).

VI. CONCLUSION

It has been the purpose of this introduction to present selected examples of theory and knowledge of drug receptors and of their interaction with drugs in the field of antimicrobial chemotherapy. From this, I hope it has become apparent that the receptor theory is well developed, at least in certain areas, and has a demonstrable relationship to structure-activity relationships. This will become even more apparent during the course of our Symposium. It also is evident that there still exist large areas of incomplete knowledge. This is especially the case when drug receptors are on biopolymers which are constituents of large and complicated organelles such as ribosomes or membranes and in which drug binding and structure-activity relationships can only be studied with intact organelles or organisms but not with isolated macromolecules of defined structure and function. To the extent that antimicrobial drug design presupposes some knowledge of drug receptors, it remains limited to DNA-binding compounds and to antimetabolites.

REFERENCES

Albert, A., S.D. Rubbo and M.I. Burvill: The influence of chemical constitution on antibacterial activity. Part IV: A survey of heterocyclic bases with special reference to benzquinolines, phenanthridines, benzacridines, quinolines and pyridines. Brit. J. Exp. Path. 30, 159 (1949).

Ciak, J. and F.E. Hahn: Mechanisms of action of antibiotics. II. Studies on the modes of action of cycloserine and its L-stereoisomer. Antibiotics & Chemother. 9, 47 (1958).

Fildes, P. and M.B. Camb: A rational approach to research in chemotherapy. Lancet 1, 955 (1940).

Guttmann, P. and P. Ehrlich: Über die Wirkung des Methylenblau bei Malaria. Berl. Klin. Wochenschr. 28, 953 (1891).

Hahn, F.E.: Complexes of biologically active substances with nucleic acids - yesterday, today, tomorrow. Progr. Mol. Subcell. Biol. 2, 1 (1971) Springer, Berlin-Heidelberg-New York.

Hahn, F.E.: Distamycin A and Netropsin. In Antibiotics III. J. Corcoran and F.E. Hahn edts. Springer, Berlin-Heidelberg-New York, 1974, p 79.

Hahn, F.E., R.L. O'Brien, J. Ciak, J.L. Allison and J.G. Olenick: Studies on modes of action of chloroquine, quinacrine and quinine and on chloroquine resistance. Military Med. 131, 1071 (1966).

Hopps, H.E., C.L. Wisseman, F.E. Hahn, J.E. Smadel and R. Ho: Mode of action of chloramphenicol. IV. Failure of selected natural metabolites to reverse antibiotic action. J. Bact. 72, 561 (1956).

Krey, A.K. and F.E. Hahn: Optical studies on the interaction of DL-quinacrine with double- and single-stranded calf thymus DNA. Molecular Pharmacol. 10, in press (1974).

Lerman, L.S.: The structure of the DNA-acridine complex. Proc. Nat. Acad. Sci. USA 49, 94 (1963).

Lerman, L.S.: Acridine mutagens and DNA structure. J. Cell. Comp. Physiol. 64, Suppl 1, 1 (1964).

Nathans, D.: Puromycin inhibition of protein synthesis: The incorporation of puromycin into peptide chains. Proc. Nat. Acad. Sci. USA 51, 585 (1964).

Newton, B.A.: A fluorescent derivative of polymyxin: Its preparation and use in studying the site of action of the antibiotic. J. Gen. Microbiol. 12, 226 (1955).

Newton, B.A.: Interaction of berenil with deoxyribonucleic acid and some characteristics of the berenil-deoxyribonucleic acid complex. Biochem. J. 105, 50 p (1967).

Newton, B.A. and R.W.F. LePage: Preferential inhibition of extranuclear deoxyribonucleic acid synthesis by the trypanocide berenil. Biochem. J. 105, 50 p (1967).

Nierhaus, D. and K.H. Nierhaus: Identification of chloramphenicol-binding protein in Escherichia coli ribosomes by partial reconstitution. Proc. Nat. Acad. Sci. USA 70, 2224 (1973).

Pachmann, U. and R. Rigler: Quantum yield of acridines interacting with DNA of defined base sequence. Expt. Cell Res. 72, 602 (1972).

Prusoff, W.H., Y.S. Bakhle and J.F. McCrea: Incorporation of 5-iodo-2'-deoxy-uridine into the deoxyribonucleic acid of vaccinia virus. Nature 199, 1310 (1963).

Strominger, J.L.: Antibiotics as inhibitors of bacterial cell-wall synthesis. Antimicrobial Agents Annual 1960, 328 (1961).

Szybalski, W. and V.N. Iyer: The mitomycins and porfiromycins. In Antibiotics I, D. Gottlieb and P.D. Shaw edts. Springer, Berlin-Heidelberg-New York, 1967, p 211.

Thomas, J.C., G. Weill and M. Daune: Fluorescence of proflavine-DNA complexes: Heterogeneity of binding sites. Biopolymers 8, 647 (1969).

Watson, J.D. and F.H.C. Crick: The structure of DNA. Cold Spring Harb. Symp. Quant. Biol. 18, 123 (1953).

Wolfe, A.D. and F.E. Hahn: Mode of action of chloramphenicol. IX. Effects of chloramphenicol upon a ribosomal amino acid polymerization system and its binding to bacterial ribosomes. Biochim. Biophys. Acta 95, 146 (1965).

Strategy of Drug-Design
William P. Purcell

I.   Introduction

Beginnings in quantitative structure-activity relationship (QSAR) studies were made about twenty years ago (Bruice *et al.*, 1956) but only in the last ten years (Hansch and Fujita, 1964; Free and Wilson, 1964) has this powerful methodology been widely applied. The realization that long waiting periods necessary for pharmacological and clinical testing along with the tremendous costs associated with synthesis have "forced" the discovery of techniques that would increase the probability of selecting useful compounds for synthesis and evaluation. When one considers that it costs about $2,000 per compound for synthesis and about $10,000,000 and 10 years to bring a new drug to the market, one must search for more effective ways to select molecules for synthesis and evaluation. QSAR techniques, while not a panacea, are now being used successfully to reach target molecules faster and at less expense. Those using QSAR thoughtfully recognize them as another tool in our background of knowledge much the way an organic chemist uses the tools of infrared and nmr in addition to elemental analysis in compound identification. QSAR should not replace existing experiences in drug design, but it should be added to them (Purcell, 1973).

As testimony to the possible success of the QSAR methodology, two examples of such applications will be presented here along with a citation to the successful prediction of the biochemical activity of a compound three years prior to its synthesis.

II.   Example: Interpretation of Antimalarial Activity

QSAR techniques were used to test a model (O'Brien and Hahn, 1965) to account for the antimalarial activity of chloroquine and its congeners (Bass *et al.*, 1971). The model proposed that (a) these compounds act as antimalarials by intercalating with the parasite DNA and that the activity is a function of the stability of this complex, (b) good activity requires an electronegative group attached to position 7 of the quinoline ring, and (c) the diamino side chain bridges the two DNA strands by electrostatic interactions between the diamino nitrogens and the DNA phosphate groups.

In order to test this model, a free-energy related expression, Eq. 1, was chosen. A is the relative antimalarial activity against

$$A = a\pi^2 + b\pi + cQ_x + dQ_{N_4} + eQ_{N_t} + f \qquad (1)$$

2

Plasmodium gallinaceum (O'Brien and Hahn, 1965), π is the octanol/water partition coefficient substituent constant (Hansch and Fujita, 1964; Fujita *et al.*, 1964; Iwasa *et al.*, 1965; Hansch *et al.*, 1968; Hansch and Helmer, 1968; Helmer *et al.*, 1968; Leo *et al.*, 1969), Q_X, Q_{N_4}, and Q_{N_t} are the net charges (from combined Hückel and Del Re molecular orbital calculations) for the substituents at position 7, the nitrogen at position 4, and the terminal nitrogen of the diamino side chain, respectively (Bass *et al.*, 1971). The constants of the regression are a, b, c, d, e, and f.

The series of compounds studied are:

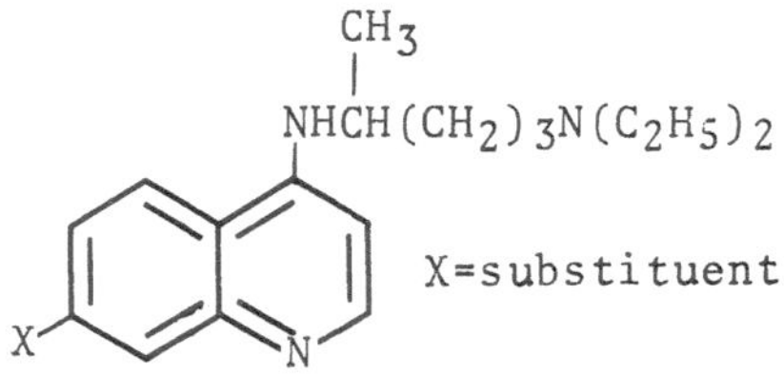

$$CH_3$$
$$|$$
$$NHCH(CH_2)_3N(C_2H_5)_2$$

X=substituent group

Series I

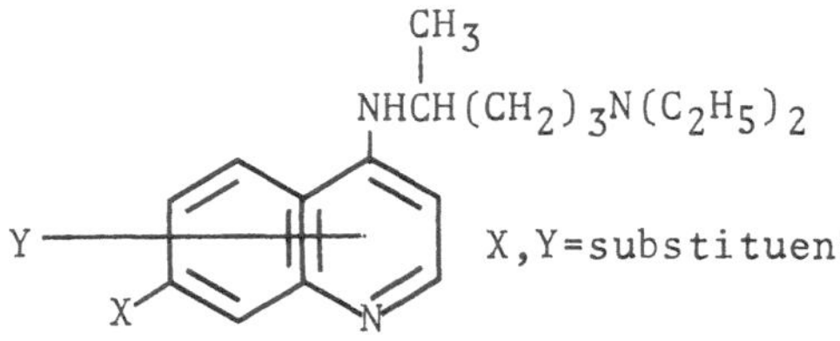

$$CH_3$$
$$|$$
$$NHCH(CH_2)_3N(C_2H_5)_2$$

X,Y=substituent groups

Series II

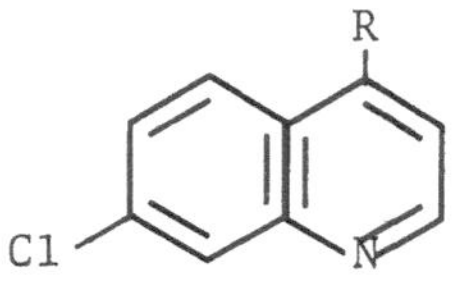

R=diamino side chain

Series III

When Eq. 1 was applied to all 33 compounds in Series I, II, and III, no correlation was found. Regression analyses on Series I alone showed reasonably good correlation with the charge on the substituent at the 7 position (Table 1). These results are in complete agreement with the model proposed by O'Brien and Hahn.

No correlation was found in the regression analyses using Series II alone. When all 14 of the molecules in Series III were analyzed, the only significant correlation was with π^2 and π. The charges on the nitrogen atoms, considered alone, could account for none of the variation in biological activity (Table 2).

To investigate the possible influence of the separation on the diamino nitrogens, the subgroups with three and four carbon separations within Series III were analyzed separately. In both examples, it was again found that the charges on the nitrogen atoms could account for none of the variance, while π did seem important. An increase in the significance in the correlation was found, however,

Table 1. *Regression analyses on series I*

$$A = cQ_X + f$$

Substituents included	r^2 [a]	Significance level (%) [a]	Explained variance[a]
H, F, Cl	0.79	<75	0.59
H, F, Cl, Br	0.80	85-90	0.70
H, F, Cl, Br, I	0.78	93-95	0.69
H, F, Cl, Br, CH_3	0.75	90-95	0.67
H, F, Cl, Br, I, CH_3	0.73	95-97	0.66
H, F, Cl, Br, I, CH_3, CF_3	0.63	95-97	0.56
H, F, Cl, Br, I, CH_3, CF_3, OCH_3	0.58	95-97	0.52

[a]Standard statistical tests (Snedecor and Cochran, 1967).

when both Q and π were used (Table 2). One might conclude that the charge on the terminal nitrogen can be correlated with antimalarial activity if it is considered along with π.

All our results are consistent with the model proposed by O'Brien and Hahn.

III. Example: Interpretation of Cholinesterase Inhibition

QSAR methods were used to come to a better understanding of the mechanism of inhibitory potencies of selected N,N-diethyl-3-(dimethyl-phenylammonium)propionamide iodides against electric eel acetylcholin-esterase, AChE, (Clayton, 1971). The study includes synthesis of the inhibitory molecules and selected congeners, electric dipole moment measurements, molecular orbital calculations, and the application of the Hansch type QSAR model (Purcell and Clayton, 1972).

1. Methods

Table 3 gives the compounds evaluated as inhibitors and their corresponding method of synthesis. Table 4 gives the congeners used for electric dipole moment measurement and molecular orbital calculation and their sources (Clayton *et al.*, 1974).

Table 2. *Regression analyses on series III*

Regression equation	Number of compounds	r^2	Significance level (%)	Explained variance
$A = b\pi + f$	14	0.24	90-95	0.17
$A = a\pi^2 + b\pi + f$	14	0.69	> 99	0.63
$A = eQ_{Nt} + f$	14	0.09	< 75	0.02
$A = a\pi^2 + b\pi + eQ_{Nt} + f$	14	0.70	> 99	0.60
$A = a\pi^2 + b\pi + dQ_{N_4} + eQ_{Nt} + f$	14	0.70	97-99	0.57
$A = b\pi + f$	9	0.44	90-95	0.36
$A = a\pi^2 + b\pi + f$	9	0.44	80-85	0.26
$A = eQ_{Nt} + f$	9	0.01	<< 75	0.00
$A = b\pi + eQ_{Nt} + f$	9	0.78	97-99	0.71
$A = a\pi^2 + b\pi + eQ_{Nt} + f$	9	0.79	95-97	0.66
$A = b\pi + f$	5	0.30	< 75	0.07
$A = a\pi^2 + b\pi + f$	5	0.64	< 75	0.28
$A = eQ_{Nt} + f$	5	0.01	<< 75	0.00
$A = b\pi + eQ_{Nt} + f$	5	0.94	90-95	0.88
$A = a\pi^2 + b\pi + eQ_{Nt} + f$	5	0.95	< 75	0.80

14 compounds: all compounds in Series III
9 compounds: 4 methylene separation
5 compounds: 3 methylene separation

The dielectric constants of the series of N,N-dimethylaniline derivatives (Table 4) were measured in benzene solution at 25°C by the heterodyne beat method using a Wissenschaftlich-Technische Werkstatten DMO1 Dipolemeter. The moments were calculated by two methods (Guggenheim, 1949; Smith, 1950).

Molecular orbital calculations were conducted at different levels of approximation. The Hückel Molecular Orbital method (Salem, 1966), the Pariser-Parr-Pople method (Pariser, 1953; Parr, 1966), the Complete Neglect of Differential Overlap method (Pople and Segal, 1965; Pople and Segal, 1966), and the Del Re Sigma-Electron method (Del Re, 1958) were used to calculate the electronic indices for the molecules in Table 4.

As a measure of the electric eel AChE inhibitory potencies of the compounds in Table 3, the relative dissociation constant, K_i, of the enzyme inhibitor complex was calculated for each congener from experimental kinetic data. The Radiometer Type RR1c automatic titrator with digital readout attachment (Beasley *et al.*, 1968) was used.

Table 3. *Inhibition of acetylcholinesterase by substituted N,N-di-ethyl-3-(dimethylphenylammonium)propionamide iodides*[a]

$$CH_3$$
$$H_3C-\overset{+}{N}-CH_2CH_2CON\overset{C_2H_5}{<}_{C_2H_5}$$
$$I^-$$
R

R^b	Relative K_i $(\times 10^4)$	Relative $I_{50}{}^d$ $(\times 10^4 M)$	Relative $pI_{50}{}^e$
H^c	5.21	22.06	2.656
m-CH_3	4.27	22.98	2.638
p-CH_3	4.78	23.50	2.629
m-OCH_3	4.62	23.37	2.631
p-OCH_3	6.31	31.03	2.508
m-Cl	1.38	6.98	3.156
p-Cl	1.85	9.96	3.001
p-NO_2	2.07	10.47	2.980

[a]Determined potentiometrically at $25.00 \pm 0.05°C$ using electric eel acetylcholinesterase.

[b]Synthesis by Purcell and Clayton, 1972.

[c]The synthesis of this compound has been reported previously (Larizza and Brancaccio, 1959).

[d]I_{50} is the molar concentration of compound necessary to elicit 50 percent inhibition of the enzyme (Bergmann and Segal, 1954).

[e]Negative logarithm of I_{50}.

2. Results

In QSAR studies one interesting by-product is the comparison between experimentally measured physicochemical properties and those calculated from molecular orbital methods. The electric dipole moments, measured and calculated from the molecular orbital methods, were therefore compared. Of all the methods used, best agreement was obtained using a combination of the simple Hückel method and the Del Re Sigma treatment (Table 4).

The results of the inhibitory potencies of the N,N-diethyl-3-(dimethylphenylammonium)propionamide iodides measured potentiometrically against electric eel AChE are given in Table 3. All eight compounds of this series exhibited purely competitive inhibition. The molar concentration of compound necessary to elicit 50% inhibition of the enzyme (I_{50}) for each compound was calculated (Bergmann and Segal, 1954).

Table 4. *Theoretical electric dipole moments of N,N-dimethylanilines calculated from the Del Re Sigma-Electron and Hückel Molecular Orbital pi-electron charges and comparison with the observed values*

R	μ_σ	μ_π (HMO)	$\mu_{\sigma+\pi}$(HMO)	μ_{obs}[c]	$\Delta\%\mu$[d]
H[a]	0.062	1.13	1.19	1.59	25
m-CH$_3$[a]	0.076	1.13	1.15	1.51	24
p-CH$_3$[a]	0.022	1.13	1.11	1.12	1
m-OCH$_3$[b]	1.429	1.16	2.12	2.18	3
p-OCH$_3$[b]	1.398	0.16	1.31	1.77	26
m-NO$_2$[a]	1.413	3.44	4.82	5.28	9
p-NO$_2$[a]	1.446	3.96	5.40	7.10	24
m-Cl[b]	1.898	0.99	2.35	3.19	26
p-Cl[b]	1.930	0.79	2.72	3.32	18

[a]These compounds were obtained from commercial sources and purified.

[b]These compounds were synthesized and purified (Billman *et al.*, 1942; Thomas *et al.*, 1946).

[c]Observed dipole moments were measured in benzene solution at 25.00±0.01°C.

$$\text{[d]}\Delta\%\mu = \frac{\mu_{obs} - \mu_{\sigma+\pi}\text{(HMO)}}{\mu_{obs}} \times 100.$$

For the QSAR studies the generalized Hansch expression (Purcell *et al.*, 1973), Eq. 2, was used.

$$pI_{50} = a\pi^2 + b\pi + c\sigma + d \qquad (2)$$

In Eq. 2 pI_{50} is -log I_{50}, π values were taken from the literature (Fujita *et al.*, 1964; Leo *et al.*, 1971), and Hammett σ values were used (Lefflet and Grunwald, 1963). The values of the electric dipole moment (Table 4) were also used as an electronic parameter (σ). There was no cross correlation between π and σ or π and μ. The values of σ and μ, however, were interdependent ($r^2 = 0.89$). The results of the regression analyses using the compounds in Table 3 and Eq. 2 are given in Table 5. One can see the importance of the hydrophobic and electronic factors in anti-AChE activity from the results in Table 5. Neither parameter alone adequately describes the activity data; however, the combination of more lipophilic (higher π values) and stronger electron-withdrawing (higher $+\sigma$ values) properties of a substituent group leads to better AChE inhibitors. Addition of the π^2 term in the equation did not increase the significance of the correlation.

Table 5. *Quantitative structure-activity analyses of* pI_{50} *values of*
N,N-diethyl-3-(dimethylphenylammonium) propionamide iodides

Equation	r^2 [a]	F[a]	Explained variance[a]	s
$pI_{50} = 0.357\pi + 0.484\sigma + 2.586$	0.866	16.12	0.81	0.10
$pI_{50} = 0.442\pi + 0.076\mu + 2.410$	0.791	9.41	0.71	0.12
$pI_{50} = 0.465\pi + 2.607$	0.403	4.05	0.30	0.19
$pI_{50} = 0.558\sigma + 2.706$	0.641	10.72	0.58	0.15
$pI_{50} = 0.079\mu + 2.560$	0.427	4.48	0.33	0.19

[a]Standard statistical tests (Snedecor and Cochran, 1967).

Table 6. *Predicted and observed butyrylcholinesterase inhibitory*
potencies

$$CH_3(CH_2)_9N \cdot HBr$$

	Predicted 1965		Observed 1968
	Free-Wilson	Hansch	
pI_{50}	4.99	5.00	5.01±0.03

IV. Example: Successful Prediction

In 1965 Purcell predicted the butyrylcholinesterase inhibitory potency of 1-decyl-3-(N-ethyl-N-methylcarbamoyl)piperdine hydrobromide, which was a nonexistent compound at that time (Purcell, 1965). In 1968 the compound was synthesized and evaluated and the prediction proved to be correct (Beasley and Purcell, 1969). The results are given in Table 6.

V. Conclusion

The point to be emphasized in the application of QSAR techniques to drug design is that it is but another tool to be added to our knowledge and experience. One approach (molecular orbital calculations, for example) may be better for specific application than another (measurement of partition coefficients, for example). Perhaps the greatest chance for the successful application of QSAR methods, however, lies in a *combined* approach as illustrated in Fig. 1. The investigator can take advantage of a number of parameters which may be important factors in considering the interaction of a molecule with a biological system while, at the same time, minimizing his chances of overlooking a rather straight-forward and simple expres-

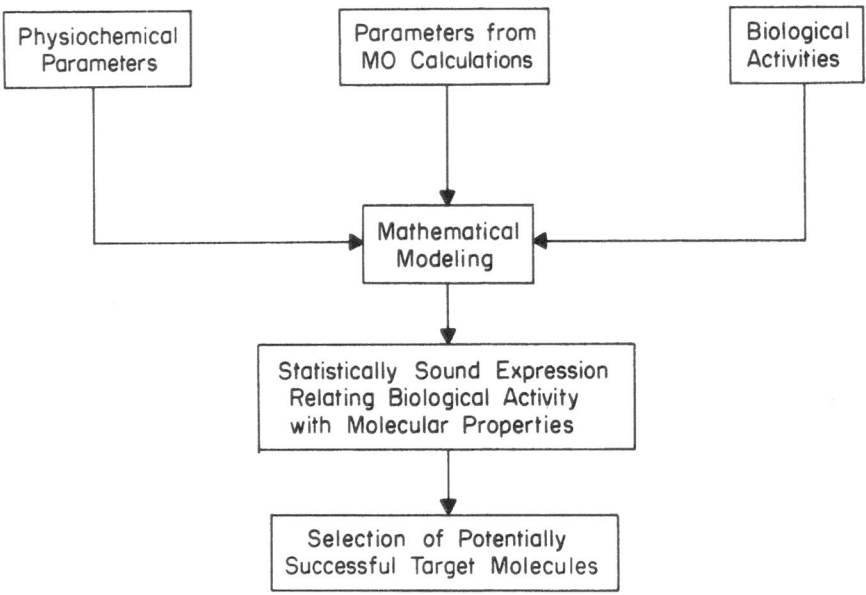

Fig. I. Combined approach using QSAR in drug design.

sion that accounts nicely for the biological variation among a series of congeners. This search for a predictive model, of course, should be carefully guided by the statistical analyses of the attempted correlations.

Acknowledgements

The author gratefully acknowledges support by Cotton Incorporated and the National Institutes of Health (Grant HE-09495).

References

Bass, G. E., D. R. Hudson, J. E. Parker, and W. P. Purcell: Interpretation of antimalarial activity in terms of regression analyses, molecular orbital calculations, and theory of DNA-drug binding. In: Prog. Molecular and Subscellular Biol. 2, pp. 126-133 (Hahn, F. E., Ed.). Berlin: Springer-Verlag 1971.

Beasley, J. G., A. C. York, S. T. Christian, and W. A. Frase: Technical note. A digital readout attachment for the radiometer syringe burette unit. Med. Biol. Eng. 6, 181-183 (1968).

Beasley, J. G., and W. P. Purcell: An example of successful prediction of cholinesterase inhibitory potency from regression analysis. Biochim. et Biophys. Acta 178, 175-176 (1969).

Bergmann, F., and R. Segal: The relationship of quaternary ammonium salts to the anionic sites of true and pseudo cholinesterase. Biochem. J. 58, 692-698 (1954).

Billman, J. H., A. Radike, and B. W. Mundy: Alkylation of amines. I. J. Amer. Chem. Soc. 64, 2977-2978 (1942).

Bruice, T. C., N. Kharasch, and R. J. Winzler: A correlation of thyroxine-like activity and chemical structure. Arch. Biochem. Biophys. 62, 305-317 (1956).

Clayton, J. M.: Application of quantitative structure-activity relationships to selected biochemical systems. Ph.D. Thesis, University of Tennessee 1971.
Clayton, J. M., G. E. Bass, W. P. Purcell, and C. C. Thompson: Comparison between theoretical and experimental electric dipole moments of selected N,N-dimethylaniline derivatives. J. Pharm. Sci.
2, 230-234 (1974).
Del Re, G.: A simple MO-LCAO method for the calculation of charge
distribution in saturated organic molecules. J. Chem. Soc. 1958,
4031.
Free, S. M., Jr., and J. W. Wilson: A mathematical contribution to
structure-activity studies. J. Med. Chem. 7, 395-399 (1964).
Fujita, T., J. Iwasa, and C. Hansch: A new substituent constant, π,
derived from partition coefficients. J. Amer. Chem. Soc. 86, 5175-
5180 (1964).
Guggenheim, E. A.: A proposed simplification in the procedure for
computing electric dipole moments. Trans. Faraday Soc. 45, 714-
720 (1949).
Hansch, C., and T. Fujita: ρ-σ-π Analysis. A method for the correlation of biological activity and chemical structure. J. Amer.
Chem. Soc. 86, 1616-1626 (1964).
Hansch, C., and F. Helmer: Extrathermodynamic approach to the study
of the adsorption of organic compounds by macromolecules. J. Polymer Sci., Part A-1 6, 3295-3302 (1968).
Hansch, C., J. E. Quinlan, and G. L. Lawrence: The linear free-
energy relationship between partition coefficients and the aqueous
solubility of organic liquids. J. Organ. Chem. 33, 347-350 (1968).
Helmer, F., K. Kiehs, and C. Hansch: The linear free-energy relationship between partition coefficients and the binding and conformational perturbation of macromolecules by small organic compounds. Biochemistry 7, 2858-2863 (1968).
Iwasa, J., T. Fujita, and C. Hansch: Substituent constants for ali-
phatic functions obtained from partition coefficients. J. Med.
Chem. 8, 150-153 (1965).
Larizza, A., and G. Brancaccio: Aniline derivatives with pharmaco-
logic activity. Gazz. Chim. Ital. 89, 2402-2420 (1959).
Leffler, J. E., and E. Grunwald: Rates and Equilibria of Organic
Reactions. New York: John Wiley 1963.
Leo, A., C. Hansch, and C. Church: Comparison of parameters cur-
rently used in the study of structure-activity relationships. J.
Med. Chem. 12, 766-771 (1969).
Leo, A., C. Hansch, and D. Elkins: Partition coefficients and their
uses. Chem. Rev. 71, 525-616 (1971).
O'Brien, R. L., and F. E. Hahn: Chloroquine structural requirements
for binding to deoxyribonucleic acid and antimalarial activity.
Antimicrobial Agents and Chemotherapy 1965, 315-320 (1966).
Pariser, R.: An improvement in the electronic approximation in LCAO
MO theory. J. Chem. Phys. 21, 568-569 (1953).
Parr, R. G.: Quantum theory of molecular electronic structure. New
York: W. A. Benjamin, Inc. 1966.
Pople, J. A., and G. A. Segal: Approximate self-consistent molec-
ular orbital theory. II. Calculations with complete neglect of
differential overlap. J. Chem. Phys. 43, S136-S151 (1965).
Pople, J. A., and G. A. Segal: Approximate self-consistent molec-
ular orbital theory. III. CNDO Results for AB2 and AB3 systems.
J. Chem. Phys. 44, 3289-3296 (1966).
Purcell, W. P.: Cholinesterase inhibitory prognoses of thirty-six
alkyl substituted 3-carbamoylpiperidines. Biochem. et Biophys.
Acta 105, 201-204 (1965).
Purcell, W. P., G. E. Bass, and J. M. Clayton: Strategy of drug
design: A molecular guide to biological activity. New York: John
Wiley 1973.

Purcell, W. P., and J. M. Clayton: An example of the application
  of quantitative structure-activity relationship models. Third
  International Symposium on Medicinal Chemistry under the sponsor-
  ship of the International Union of Pure and Applied Chemistry,
  Milan, Italy: 1972.
Salem, L.: The molecular orbital theory of conjugated systems. New
  York: W. A. Benjamin, Inc. 1966.
Smith, J. W.: Some developments of Guggenheim's simplified proce-
  dure for computing electric dipole moments. Trans. Faraday Soc.
  46, 394-399 (1950).
Snedecor, G. W., and W. G. Cochran: Statistical Methods, pp. 386-
  402. Ames, Iowa: Iowa State University Press 1967.
Thomas, D. G., J. H. Billman, and C. E. Davis: Alkylation of amines.
  II. N, N-dialkylation of nuclear substituted anilines. J. Amer.
  Chem. Soc. 68, 895-896 (1946).

Physicochemical Factors in Drug-Receptor Interactions Demonstrated on the Example of the Sulfanilamides*

Joachim K. Seydel

At the beginning of my lecture I would like to make the following statement: The relation between physicochemical parameters in a homologous series of biologically active compounds and the exerted biological response can quantitatively be described by suitable mathematical and statistical treatment of the data. I hope that during my lecture I can convince you that this statement holds. It seems obvious that we can expect very close relations between the chemicals used as a drug and the biological system which acts as a receptor. Both consist of molecules. The interactions between the chemical substance and the biological systems are responsible for the effect in the organism. The reactions of enzymes or receptor systems obey the law of mass action, even if we do not yet fully understand how. If we can explore the type of interaction between the drug molecule and the receptor molecules of the target cells then we can understand the mech-anism of action on a molecular level.

The different processes in which the drug is involved before the biological response is released may be divided into three main steps: "pharmaceutical", "pharmacokinetic" and "pharmacodynamic" processes, where the pharmaceutical properties determine the rate and the amount absorbed, the pharmacokinetic properties govern the action of the microorganism on the drug molecule, and the pharmacodynamic properties determine the interaction of the drug molecule on the receptor site.

As physicochemical parameters are involved in these correlations, I have to refer to the literature (Craig, 1971a,b; Fujita & Hansch, 1964; Seydel, 1971a) and to the foregoing paper of Dr. Purcell.

Today we shall restrict our discussion to possible relations between physicochemical parameters of the drug molecule and interaction processes at the receptor site.

The sulfanilamides played a leading role in our current understanding of the relationship between chemical structure of medicinal agents and their biological activity (Woods, 1940; Bell & Roblin,1942; Cowles, 1942; Brueckner, 1943). As already mentioned there are at least two essential structural preconditions for the biological action of a chemical agent: Those connected with the pharmacokinetic behaviour and those connected with the reaction at the receptor site. This discussion is restricted to those suppositions necessary for and re-

---

* Essential parts of this lecture are taken from papers published together with my colleagues G.H. Miller, P.H. Doukas, K.-J. Schaper and L. Bock.

lated to the biological response at the receptor site. A chemothera-
peutically active sulfanilamide consists of a sulfanilamide molecule
in which the N^1-nitrogen atom can carry different substituents. The
basic idea was that the antibacterial activity of sulfanilamide can
be altered by a change in these substituents at the N^1-nitrogen atom
(Bell & Roblin, 1942). Normally these substituents are aromatic or
heteroaromatic ring systems, which carry various substituents.

$$H_2N-\overset{4}{\bigcirc}-SO_2\cdot NH-\overset{1}{\bigcirc}^{R'}$$

The influence of the substituent is spread all over the molecule. However, it is much more convenient to study the influence of the substituents on a functional group rather than on the ring system. Therefore we have studied the influence of the various substituents on the
primary amino group of the basic amines used for the synthesis of
sulfanilamide (Seydel, 1966a,b; 1971b). The influence on electron
distribution was studied by nuclear magnetic resonance, the sulfanilamide was synthesized and its biological activity determined. An
example is given in Fig. 1. A linear correlation is found between the

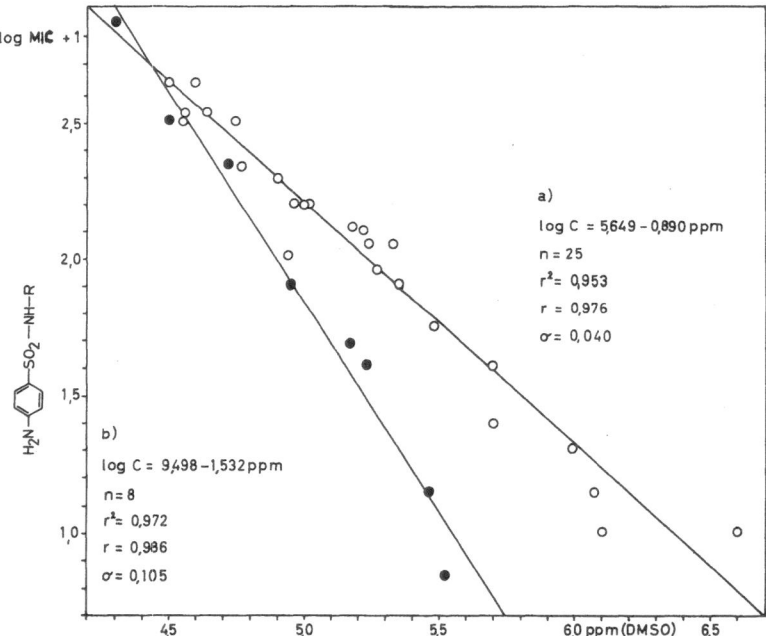

Fig. 1. Relation between whole cell activities (log MIC) of sulfanilamide and the chemical shift (ppm) of the corresponding anilines (a)
and 3-aminopyridines (b) (Seydel, 1971a).

chemical shift of the amino group protons of the basic amines and the
logarithm of the minimal inhibition concentration (MIC) of the complete
sulfanilamide. This result allows the evaluation of the activity of
a sulfanilamide within a homologous series before its synthesis. Decrease in the shielding of the amino group protons causes an increase
in the biological activity of the sulfanilamide. Too strong a decrease

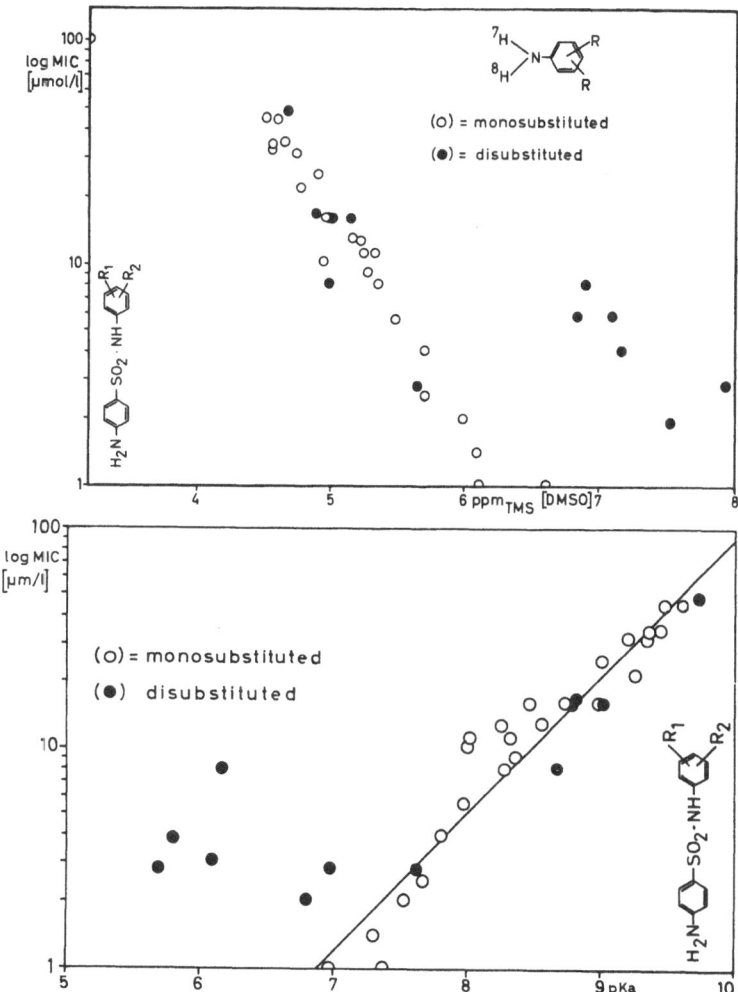

Fig. 2. Relation between whole cell activities (log MIC) of mono- and disubstituted N^1-phenylsulfanilamides and (a) the chemical shift (ppm) of the corresponding precursor anilines and (b) the N^1-pKa of the N^1-phenylsulfanilamides (Seydel, 1971a).

of the basicity of the amines, however, is reflected in a decrease of the biological activity (Fig. 2). This observation has already been described by different theories of Bell and Roblin (1942), Brueckner (1943), and Cowles (1942) using the pKa as indicator.

The result which enables one to predict the biological activity of sulfanilamide before its synthesis gives no information concerning the mode of action of this compound. It means only that there is a correlation but it does not necessarily mean that the electron density at the N^1-nitrogen atom is directly involved in the center of action, i.e. in the interaction with the receptor.

Recognition of the importance of para-amino benzoic acid (PABA) in folic acid metabolism and the ability of certain folate derivatives and/or products to reverse the effect of sulfanilamide has led to a general theory of sulfanilamide action. In principle this theory states that sulfanilamides are competitive inhibitors of the enzymatic incorporation of PABA into folic acid.

The sequential pathway of folic acid synthesis has been evaluated by Jaenicke and Chan (1960), Brown (1962, 1964), Shiota *et al.* (1964), and Ortiz and Hotchkiss (1966) and it has been shown that bacterial cell-free folate synthesizing extracts are inhibited by sulfanilamide

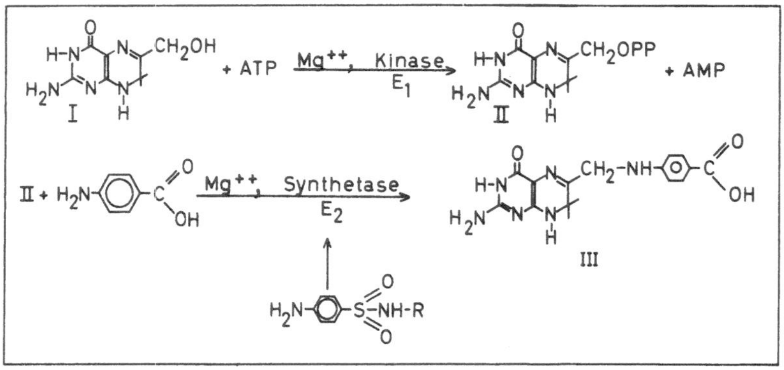

Fig. 3. Scheme of the biosynthetic pathway of folate synthesis.

(Fig. 3). In general, the mechanism of enzyme function can be described with the following scheme:

$$E + S \underset{k_{-1}}{\overset{k_1}{\rightleftharpoons}} E...S \xrightarrow{k_2} E + P$$

The biological specificity is dependent on the formation (or the lack of formation) of the enzyme substrate complex E...S. If a further reaction occurs the functional groups on the enzyme and the substrate must be suitably positioned in the E...S complex so that a reaction to products (P) can occur. In the formation of the complex E...S only such noncovalent binding forces as charge-charge transfer, ionic, hydrophobic or hydrogen bonding are involved. These forces together with the stereochemical relation of different types of interaction forces determine whether the formation of the complex is possible. In addition, the proper positioning of the functional groups involved is essential for the subsequent chemical reaction to occur.

If an inhibitor and the substrate have similar binding groups and the inhibitor forms complexes with the same sites on the enzyme the complex should not be significantly stronger than the one with the substrate. The dissociation constant of the enzyme inhibitor complex should therefore be equal to or larger than the substrate enzyme complex.

Certain enzymes can use different small molecules as substrate if there is a close similarity in structure, i.e. the binding is not absolutely specific. A reversible complex can be formed which does not lead to the formation of products, but to an inhibition of enzymatic reaction. In this case the equation reduces to

$$E + I \underset{k_{-1}}{\overset{k_1}{\rightleftharpoons}} E I$$

Reversible inhibitors may act competitively or noncompetitively. Competitive inhibitors react reversibly with the enzyme to form the complex so that the substrate cannot react with the enzyme. This does not necessarily mean, that the competitive inhibitor and the substrate might complex at the same site of the enzyme. It says, however, that inhibitor and substrate exclude each other from binding.

To gain more information about the structural supposition, and the physicochemical forces which are directly related to the enzyme sulfanilamide interaction and to find an explanation for the observed maximum in whole cell activity we have studied the inhibitory activity of sulfanilamide in a cell-free system. The extract proteins were prepared from *E. coli* according to Brown (1962) with minor modifications (Miller *et al.*, 1972; Bock *et al.*, 1974). Using this cell-free system we were able to evaluate the possible role of ionization and lipid partitioning for the permeation and the role of ionic and steric factors as well as lipid partitioning in the interactions with the receptor.

Some typical single point method experiments were conducted to determine the inhibitory activities of several N^1-phenyl- and N^1-pyridyl sulfanilamides. The results in Fig. 4 (Miller *et al.*, 1972) show a plot of the fractional inhibition of folate synthesis against the logarithm of the sulfanilamide concentration used. From such plots the sulfanilamide-concentration which causes 50 % inhibition was determined. The synthesized amount of folate was determined bacteriologically (growth of *Streptococcus faecalis*). The incubation time was 3 hours.

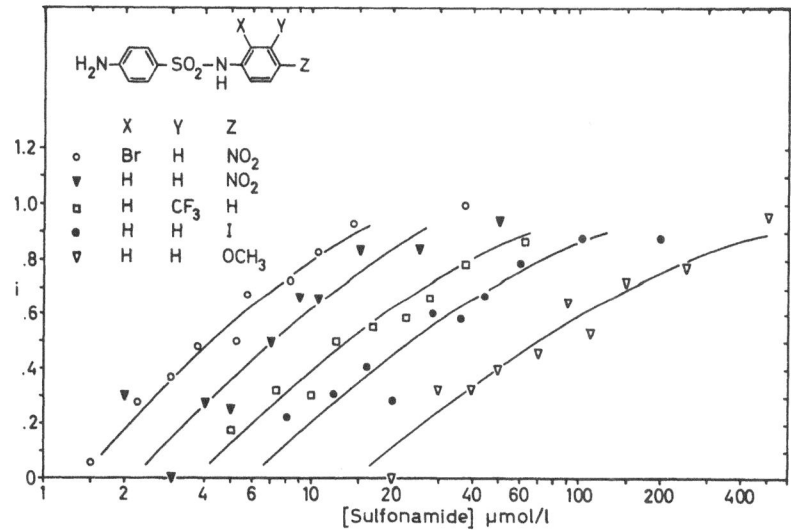

Fig. 4. Determination of sulfanilamide inhibitory activities. The fraction of inhibition, i, of cell-free folate synthesis versus log of sulfanilamide concentration (Miller *et al.*, 1972).

It may be of interest to note the nature of the dose-response curve obtained. There is a small range of inhibitory concentrations, i.e. the ratio of the concentration causing 10 % inhibition to that causing a 90 % inhibition falls between 1:5 and 1:20, usually it is 1:50 to 1:100. Such a narrow range may often be associated with inhibition caused by depletion of substrate (Webb, 1966). We shall come back to this point later on.

The tested sulfanilamide showed a wide range of physicochemical properties and exhibited an approximately twenty-fold variation in inhibitory activities.

If the inhibitory activity in whole cell systems (MIC) is plotted against the activity obtained in the cell-free system (i_{50}) in a double logarithmic graph a linear correlation is obtained (Fig. 5). This is very surprising because the sulfanilamides tested belong to different

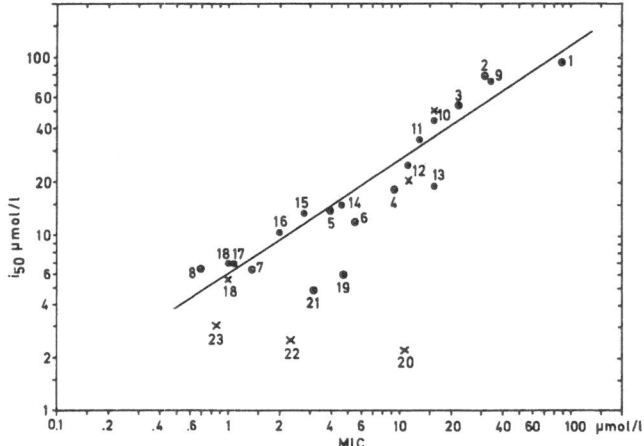

Fig. 5. The relationship of cell-free inhibitory activities to whole cell inhibitory activities (● single point method, x kinetic method) (Miller *et al.*, 1972).

homologous series with very different inhibitory activities. It is apparent that with the exception of 5 compounds all the sulfanilamides fit a single line, whose equation is:

log i_{50} = 0.633 log MIC + 0.779; n = 18, r = 0.95, s = 0.051

The result indicates that the differences in MIC values obtained are paralleled by differences in cell-free activities. Therefore these differences cannot be attributed to permeation but must be associated with the interaction and reaction of sulfanilamide with the extract protein. It seems most likely that permeation factors do not contribute substantially to the antibacterial activity of these 18 compounds *in vitro*. It should be pointed out that the occurrence of a relationship of the type shown in Fig. 5 between whole cell activities and cell-free activities is good evidence that the rate determining step in both systems is similar. While there is no definite proof that these reactions are the same there is nothing in our data to contradict such a conclusion. A plot of log i_{50} vs. log MIC is a plot of two free energies. In a previous paper (Seydel, 1971) we were able to show that the MIC data can be considered as a reflection of the generation rate constants of the growth of *E. coli* in the presence of sulfanilamide. A plot of log MIC or log i_{50} versus such physicochemical parameters as chemical shift, pKa, or σ-Hammett data is therefore a free energy relationship. Four of the drugs which do not fit this singular relationship between MIC and cell-free inhibitory activity are compounds whose pKa values are such that under the experimental conditions they are at least 90 % ionized. It might reasonably be expected that under such conditions the permeation of the ionized form into the cell might be the rate determining step in the whole cell activity determination. These compounds were also exceptions in the linear relation between ppm or pKa and whole cell activity (MIC) as mentioned before (Fig. 2). Indeed they all exhibit lower than expected activities in the whole cell system and very high (but not as high as expected) activities in the cell-free system. The deviation of these four compounds from the singular relationship of i_{50} values to MIC values can then most probably be assigned to their poor permeation into bacterial cells, i.e. a decrease in the effective concentration of the drug. This argument is supported by the high activity found for sulfanilic acid in cell-free systems (Brown, 1962; McCullough & Maren, 1973; Seydel, unpublished data) which is comparable to the activity of highly active sulfanilamide. In contrast, in whole cell systems no inhibitory activity of sulfanilic acid can be detected, the pKa is 3.12, i.e. the compound is totally ionized under the conditions of the experiment (Table I). In an additional experiment the cell-free and whole cell activity of two series of closely related sulfanilamide derivatives namely sulfadimethoxazole and 2-chloro-4-nitro-N^1-phenylsulfanilamide and their corresponding N^1-acetyl- and N^1-methyl derivatives are compared. The parent compounds and the acetyl derivatives which are rapidly hydrolyzed to the parent compounds possess highly inhibitory activities in the cell-free system. In the whole cell system the N^1-acetyl derivatives are more potent inhibitors than the parent compounds. In contrast the N^1-methyl derivatives do not possess any inhibitory activity at the highest testable concentration. Since the N^1-methyl compound has not the ability to form the sulfanilamide anion these results would be expected if the ionic form is necessary for activity. We have, however, to consider that the inactivity of the N^1-methyl compound might be due to steric hindrance of receptor approach, but in view of the evidence presented, this is unlikely.

Table I

INFLUENCE OF IONIZATION ON WHOLE CELL (*E. COLI*) AND CELL-FREE INHIBITORY ACTIVITIES OF SOME SULFANILAMIDES

	N^1-pKa	MIC (*E.coli*) [μM]	i_{50} (cell-free system [μM]
H₃C, CH₃ structure: H_2N-⟨⟩-$SO_2 \cdot$ N(R)-⟨⟩-O (isoxazole)			
H	4.9	4.0	16
-COCH₃..	-	0.5	16
-CH₃	-	no inhibition	no inhibition
H_2N-⟨⟩-$SO_2 \cdot$ N(R)-⟨⟩(Cl)-NO_2			
H	6.17	2.8	6
-COCH₃	-	0.5	10
H_2N-⟨⟩-SO_3H	3.12	no inhibition	5

A more direct approach to this problem would be to show that the
activity of a compound in test systems maintained at different pH-
values is directly related to the concentration of the ionic form present. Several single point method experiments have been performed in
an attempt to verify this theory. Table II shows the results of these

Table II

THE OBSERVED DEPENDENCY UPON pH OF "FOLATE" SYNTHESIS INHIBITION BY
N^1-PHENYLSULFANILAMIDE (pKa 9.0, 37.5 °C)

initial pH of buffer at 20°C	final pH of reactions at 37.5°C	% of sulf-anilamide present in ionic form	observed i_{50} [μM]	"folate" produced in the control
8.75	7.9 - 8.0	8.20	25	325 mμg
8.60	7.8 - 7.9	6.65	39	310 mμg
7.9 - 8.0	7.5	3.07	46	230 mμg
7.60	7.2	1.56	45	230 mμg

experiments in which the i_{50} values of N^1-phenylsulfanilamide (pKa
9.0, 37.5 °C) were determined in reaction mixtures prepared at different pH values. The range of pH values obtainable was limited by the
temperature coefficient of the Tris buffers employed. It can be seen
that there is an increase in inhibitory activity associated with an
increase in the percent of sulfanilamide present in the ionic form.
The increase is not, however, as large as it would be expected. A
possible explanation for this result may lie in the increased activity of the enzyme preparation at higher pH-values. Such an increase in
activity could quite easily lead to the occurrence of the type of non-
linear kinetics as seen in Fig. 6. If this does indeed occur at higher
pH values, then the result obtained from a single point experiment of
5 hours duration may be too low.

The results presented so far would then support the Brueckner- and
Cowles-theory of sulfanilamide-activity (Cowles, 1942; Brueckner, 1943)
which stated that only the ionized form is active. However, the ionized
form cannot permeate the bacterial cell wall.

Let us come back to the correlation found between MIC and cell-free
activity (Fig. 5). In view of this relationship we would expect all
physicochemical parameters describing electronic influences of the
various substituents (NMR-data (ppm), pKa and σ-Hammett) which gave
successful correlations with MIC data to be equally successful with
cell-free activities. In addition, those exceptions to correlation
of MIC data with physicochemical parameters should not be exceptions
when cell-free activities are compared. This, indeed, appears to be
the case as can be seen from Fig. 7, where i_{50} values and MIC values
are plotted against the pKa of the sulfanilamide. The deviation from
linearity which occurs for substance 20 and 22 in the whole cell
system (compounds with pKa less than 7) does not occur in the cell-
free system. It is however remarkable that these compounds, which are
highly active in the cell-free system, are less active than expected.

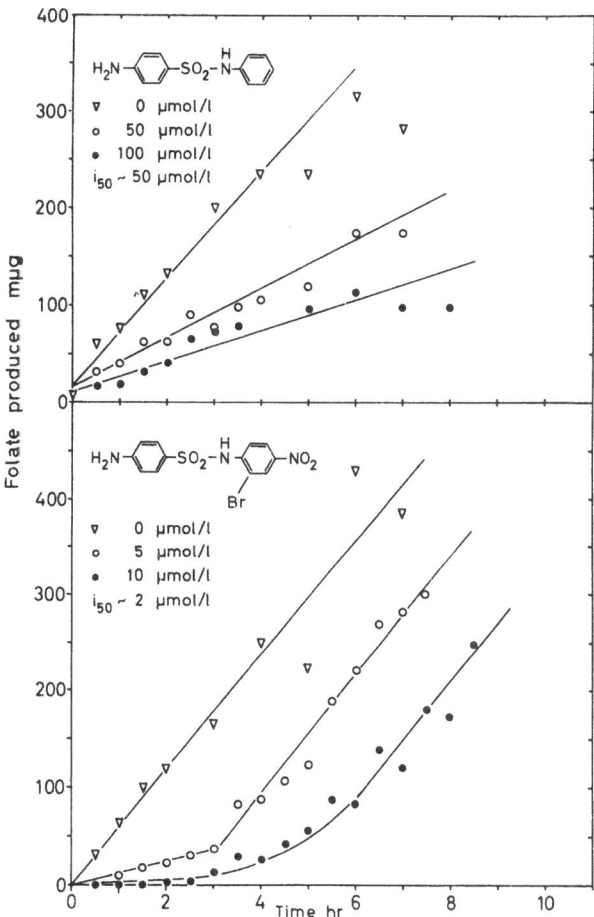

Kinetics of Inhibition of Folate Synthesis by a Sulfonamide
with a very high i_{50} (~50 µmol/l), and by a Sulfonamide
with a very low i_{50} (~ 2 µmol/l).

Fig. 6. The kinetics of inhibition of folate synthesis by N^1-phenyl-
sulfanilamide and by 2-bromo-4-nitro-N^1-phenylsulfanilamide. The
kinetics of inhibition exhibited by N^1-phenylsulfanilamide were found
to be pseudo-zero-order throughout the experimental period. In contrast, the highly active compound, 2-bromo-4-nitro-N^1-phenylsulfanil-
amide, only exhibited pseudo-zero-order kinetics for a short initial
time. After this time the rate of folate synthesis is similar to that
seen in the control (Miller *et al.*, 1972).

These activities have been determined with single point method experiments. The inhibition of folate synthesis was determined after
5 hours of incubation. To gain a better insight into the time dependency of the inhibition reaction, kinetic experiments were performed.
Fig. 8 shows a typical kinetic experiment in which the amount of folate-
like material produced in the reaction mixture was determined for
several sulfonamide concentrations as a function of time. From such
plots the sulfanilamide-concentration which causes 50 % inhibition
(k_{50}) was determined.

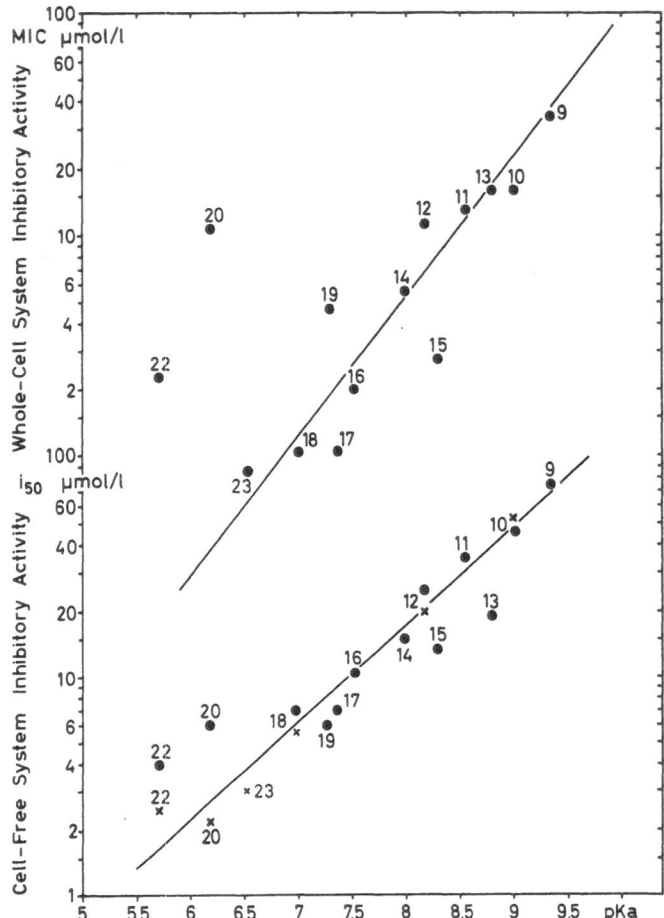

Fig. 7. Relation of inhibitory activities (whole cell and cell-free system) to the pKa of substituted N^1-phenylsulfanilamides ($\bullet$ single point activity determination, x kinetic activity determination) (log MIC = -4.2 + 0.62 pKa, n = 36, r = 0.93, only those compounds which were also tested in the cell-free system are indicated; log i_{50} = -2.1 + 0.41 pKa, n = 13, r = 0.96) (Miller *et al.*, 1972).

Fig. 6 shows that the kinetics of inhibition for a less active sulfanilamide, N^1-phenylsulfanilamide, is pseudo zero order throughout the entire time period, and for most of the compounds studied the activities were the same as those obtained with the single point method. However, in case of highly active compounds a different picture was observed. This is also demonstrated in Fig. 6 for the highly active sulfanilamide 2-bromo-4-nitro-N^1-phenylsulfanilamide. The reactions were only linear during the initial time period (approx. 2 - 3 hr). After this time the reaction returned to a rate of folate synthesis similar to that seen in the control. Because of this effect, the amount of folate synthesized after 5 hours in the presence of the sulfanilamide was 50 % less than that of the controls despite the inhibition of the initial rate of 70 %. For these compounds, if the k_{50} values

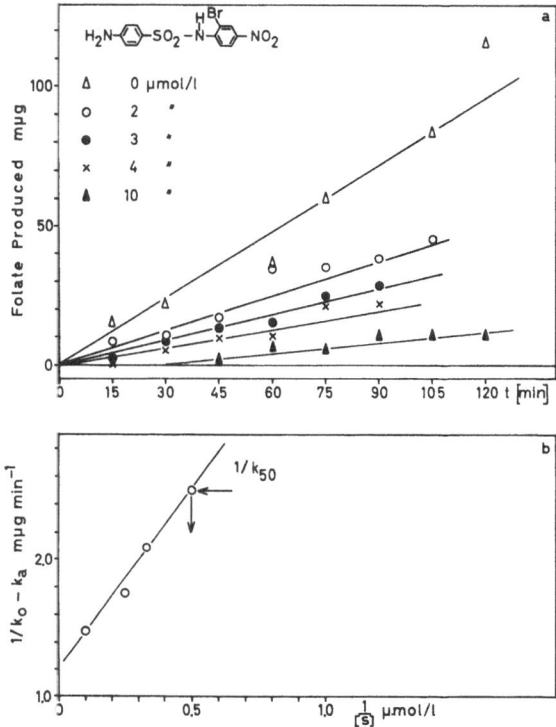

Fig. 8. Determination of the inhibitory activity of 2-bromo-4-nitro-N^1-phenylsulfanilamide by the kinetic method. Rate constants for folate synthesis in the presence of several concentrations of 2-bromo-4-nitro-N^1-phenylsulfanilamide were obtained from kinetic experiments (a) and used in Lineweaver-Burke type plots (b) to obtain estimates of k_{50} (Miller *et al.*, 1972).

are used instead of the i_{50} values (which are identical for less active sulfanilamides) the correlation between the log of biological activity and the physicochemical parameters becomes more significant (Fig. 9). A likely reason for such behaviour is depletion of the inhibitor, presumably due to its utilization as a false substrate. In addition to other indirect evidence for the formation of a sulfanilamide-containing folate analogue in the cell-free experiments, Brown (1962) has already shown that sulfanilic acid is incorporated by *E. coli* extract intc a new compound of unknown structure in the presence of 7,8-dihydro-6-hydroxymethylpterin and ATP-Mg^{2+}. The synthesis of a sulfanilamide-containing pteroate analogue could proceed according to the following scheme (Fig. 10). To prove this hypothesis we have synthesized the expected analogue (Bock *et al.*, 1974) (Fig. 11) and performed experiments in cell-free systems using [^{35}S]sulfamethoxazole. We were able to demonstrate the production of a radioactive product in the cell-free systems which shows identical R_f values on different thin layer plates and in different solvent systems (Fig. 12). The same product could be detected in whole cell systems after incubation with [^{35}S]sulfamethoxazole (Table III). This demonstrates that sulfanilamides do compete with PABA not only for receptor binding sites but also for the natural substrate 7,8-dihydro-6-hydromethylpterin.

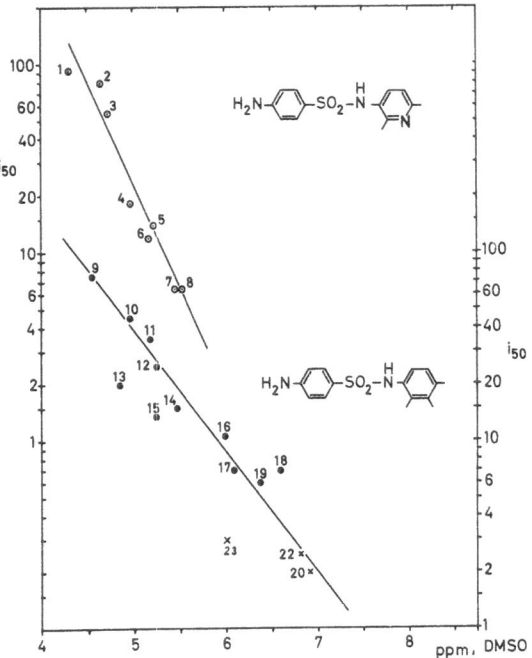

Fig. 9. The relation of cell-free inhibitory activities, i_{50}, to chemical shift, ppm, of sulfanilamide precursor amines (Miller *et al.*, 1972).

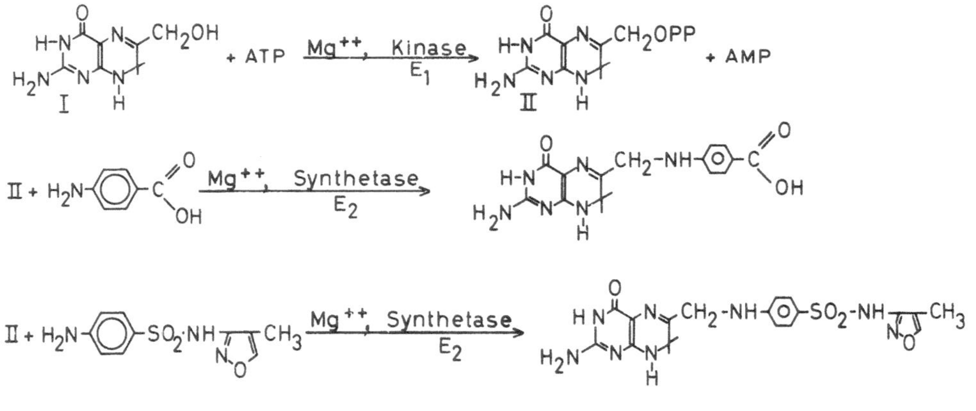

Fig. 10. Reaction scheme for the enzymatic synthesis of the sulfanilamide containing folate analogue.

If we consider the correlation between one physicochemical parameter and the cell-free activities more closely, a deviation of compounds 13, 15, and 23 can be noticed in spite of the fact that we have corrected the biological activity data using the k_{50} values for highly active compounds. Again we are confronted with exceptions, whose activity seems to be shifted parallel to the linear regression line. These three compounds are N^1-phenylsulfanilamides substituted in o-position

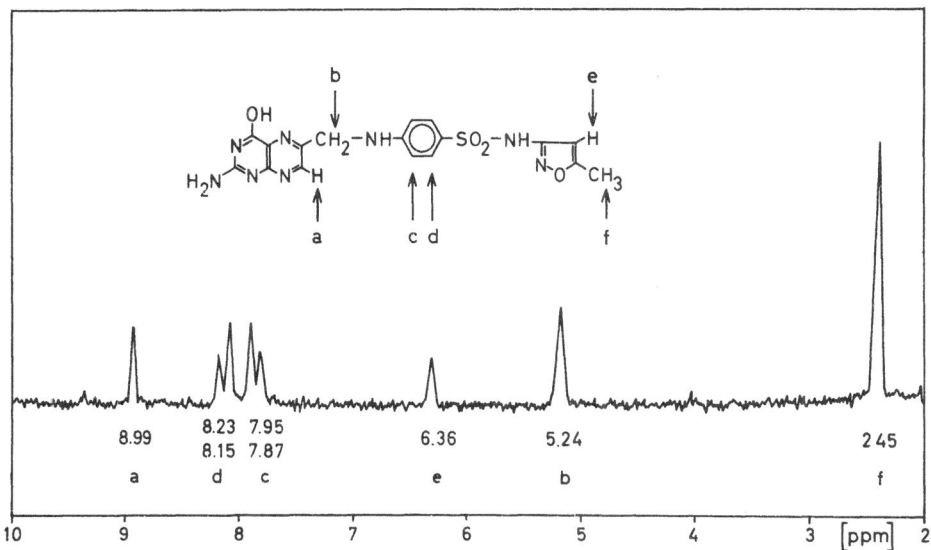

Fig. 11. NMR spectrum of N^1-3-(5-methylisoxazolyl)-N^4-(6-pterinyl-methyl)sulfanilamide in CF$_3$COOD, 100 MHz; tetramethylsilane used as internal standard (Bock *et al.*, 1974).

of the phenyl ring and possess higher activities than predicted from their physicochemical parameters (ppm, pKa). The reason for this be-haviour is not fully understood. Large scale studies, however, reveal that a general rule seems to be operative. Even in the whole cell studies all o-substituted and some m-substituted sulfanilamides show a higher activity than expected from their physicochemical parameters. This enables one to conclude that permeation factors are not the reason for the observed higher activity. The kinetics of inhibition for these compounds in cell-free systems demonstrate a certain difference in in-hibitory action. After three hours of incubation a nearly complete cessation of folate synthesis in a cell-free extract is observable if only a small excess of 7,8-dihydro-6-hydroxymethylpterin (compared to sulfanilamide concentration) is used (Fig. 13). This phenomenon is not observed for the p-substituted isomer with the same activity (Fig. 14). The inhibition type observed seems to be "irreversible" to a certain extent. The observed kinetics are not pseudo first order for the first 3 - 4 hours. There is a decrease in inhibition with time and suddenly the curve bends over indicating a complete stop of folate synthesis. This could mean the production of an analogue which, in contrast to the p-substituted derivatives, is an inhibitor itself and which stops synthesis after a certain concentration is reached. The decrease of inhibition with time during the first time interval is, however, difficult to explain. Another explanation would be a strong increase in the reaction rate of analogue formation. By this the amount of 7,8-dihydro-6-hydroxymethylpterin in the reaction mixture is depleted and a further synthesis of folate like material is stopped. If this were true the addition of 7,8-dihydro-6 hydroxymethylpterin after 4 hours should lead to a normal rate of folate production because all sulf-anilamide has been used up by analogue production. This is indeed ob-served (Fig. 15). Possibly upon o- or m-substitution a conformational change in sulfanilamide conformation takes place which increases its affinity for the receptor and the rate of analogue synthesis. This seems to be independent of the ring system and the o-substituents of

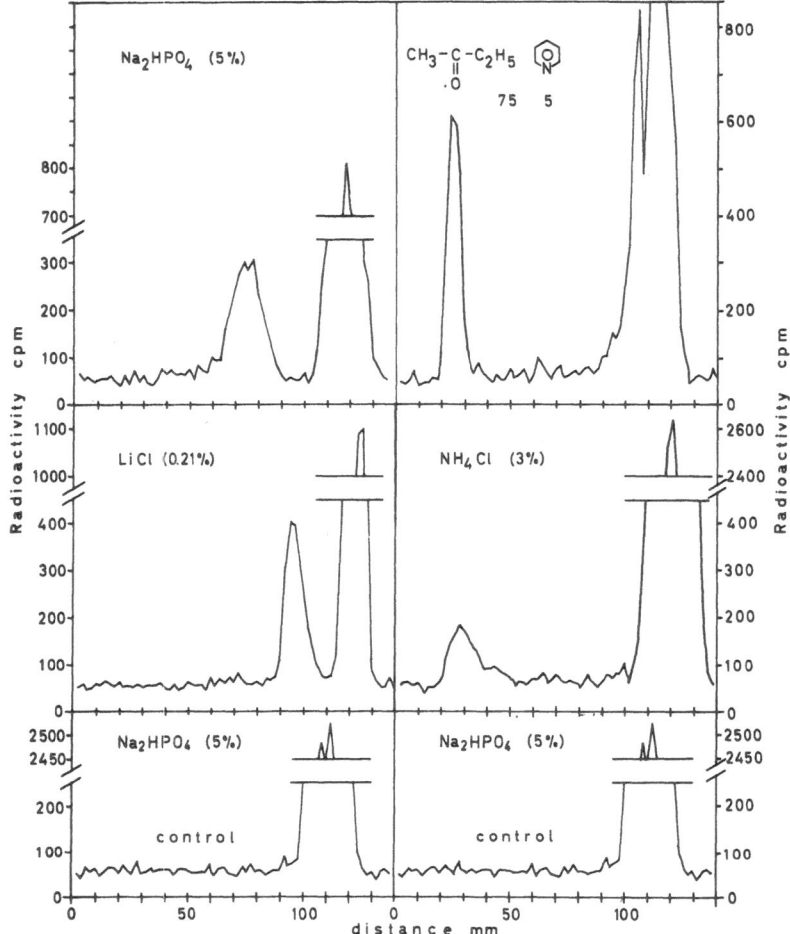

Fig. 12. Thin-layer radiochromatogram of cell-free folate synthesizing
reaction mixtures containing [^{35}S]sulfamethoxazole. The solvent systems
used were: Na_2HPO_4 (5 %), LiCl (0.21 %), NH_4Cl (3 %) on cellulose layers,
and methyl ethyl ketone and pyridine (75 and 5 v/v) for silica gel.
The radiochromatograms demonstrate the separation of an additional
radioactive spot. The R_f values are identical with the R_f values found
for N^1-3-(5-methylisoxazolyl)-N^4-(7,8-dihydro-6-pterinylmethyl)sulf-
anilamide under the same conditions. The control reaction mixture,
which did not contain the pterin substrate, shows the normal position
of sulfanilamide in the chromatographic system (Bock *et al.*, 1974).

the N^1-substituent of the sulfanilamide (Fig. 14). The results of
regression analysis are summed up in Fig. 16. Two parallel lines are
obtained if the logarithms of the biological activities in a cell-free
system (i_{50}) are plotted against the pKa's of the p-substituted and
o- and m-substituted sulfanilamide. The result supports the assumption
that the difference of the steric parameters for the different substituents in o- and m-position is not responsible but that the presence

Table III

IDENTIFICATION OF A SULFAMETHOXAZOLE-CONTAINING PTEROATE ANALOGUE FROM
E. coli

Thin layer chromatography, cellulose layer, solvent: 5 % aqueous Na_2 HPO_4 (Bock *et al.*, 1974).

substance	R_f	
	products of chemical synthesis	^{35}S-radioactive compounds from whole cell system of E. coli
H_2N—◯—SO_2—NH — N—O—CH_3	0.87	0,91
O HN N—CH_2—NH—◯—SO_2—NH — O—CH_3, H_2N N N	0.385	0.37
O HN N—CH_2—NH—◯—SO_2—NH — N—O—CH_3, H_2N N N—H	0.262	0,24

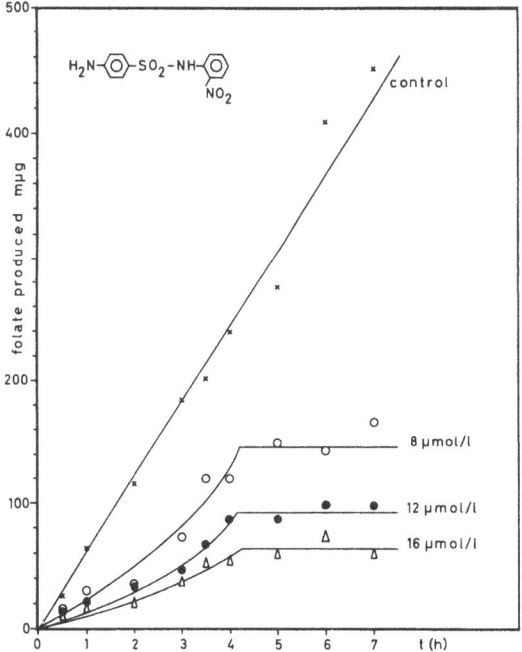

Fig. 13. Kinetics of inhibition of folate synthesis by 2-nitro-N^1-phenylsulfanilamide demonstrating a "mixed" type of inhibition. After 3 - 4 hr a complete stop of folate synthesis in a cell-free extract is observable (Seydel *et al.*, 1973).

40

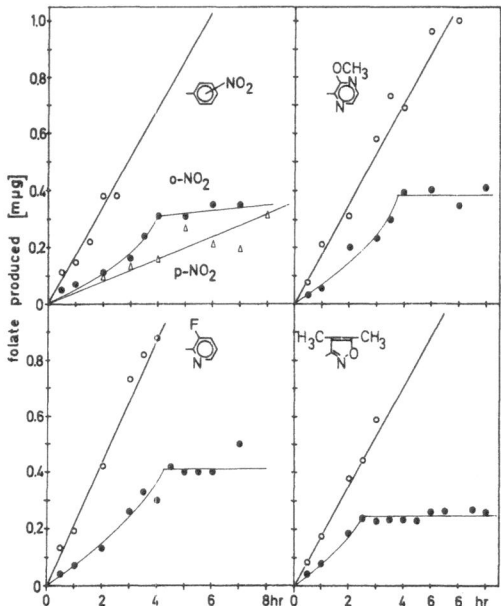

Fig. 14. Some o-substituted sulfanilamide with "ortho"-effect type inhibition of folate production in a cell-free system (*E. coli*) (Seydel
et al., unpublished data).

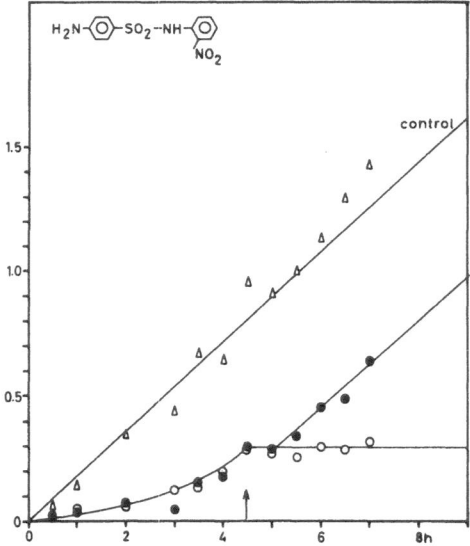

Fig. 15. The total inhibition of folate synthesis by 2-nitro-N[1]-phenyl-
sulfanilamide after 4 hr is completely reversed by the addition of
5 µl (0.01 µM) 7,8-dihydro-6-hydroxymethylpterin. The concentrations
of 7,8-dihydro-6-hydroxymethylpterin and the sulfanilamide are approximately equimolar in the incubation mixture (Seydel *et al.*, unpublished
data).

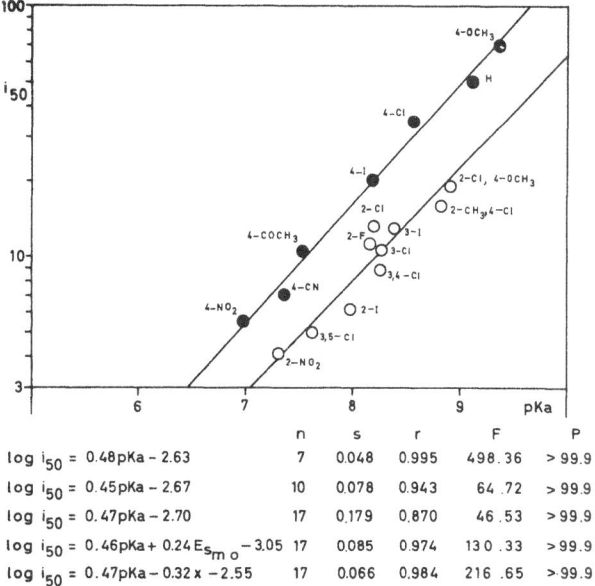

	n	s	r	F	P
$\log i_{50} = 0.48 pKa - 2.63$	7	0.048	0.995	498.36	> 99.9
$\log i_{50} = 0.45 pKa - 2.67$	10	0.078	0.943	64.72	> 99.9
$\log i_{50} = 0.47 pKa - 2.70$	17	0.179	0.870	46.53	> 99.9
$\log i_{50} = 0.46 pKa + 0.24 E_{s_{m o}} - 3.05$	17	0.085	0.974	130.33	> 99.9
$\log i_{50} = 0.47 pKa - 0.32 x - 2.55$	17	0.066	0.984	216.65	> 99.9

Fig. 16. Log i_{50} versus pKa of some o- and m-substituted N^1-phenyl-sulfanilamides which show a "mixed" inhibition type and exert an activity higher than expected from their pKa, compared to the general correlation curve obtained with p-substituted derivatives. If a steric (E_s) or a dummy parameter is included for the o- and m-substitution in the equations, o-, m-, and p-substituted sulfanilamide can be described in one equation (Seydel *et al.*, 1973).

of a substituent in the o- or m-position causes a change in conformation of the sulfanilamide molecule.

From crystallographic studies of Shefter (1972) and HMO-calculations of Peradejordi (personal communication) a change from cis to configuration is likely. If this is considered as a dummy parameter in the regression a highly significant correlation between "electronic" and a "conformation" parameter and the log of the biological response is obtained (Fig. 16).

In contrast there is no significant contribution of lipophilic/hydrophilic forces on permeation and on receptor interaction in sulfanilamide (Fig. 17).

CONCLUSION

I hope that I have been able to convince you that the statement I made at the beginning of my lecture is justified. It is possible to quantify the relation between physicochemical parameters of a drug molecule and the biological response released by its interaction with the receptor site.

Besides the possibility of rationally designing new sulfanilamides, we were able to show that ionic forces and steric parameters play the major role in the interaction with the receptor and in inhibition of folate synthesis by sulfanilamide. The type of inhibition is more complex than previously assumed. There is not only competition for

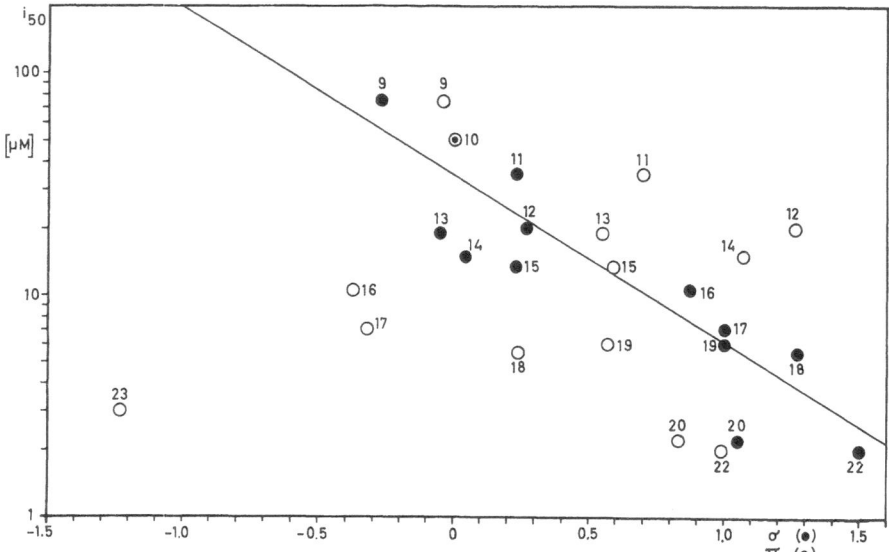

Fig. 17. The relationship of cell-free activities to Hammet σ and π values. Regression analysis for the correlation to Hammet σ and π : log i_{50} = 1.54 - 0.75 σ , n = 13, r = 0.95, s = 0.076; log i_{50} = 1.02 + 0.038 π, n = 14, r = 0.05, s = 0.21. As far as available k_{50} values are used instead of i_{50} (Miller *et al.*, 1972).

binding sites on the synthetase enzyme between PABA and sulfanilamide but also for the substrate (7,8-dihydro-6-hydroxymethylpterin). Hydrophobic forces play no significant role, either in permeation of the bacterial cell wall or in the interaction with the receptor site. Ionic forces do play a role in permeation if the ionized fraction increases to more than 90 %.

We have to realize, however, that the structure-activity correlations evaluated are of statistical nature. Therefore all statements and predictions based on these correlations are probability statements which have to be proved by experiments. In a certain percentage of the cases we have to take into account deviations from this correlation. In many cases, however, these deviations are caused by substances with different chemical or biological properties. A detailed study of these deviating compounds can contribute essentially to the evaluation of their mode of action and to the development of new inhibitors. The results presented are an example.

An essential precondition for the further development of these techniques is an increase in our knowledge in the field of molecular biology and the development of more sophisticated biological tests.

REFERENCES

BELL, P.H., and R.O. ROBLIN: A theory of the relation of structure to activity of sulfanilamide type compounds. J. Am. Chem. Soc. 64, 2905-2917 (1942).

BOCK, L., G.H. MILLER, K.J. SCHAPER, and J.K. SEYDEL: Sulfonamide structure-activity relationship in a cell-free system. II Proof for the formation of a sulfonamide containing folate analogue. J. Med. Chem. 17, 23-28 (1974).

BROWN, G.M.: The biosynthesis of folic acid. II Inhibition by sulfonamides. J. Biol. Chem. 237, 536-540 (1962).

BROWN, G.M.: Methods for measuring inhibition by sulfonamides of the
enzymatic synthesis of dihydropteroic acid. Methods Med. Res. 10,
233-238 (1964).

BRUECKNER, A.H.: Sulfonamide activity as influenced by variation in
pH of culture media. Yale J. Biol. Med. 15, 813-821 (1943).

COWLES, P.B.: The possible role of ionization in the bacteriostatic
action of the sulfonamides. Yale J. Biol. Med. 14, 599-604 (1942).

CRAIG, P.N.: Interdependence between physical parameters and selection
cf substituent groups for correlation studies. J. Med. Chem. 14,
680-684 (1971).

CRAIG, P.N., C.H. HANSCH, J.W.McFARLAND, Y.C.MARTIN, W.P. PURCELL,
and R. ZAHRADNIK: Minimal statistical data for structure-function
correlations. J. Med. Chem. 14, 447 (1971).

FUJITA, T., J. IWASA, and C. HANSCH: A new substituent constant, π,
derived from partition coefficients, J. Am. Chem. Soc. 86,
5175-5180 (1964).

JAENICKE, L., and P.C. CHAN: Die Biosynthese der Folsäure. Angew.
Chem. 72, 752-753 (1960).

McCULLOUGH, J.L., and T.H. MAREN: Inhibition of dihydropteroate synthetase from Escherichia coli by sulfones and sulfonamides. Antimicrob.
Agents Chemother. 3, 665-669 (1973).

MILLER, G.H., P.H. DOUKAS, and J.K. SEYDEL: Sulfonamide structure-
activity relationships in a cell-free system. Correlation of inhibition of folate synthesis with antibacterial activity and
physicochemical parameters. J. Med. Chem. 15, 700 - 706 (1972).

ORTIZ, P.J. and R.D. HOTCHKISS: The enzymatic synthesis of dihydrofolate and dihydrophteroate in cell-free preparations from wild-
type and sulfonamide-resistant pneumococcus. Biochemistry 5, 67-74
(1966).

SEYDEL, J.K.: Prediction of in vitro activity of sulfonamides using
Hammett constants or spectrophotometric data of the basic amines
for calculation. Mol. Pharmacol. 2, 259-265 (1966).

SEYDEL, J.K.: Molekulare Grundlagen der Sulfonamidwirkung. Arzneim.-
Forsch. 16, 1447-1453 (1966).

SEYDEL, J.K.: Physicochemical approaches to the rational development
of new drugs. Drug Design (Ariens, Edt.) Vol. 1, 343-379 (1971).

SEYDEL, J.K.: Prediction of the in vitro activity of sulfonamides
synthesized from simple amines by use of electronic data obtained
from the simple amines. J. Med. Chem. 14, 724-729 (1971).

SEYDEL, J.K., G.H. Miller, and P.H. DOUKAS: Structure-activity correlations of sulfonamides in cell-free systems compared to correlations
obtained in whole cell systems and in vivo. (P. Pratesi, Edt.)
Medicinal Chemistry, Butterworth, London 1973.

SHEFTER, E., Z.F. CHMIELEWICZ, J.F. BLOUNT, T.F. BRENNAN, B.F. SACKMAN
and P. SACKMAN: Biological implications of molecular and crystal
structures of sulfadimethoxine, sulfadoxine, and sulfisoxazole.
J. Pharm. Sci. 61, 872-877 (1972).

SHIOTA, T., M.N. DISRAELY, and M.P.McCANN: The enzymatic synthesis of
folate like compounds from hydroxymethyldihydropteridine pyrophosphate. J. Biol. Chem. 239, 2259-2266 (1964).

WEBB, J.L.: Enzyme and Metabolic Inhibitors. Vol. II, Academic Press,
New York, London, 1966.

WOODS, D.D.: The relation of p-aminobenzoic acid to the mechanism of
the action of sulphanilamide. Brit. J. Exp. Path. 21, 74-90 (1940).

Quantitative Structure-Activity Relationships in Drug-Design

Albert J. Leo

If it is our goal to make structure-activity relationships quantitative, then it necessarily follows that we must strive to obtain the most significant measures of both the *perturbation*--i.e., the action observed in the biological system--and the changes in *structure* in the chemicals which bring them about. There certainly is no unanimous agreement in an 'ideal' means of recording either perturbation or structural change, and if we introduce the further requirement that such measurements should be suitable to computer storage and manipulation, an even smaller fraction of today's flood of data manages to qualify.

A simple statement of the principles underlying the relationships we wish to establish greatly helps to clarify what needs to be quantified and how this can be accomplished. These principles can be expressed in two deceptively simple equations (Hansch, 1972).

$$\text{System}_i + (\text{Drug-X}_j) \rightarrow \text{Perturbation}_{ij} \tag{1}$$

$$\text{Perturbation}_{ij} = f(\text{Parameters of } -X_j) \tag{2}$$

For example: (Graham and James, 1961)

$$\text{Rat} + C_6H_5CHBrCH_2-N\begin{smallmatrix}R_1\\R_2\end{smallmatrix} \rightarrow \text{Blood pressure decrease vs std. dose adrenaline} \tag{1}$$

$$1/C \text{ (for ED50)} = f(E_s^c, \sigma^*, \#H) \tag{2}$$

$$\text{Log } 1/C = 9.86 + 0.90 \ E_s^c + 0.83 \ \sigma^* - 3.08 \ \#H \tag{2}$$

Our biological data file presently contains over 1,500 studies where the system varies in complexity from a purified macromolecule, such as serum albumin, to an organelle, to an intact plant or animal.

The term 'Drug-X' usually is a member of a chemically-related set (e.g. the phenethylamines or barbiturates), but it may be in a miscellaneous group, each of which perturbs the system in a way which appears identical. A complete record of the structural variations in the drugs appearing in the file involves construction, storage, and ability to manipulate connection tables wherein not only the bond types are indicated but also the stero-relationships of appropriate atoms. This is a task of no small magnitude and is, at present, very slow and cumbersome to use even if one has the funds to operate it.

On the other end of the spectrum is the use of a 'fragment code' which requires only the entry, for each drug, of any of a pre-selected list of sub-structures it may contain. The obvious shortcomings of this system are: first, as soon as the 'significant fragments' are selected, the system is closed; second, any fragments which ajoin others can create new fragments but these go unrecognized.

For our system, we have chosen to encode all drugs in Wiswesser Line Notation which combines most of the advantages of the two previous methods: structure-searching can be as thorough as with a connection table when needed, or as rapid as with fragment code. (Granito and Garfield, 1973) It is true that fragment specification with WLN must be made with great care in some instances, but it is, nevertheless, open-ended.

The 'perturbation', i.e. the biological response, should be registered in quantitative terms. Only in rare instances have we considered data of sufficient interest that we attempt to apply our approach to results reported as: 0 = inactive; + = active; ++ = very active etc. The great majority of the actions in our file are expressed as log 1/C, where C = moles/liter of drug needed to elicit a specified response, such as a certain degree of muscle contraction, or a given millivolt decrease in membrane potential (accepting the approximation that a kilogram of animal is equivalent to one liter).

Measurements of a variable response caused by a constant dose of a series of drugs, while useful for study of one particular system, has little value when a wide variety of systems are being compared in the search for common mechanisms of action. 'Relative biological response', if expressed in a concentration which gives a response equal to a unit concentration of a standard drug (say, atropine), is a useful measure, but must be separated from the more common 1/C for comparitive purposes. In cancer chemotherapy, the most common measure is (T/C)-150, which is the concentration needed to increase the lifespan of the treated vs control animals by 50% when both are given a standardized tumor challenge. It, too, forms a category by itself.

In Dr. Hansch's group, we have concentrated on the attempt to explain the perturbation as a linear function of parameters which are derived from physical chemistry; that is, from model reactions in homogenous solution, or from spectral data. Of course nothing in Eq. (2) limits us to physical-chemical parameters, and it is often advantageous to combine them with those calculated *de novo* (Craig, 1972) or from Molecular Orbital theory (Kier, 1971).

If we postulate that the observed response arises from the influence of the drug upon a single reaction which is rate-controlling, then the expressions are likely to resemble either those for reaction rates or for equilibria. Since both of these are free-energy related, the activity and the parameters are usually expressed in log terms to correspond to the Gibbs expression: $\Delta G = -RT\ln K$.

This 'single reaction' postulate is not as difficult to accept as it first seems. No doubt the majority of *random chemicals* would elicit many separate but conflicting responses, and the specific mechanisms would be hopelessly obscured. But the really effective *drugs* generally have both of the following characteristics: first, they possess a pharmacophore unusually well-suited to interact with an enzyme or co-factor; and second, the immediate target often acts through some amplification process. Of course in a chain reaction, such as the action of guinea pig complement on red cells to be dealt with later it is not possible in the early stages to say which of the nine enzymes in the chain is actually being inhibited, but considerable improvement in drug design can be made without ever finding this out.

Two objectives can be set for this system. It has already demonstrated its capability of meeting the first, short-range objective: that of 'zeroing in' more quickly on the optimal derivative of a particular pharmacophore which was discovered earlier by other means. The second objective, that of providing leads to new pharmacophores, will undoubtedly be a long time in coming, but may be reached when there are a sufficient number of pertinent equations to enable the responses in the more complex systems to be reliably related to those in the more simple ones--a step which can be critical in establishing a mechanism of action. Being able to clearly separate out non-specific influences, such as generalized hydrophobic bonding, from those which are explicitly affecting the active site is an obvious prerequisite to this task.

In designing a computerized data management system which would respond effec- tively in the type of search questions we wanted to ask, we had no clear precedent to follow. Our present system has evolved while keeping the following two problems foremost in our minds: 1) How could we *unify* the 'systems' and 'activities' of the biological reports without undue loss of *flexibility*? and 2) How should the data files be structured so that the meaningful characteristics of the regression equations could most effectively be compared? A brief summary of our file structure and content follows, and further details can be found in the recent literature (Hansch, et.al., 1974)

DESCRIPTOR DATA

1. System name and number.
2. Compound class & WLN superscreen.
3. Action.
4. Reference.
5. Dependent variable name.
6. Independent variable names.

COMPOUND DATA

1. Biological activity.
2. Parameter values (π, σ etc.)
3. Compound name & WLN
4. Deviation from regression.
5. WLN screen.

EQUATION DATA

1. Regression equation.
2. Correlation coeff. (R).
3. Standard deviation.
4. Confidence intervals etc.
5. Optimal P value (if any).

Fig. 1.'Set' Contents

A 'Set' contains three types of information: descriptive, in text; structural, i.e., topological (in Wiswesser Line Notation); and numeric. Searching the file will, at times, use Boolean *and/or* logic with combinations of all three types of information. With certain modifications, ordinary PL/I is suitable.

The 'descriptor data' file consists largely of text, but does contain the WLN 'superscreen' for more efficient searching. The 'compound' file is split equal- ly between numeric and topological information, while the 'equation' file is all numeric.

Some unification and simplification of the 'system' file is achieved through the assignment of a System Number, which can be employed in combination. For ex- ample as is shown in Fig. 2, all experiments on bacteria *in vitro* can be surveyed by specifying Sys#(04B), while those *in vivo* will be found by specifying (04B,06A).

Some of the 'workings' of our approach are best explained by examining a typical computer report of a regression analysis. The system in this set is 'E. Coli', and the compound class name is 'RCONH-Chloramphenicol'. Note that this class name need not be systematic since all structure searching is done via WLN. The action in this case is 'Growth Inhibition, Kinetic', which is different in in- trinsic sensitivity than the more common 'Growth I50'. It is important, therefore, that the dependent variable, designated 'K-App' in this case, <u>not</u> be retrieved when it is desired to compare intrinsic activity of pharmacophores by comparison of the intercepts of appropriate equations.

48

01_ Non-enzymatic macromolecules: e.g. albumin, fibrinogen.

02_ Enzymes:
  A = Oxido-reductases   D = Lyases
  B = Transferases   E = Isomerases
  C = Hydrolases

03_ Organelles: mitochondria, chloroplasts, etc.

04_ Single Cell Organsims
  A = Algae   P = Protozoa
  B = Bacteria   T = Tumor cells
  C = Cells (in culture)   V = Virus particles
  E = Erythrocytes   Y = Yeasts
  F = Fungi (molds)

05_ Isolated Parts or Organs: e.g. lobster axon, frog heart.

06_ Large Functioning Organism
  A = Animal
  B = Plant
  H = Human
  S = 'Sectionized' animal: e.g. thyroidectomized dog.

Fig. 2. System Numbers

    The variable structure of each of the compounds tested appears in the usual
chemical notation along with the cannonical WLN for the entire compound for exact
structure verification. The parameters in this study are: partition coefficient,
Taft's electronic sigma star, and molar refractivity. The activities, observed and
calculated, are in terms of log 1/C and the deviations between the two are listed.

    An asterisk can be used to prevent an 'outlier' from influencing the regression
line, but one can still keep track of its activity and the extent of its deviation.
The 'best' equation for each set is not automatically chosen on the basis of some-
one's favorite statistical criterion. Statisticians can be found who champion very
different tests of quality. We often use an option to examine the equations and
statistical summaries of all combinations of parameters. Of course 10 parameters
produce 1,000 equations, but these are quickly narrowed down by their standard
deviations, S, and correlation coefficients, R, to a manageable size for closer
scrutiny.

    It certainly would be more satisfying if we were able to make do with only
three parameters: one for hydrophobic bonding, one for electronic effects, and
one expressing variations in substituent volume to reflect a steric effect. Even
if this ideal were attained, it still would be frequently necessary, especially
in studies of purified enzymes, to factor each of these for positional variations,
because they may not be the same in all portions of the molecules being tested.
Positional effects are, of course, already considered in the electronic terms, σ-
meta and σ-para, but each of these might carry different coefficients if the substitutions are made on more than one ring.

    Π-sum is frequently pertinent in describing a random walk process of binding-
desorption required to reach the active site. But an additional π-term for substituents in a particular position can become significant to account for *oriented*
on-site binding. A case where both π and σ are apparently position-dependent is
found in the phenanthreneaminoalkylcarbinol antimalarials as shown in Fig. 4 (Craig
and Hansch, 1973).

Descriptor Data

Compound Data

Regression Analysis Data

E.COLI*RCONH-CHLORAMPHENICOL*GROWTH INH.KINETIC*GARRETT UNPUB*K-APP*ES*P*S'*
ES'*ES-S*ES-2L*S-SUM*PE*$HANSCH POMONA COLLEGE   SYS#(04B)   W$

H3AA. DOUBLE PRECISION MATRIX INVERSION. 95% CONFIDENCE INTERVALS DELTA=0.1D-09
THIS RUN DATED 11/28/73
1)

NO.	P	S'	PE	K-APP (OBS)	K-APP (PRED)	DEV	GROUP	WLN
1	1.070	2.610	5.690	2.240	2.743	-0.503	CF3	WNR DYQY1QMVXFFF
2	1.150	1.940	15.440	2.000	1.821	0.179	CHCL2	WNR DYQY1QMVYGG
3	1.360	1.940	21.240	1.840	1.409	0.431	CHBR2	WNR DYQY1QMVYEE
4	0.590	1.050	10.580	1.710	1.439	0.271	CH2CL	WNR DYQY1QMV1G
5	0.980	1.000	15.200	1.470	1.289	0.181	CHCLCH3	WNR DYQY1QMVYG
6	0.660	1.000	13.480	1.380	1.306	0.074	CH2BR	WNR DYQY1QMV1E
7*	0.420	2.050	5.700	1.300	2.164	-0.864	*CHF2	WNR DYQY1QMVYFF
8	0.150	1.100	5.710	1.160	1.242	-0.082	CH2F	WNR DYQY1QMV1F
:	:	:	:	:	:	:	:	:
19	→	→	→	→	→	→	→	→
MEAN	1.063	1.020	17.701	0.793				
SD	0.646	0.990	8.623	0.858				

DF1 = 18   SS1 = 13.2470   VAR1 = 0.7359   DEV+ = 11
DF2 = 14   SS2 = 1.9022   VAR2 = 0.1359   DEV- = 8
N = 19   S = 0.3686   R2 = 0.8564   R = 0.9254   EMAX = 0.2E-12

1) $K-APP = 0.5947 + 1.7570*P + 0.6228*S' - 0.0490*PE - 0.9417*P**2$

95 PERCENT CONFIDENCE INTERVALS
     0.5628   0.8473   0.2233   0.0377   0.4173

           IDEAL P = 0.9329
CON INT FOR IDEAL P = 0.6528   TO   1.2732

Fig. 3. Computer Report of Regression Analysis

PHENANTHRENEAMINOALKYLCARBINOL

Antimalarials

$x = 1\text{-}4$
$y = 5\text{-}8$

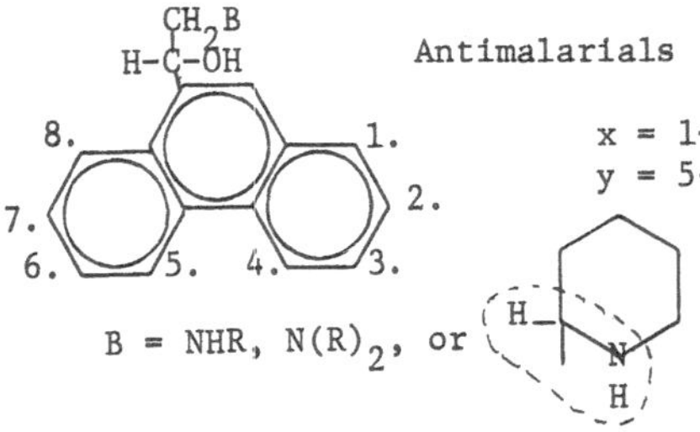

$B = NHR, N(R)_2,$ or

$$1/C = 2.355 + .270\,\pi_x + .396\,\pi_y +$$
$$.654\,\sigma_x + .878\,\sigma_y + .137\,\pi_{sum} - 0.15\,\pi^2_{sum}$$

$n = 102$ (out of 107); $S = .258$; $R = .913$

Fig. 4. π and σ Position-Dependent

There is an optimal hydrophobicity for the entire molecule, as might be expected. Hydrophobic substituents on each of the side rings increase activity in
linear fashion, but in each ring to a different degree. The activating effects of
σ in the 1-4 positions are likewise only about 70% as great as in the 5-8 positions.

At the present 'state of the art', one can be mislead by putting too much faith
in the absolute separation of effects by the various parameters. For instance, the
steric parameter, E_s, definitely appears to reflect a considerable electronic influence as well (Unger and Hansch, 1975). Of course, even if the parameters are
theoretically capable of a good separation of effects, a given set of substituents
may not show this (Hansch and Unger, 1973). For this reason, our program prints
out the R^2 between each of the parameters as well as a 'T-matrix'(Farrar and Glauber,
1967).
In casting about for a substitute parameter which would be at least as effective as E_s for bulk effects, but one which could be applied to a broader range of
substituent groups--groups for which no E_s can be measured--we are currently encouraged by results using Molar Refractivity, MR. For liquids whose index of refraction is known, MR can be calculated using molecular weight and density by way
of the Lorentz equation:

$$MR = M.W.(\eta^2 - 1)/d(\eta^2 + 2)\ ml/mol \qquad (3)$$

where:

M.W. = molecular weight
η = index of refraction (20° Na-D line)
d = density

Using these 'measured' values as a base, it is possible to extend the calculations to compounds not normally liquid by assigning refractivities to either
atoms or bonds (Vogel et. al., 1952). Molar refractivity is expressed in units
of volume and may indicate, for example, the ability of the bulk of a substituent
to distort the enzyme to which it is bound and thereby affect a reaction rate. On
the other hand, as has been noted (Agin and Hersch, 1965), there is good reason to
expect that, as a sum of electronic polarizabilities, MR can serve as a measure of
the binding arising out of dispersion forces.

In an earlier study of biological activities, which may have been somewhat
weighted in favor of membrane binding effects, we concluded that polarizability
(and therefore MR) was not as effective as log P (Leo et. al., 1969). Since then
we have studied more systems which involve binding of substrates to more polar
macromolecules, and especially in studies of purified enzyme systems, we find instances where MR is superior to log P. Two examples are shown by the following
equations:

System: Concanavalin + β-phenylglucosides

A. n = 17 (of 19 tested)

$$1/C = 2.231 + 0.0186 \text{ MR} \quad S = .033; R = .964 \quad (4)$$
$$1/C = 2.367 + 0.0991 \text{ Pi} \quad S = .100; R = .585 \quad (5)$$

B. n = 16 (of 16 tested)

$$1/C = 5.206 + 0.0249 \text{ MR} \quad\quad S = .097; R = .920 \quad (8)$$
$$1/C = 5.479 + 0.2192 \text{ Pi} \quad\quad S = .098; R = .919 \quad (9)$$
$$1/C = 5.135 + 0.0238 \text{ MR} + 0.095 \text{ E}_s \quad S = .085; R = .945 \quad (10)$$
$$1/C = 5.467 + 0.2165 \text{ Pi} + 0.013 \text{ E}_s \quad S = .101; R = .920 \quad (11)$$

The clear superiority of MR over Pi in the 'A' set may be an artifact, for a warning accompanies this report: "Poor data; range of dependent variable = 0.41." In the second set, 'B', another investigator studied the same basic system with derivatives producing a wider range of activities, and a comparison of Eq. (8) with (9) shows that MR and Pi are essentially equal as single parameters. In Eqs. (10) and (11) it can be seen that the addition of a steric parameter for the ortho position does not significantly improve the equation with Pi (F = .07) but it does improve the one with MR (F = 5.46). This is unexpected and does not support the view that MR can measure a steric effect to a greater degree than does log P. For the substituents used in this particular experiment, at least, log P is more closely related to the E_s-2 parameter, as is indicated in their R^2. As expected, there is a great overlap between log P and MR.

Recently Dr. Yoshimoto of the Sankyo Co., who is presently working in our laboratories at Pomona College, developed an interesting correlation of the activities of 108 benzamidine derivatives acting as inhibitors of Guinea pig complement. These compounds were synthesized and tested by Dr. Baker's group at the University of California, Santa Barbara, and were thought to fall into several distinct categories (Baker et. al., 1969, 1971). The manner in which Yoshimoto and Hansch treated the data so that the activities of all 108 derivatives could be rationalized with a single equation, is rather instructive. (Hansch and Yoshimoto, 1974)

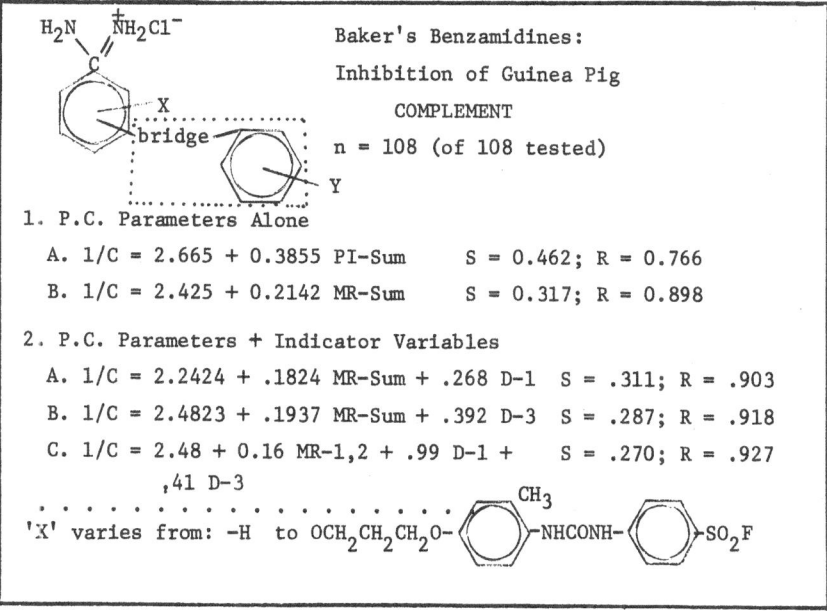

Baker's Benzamidines:

Inhibition of Guinea Pig

COMPLEMENT

n = 108 (of 108 tested)

1. P.C. Parameters Alone

  A. $1/C = 2.665 + 0.3855$ PI-Sum $S = 0.462; R = 0.766$

  B. $1/C = 2.425 + 0.2142$ MR-Sum $S = 0.317; R = 0.898$

2. P.C. Parameters + Indicator Variables

  A. $1/C = 2.2424 + .1824$ MR-Sum + .268 D-1 $S = .311; R = .903$

  B. $1/C = 2.4823 + .1937$ MR-Sum + .392 D-3 $S = .287; R = .918$

  C. $1/C = 2.48 + 0.16$ MR-1,2 + .99 D-1 + $S = .270; R = .927$
     .41 D-3

'X' varies from: −H to $OCH_2CH_2CH_2O$-⬡-CH_3-NHCONH-⬡-SO_2F

Fig. 5 Use of Indicator Variables

The first problem to overcome was posed by the range in size and complexity of the substituents. Not long ago we felt that to find parameter values for substituents varying all the way from 'H' to $C_{17}H_{18}FN_2O_5S$ was beyond our capability. But we are steadily increasing the reliability of our calculated π-values, because our data pool project is continually adding log P values of compounds which serve as closer models to any desired substituent. The new log P values are also providing refinements to the calculation of proximity effects, and of folding etc. Before the regression was attempted, it was deemed prudent to measure partition coefficients for benzamidine and four of its key derivatives. With these in hand, a hydrophobic parameter for all 108 derivatives could be calculated with confidence.

E_s values for only a few of the 108 substituents were available, and calculation of the remainder seemed fruitless; therefore MR was tried. Conceivably it could reflect both a bulk effect and a binding effect due to dispersion forces in a manner different from log P, especially if the enzyme surface surrounding the active site was not particularly conducive to hydrophobic binding.

Of course sigma values were also available for only a few of the 108 derivatives. However, these can be estimated with a greater degree of confidence, and values from similar functions established with little doubt that electronic forces play but a minor role in this type of inhibition

With sigma out of the running, it would seem hopeless to explain the wide variance in activity of these complex derivatives with log P or MR alone, or with a combination of the two, since we expect a high degree of collinearity between them. Actually, MR alone does surprisingly well, but still produced a rather high standard deviation:

$$1/C = 2.665 + 0.3855 \text{ Pi-Sum} \qquad S = 0.462; \ R = 0.766 \qquad (12)$$
$$1/C = 2.425 + 0.2142 \text{ MR-Sum} \qquad S = 0.317; \ R = 0.898 \qquad (13)$$

From these preliminary equations, one could surmise that hydrophobic bonding was probably not equally effective in all parts of the molecule in promoting inhibition, while molar refractivity, if it is modeling binding through dispersion forces in this case, was not as position dependent. But the pattern of 'outliers' with MR seemed to indicate that no continuous function was likely to prove greatly superior to it. In this type of situation we believe that the use of 'indicator variables can increase our understanding of the structure-activity relationship. This amounts to combining the 'Free-Wilson' with the 'Hammett' approach, except that at the time the indicator variables are assigned, only a small number of structural variations need be considered, and a possible mechanistic role for them may already be surmised.

In the case of Baker's benzamidines, the 'indicator variable' appeared to be required to distinguish between two types of structures: (1) where 'X' is a side chain of any length which contains no aromatic ring; or when it contains a ring but the connecting bridge is less than four atoms long; or (2) where 'X' is a chain of at least four atoms in length connected to a second aromatic ring, with the chain being hydrophobic (all alkyl) or mixed (ethers and/or aminos). In case (1), D = 0; in case (2), D = 1.

If Pi-Sum and MR-Sum are calculated to include both the bridge and second ring, MR remains superior to log P. But if the indicator variable is allowed to include any binding effect of the optimal bridge and ring (with Pi and MR calculated for only the ring substituents on Rings #1 and #2) then the parameters are essentially equal in predictive capability. These results are consistent with a mechanism whereby the side chain on Ring #1 (i.e. 'X') is contributing only a small inhibitory effect by way of stronger hydrophobic bonding. But if this chain serves to extend a second aromatic ring into a suitable area at an appreciable distance from the active site, bonding by that ring can be highly inhibitory.

A second indicator variable denoting the presence or absence of a pyridine ring on the 'X' side chain also proved to be significant. The final 'best' equation was:

$$\log 1/C = 0.99 \text{ D-1} + 0.16 \text{ MR-1,2} + 0.41 \text{ D-3} + 2.48; \quad S=0.27; \quad R=0.927 \qquad (14)$$
$$\pm (0.13) \qquad (0.03) \qquad (0.15) \qquad (0.12)$$

Since there was over a 1,000-fold variance in the activities in these 108 benzamidines, any equation which can predict them within a factor of 1,8 (on the average) is quite impressive.

Structure Searching

We have just recently completed an extensive revision of our data files which now allows us to ask of them a full range of structure-activity questions. Preliminary results are certainly encouraging, but at the same time we think they carry a note of caution.

A computer can be very impressive in how quickly it can search, sort, tabulate and type up a report, performing in a few seconds a task that might take the human researcher a week of hard effort. Perhaps because of this type of performance there can be a tendency to attach some special importance--an aura of infallibity-- to the results so derived. This can be a very insidious trap. One must always scrutinize the search reports to make sure he has not used an elaborate scheme just to confirm a particular *bias* he has unwittingly built into his data file. Perhaps the following two examples may serve as an illustration of this point, but, then again, they may be conveying some real message.

The curves in Fig. 6 summarize the results of a search of our file for compounds whose activity was expressed as either $1/C$ or K_m. Their activities should, therefore, be on a comparable scale but the type of action could vary all the way from non-specific narcosis to inhibition of a particular enzyme. In curve I. the search specification was for the structure to contain an amide group both in a ring *and* in a chain attached to the ring, while for curve II. the specification was merely an amide group in either chain *or* ring. For this search we defined an 'amide' as any nitrogen adjacent to a carbonyl, and thus the structure $=\text{N-C}=\text{O}$ qualified.

At first glance the results appear to be very significant. The diamides as a group are about a thousand-fold more active than the mono-amides. Closer inspection reveals, however, that the ring-chain diamides were very heavily represented by rifamycins, penicillins and cephalothins. Granted, they are vastly more potent bacterial growth inhibitors than, say, butyramide or methyl urethane, and the ring-chain di-function may play a role in this antimicrobic action. But few people try these more esoteric structures in the experiments commonly performed with simpler molecules, that is, in tests such as tadpole narcosis or DNA denaturation. If each molecule in our file had been subjected to the same battery of test systems, then the activity curves could truly be a result of the difference in the structures as specified.

The results of a second search are summarized in Fig. 7. The same activity selection of either $1/C$ or K_m was made, but the structure variation was:
(1) Complex = a 6-membered ring containing at least two 'N' atoms + a side-chain with a carbonyl.
(2) Simple = same as (1) but only one 'N' atom in ring.

In this case the difference in structural complexity is not nearly as great. In fact, morpholines might be considered as equal in complexity to pyrimidines. Furthermore the type of test systems in which the two classes appeared were not that different in sensitivity. Yet the compounds in class (1) were again almost a thousand-fold more active than those in class (2).

We feel that we still may uncover a hidden bias which will partly explain these results, but meanwhile we plan to extend these rather 'simplistic' searches,

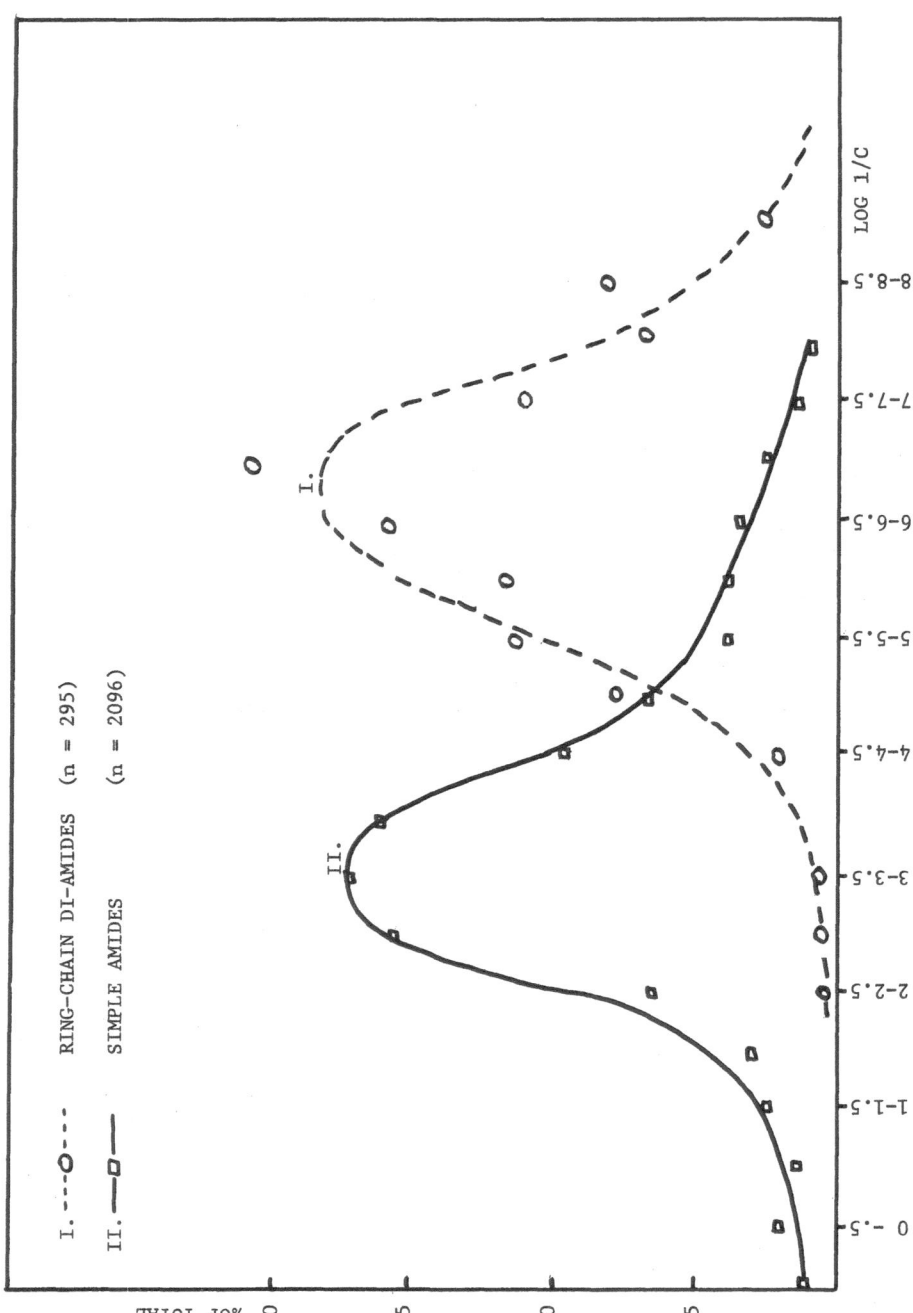

Fig. 6.

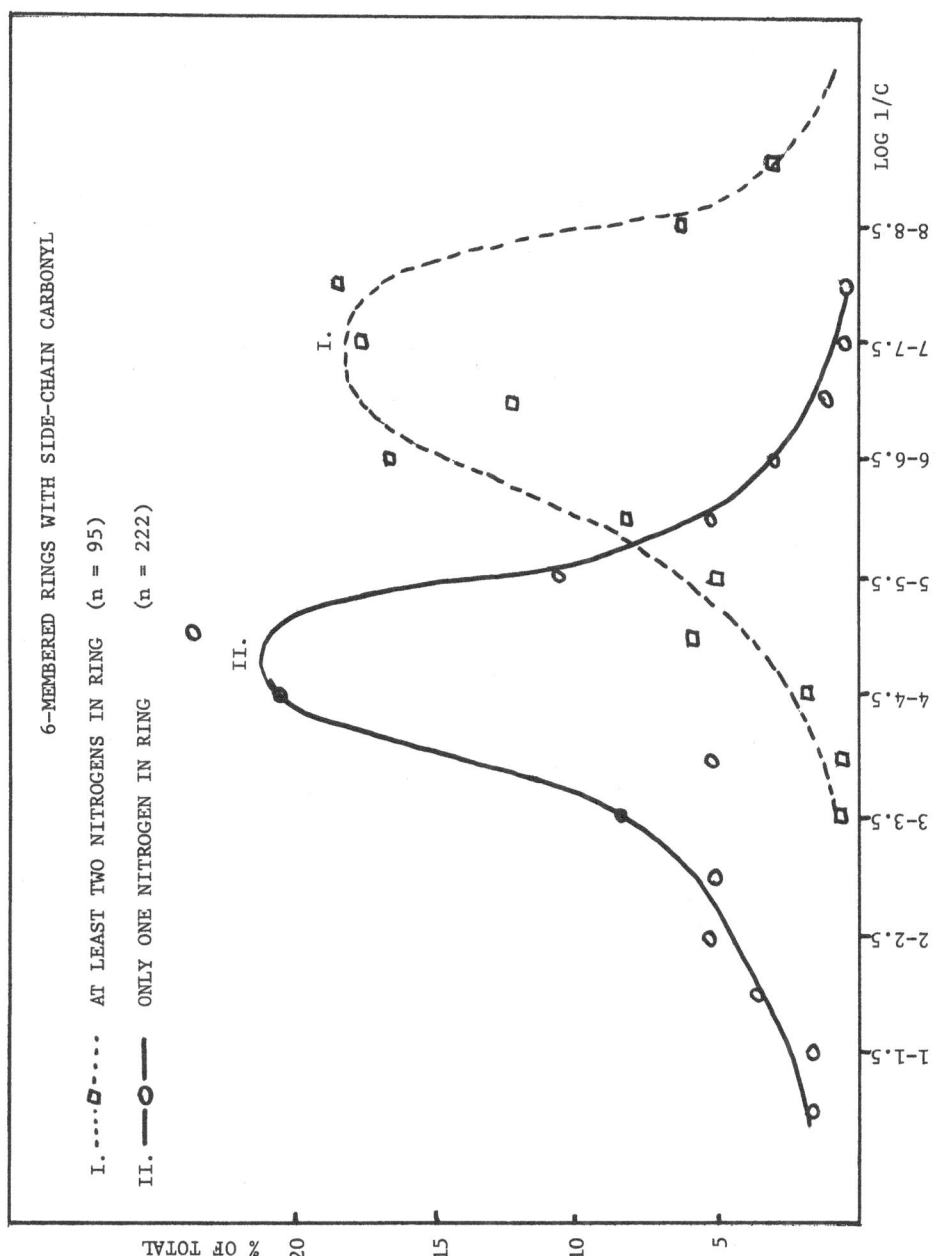

Fig. 7.

while we are learning how to operate our structure-searching tools at a more sophisticated level -- that is, somewhere between a string-search on the WLN and one using connection tables.

References

AGIN, D., L. HERSCH and D. HOLTZMAN: The action of Anesthetics on Excitable Membranes: A Quantum-Chemical Analysis. Proc. Nat. Acad. Sci. U.S., 53, 952 (1965).

BAKER, B. R. and E. H. ERICKSON: Irreversible Enzyme Inhibitors. CLII. Proteolytic Enzymes X. J. Med. Chem., 12, 408 (1969).

BAKER, B. R. and M. CORY: Irreversible Enzyme Inhibitors. 186. Ibid. 14, 805 (1971).

CRAIG, P. N.: Comparison of the Hansch and Free-Wilson Approaches to Structure-Activity Correlation. Advances in Chemistry Series No. 114, 115 (1972).

CRAIG, P. N. and C. HANSCH: Structure-Activity Correlation of Antimalarial Compounds. 2. Phenanthreneaminoalkylcarbinol Antimalarials. J. Med. Chem., 16, 661 (1973).

FARRAR, D. E. and R. R. GLAUBER: Multicollinearity in Regression Analysis: The Problem Revisited. Rev. Econ. Stat., 49, 92 (1967).

GRAHAM, J. D. P. and G. W. L. JAMES: The Pharmacology of a Series of Substituted 2-Halogenoalkylamines. J. Med. and Pharmaceut. Chem., 3, 489 (1961).

GRANITO, C. E. and E. GARFIELD: Substructure Search and Correlation in the Management of Chemical Information. Naturwissenschaften, 60, 189 (1973).

HANSCH, C.: A Computerized Approach to Quantitative Biochemical Structure-Activity Relationships. Advances in Chemistry Series No. 114, 20 (1972).

HANSCH, C., S. H. UNGER and A. B. FORSYTHE: Strategy in Drug Design; Cluster Analysis as an Aid in the Selection of Substituents. J. Med. Chem., 16, 1217 (1973).

HANSCH, C., A. LEO, and D. ELKINS: Computerized Managemennt of Structure-Activity Data. I Multivariate Analysis of Biological Data. J. Chem. Doc., 14, 57 (1974)

HANSCH, C. and M. YOSHIMOTO: Structure-Activity Relationships in Immuno-Chemistry II. Inhibition of Complement by Benzamidines. J. Med. Chem. 17 Nov. (1974).

KIER, L. B.: Molecular Orbital Theory in Drug Research. Academic Press, N.Y. (1971).

LEO, A., HANSCH, C. and C. CHURCH: Comparison of Parameters Currently Used in the Study of Structure-Activity Relationships. J. Med. Chem., 12, 766 (1969).

UNGER, S. and C. HANSCH: Quantitative Models of Steric Effects. In Press (1975).

VOGEL, A. I., W. T. CRESSWELL, G. H. JEFFREY and J. LEICESTER: Physical Properties and Chemical Constitution Part XXIV. Bond Parachors and Bond Refractions. J. Chem. Soc. 514 (1952).

II. DNA as a Drug-Receptor

The Ecological Significance of R Factor Activity

E. S. Anderson

INTRODUCTION

The long disputes over the ecological significance of R factor activity
have in the course of time resolved themselves by the significance declaring
itself. The protagonists in the debate could be broadly assigned to two camps:
those who had believed from the earliest days of the studies of transferable
drug resistance that the appearance of R factors in pathogens was a direct
indication of their importance to clinicians, and those who believed that the
phenomenon, though of great theoretical interest, was relatively unimportant
in the ecology of the enterobacteria and related species.

Those who were convinced of the ominous significance of R factors produced
evidence that established that their appearance was a response to antibiotic
pressure in animals and man, and called for a reduction in the use of antibiotics
in order to ease that pressure, in the hope that the incidence of R factors in
pathogens would thereby diminish. (see, for example, Anderson, 1965a, 1968a, b;
Anderson & Lewis, 1965a, b.)

Those who favoured the view that the importance of R factors was being
exaggerated called for calm in the face of the observations. They indicated
the hazards of abandoning the protection of the antibiotics (in which term I
shall include synthetic antibacterial drugs) for prophylaxis and treatment of
bacterial infections of both man and animals. Moreover, a serious reduction of
protein production was forecast if antibiotics such as penicillin and the
tetracyclines were withdrawn from use as feed additives for growth promotion of
livestock (Office of Health Economics, 1969).

In this paper I shall endeavour to outline these subjects in perspective,
to describe work that has clarified the modus operandi of R factors and other
bacterial plasmids, and to present a statement of the present situation relating
to transferable resistance throughout the world.

THE OPERATION OF R FACTORS

Watanabe (1963) postulated a linear structure for R factors. On this
structure were distributed the determinants for drug resistance. Transfer of
the complex depended on a region designated the Resistance Transfer Factor (RTF).
Watanabe pointed out that the whole structure could be rectilinear or circular.
The analogy between the RTF and the F (sex) factor of Escherichia coli was
recognised, and many operational similarities between the F factor and R factors
were demonstrated. In fact, as we now know, the F factor, R factors and many

other bacterial extrachromosomal genetic elements or plasmids, composed of DNA, some auto-transferable, others devoid of this character, constitute a number of plasmid "families" or groups in the enterobacteria.

The R factors originally discovered in Japan were initially all transferable to new bacterial hosts as single units carrying all their resistance determinants and the RTF. They therefore remained transferable in the new hosts. They were transduced as complete linkage groups by phage P1 in E.coli K12 (= K12), but segregation of resistance markers usually occurred during transduction by phage P22 in Salmonella typhimurium strain LT2 (review: Watanabe, 1963) and many such segregant resistances had lost the ability to transfer. Watanabe noted, however, that when an R factor coding for resistance to chloramphenicol (C), streptomycin (S), sulphonamides (Su) and tetracyclines (T) was transduced by P22, segregation followed the pattern CSSu and T. The CSSu segregants were non-transferable, but the T remained transferable and could also restore transferability to the CSSu fragment. These and related findings were used by Watanabe to construct a tentative linkage map for the R factor concerned (Watanabe, 1963).

The R factors discovered in Japan were prevalent in shigellae and E.coli, and salmonellae did not at that time appear to be contributing to the R factor problem. Indeed, because shigella R factors were difficult to transfer to S.typhimurium and were rather unstable in that host, it was assumed that salmonellae were poor hosts for R factors (Watanabe, 1963). In fact, salmonellae are excellent and unfortunately important hosts for R factors, but the R factors found in them are better suited than those from shigellae to enter and to survive in salmonellae. This form of ecological resolution can be generally and simply stated as follows: in the long term, particular R factors or R factor groups predominate in those members of the enterobacteria they are best equipped to inhabit. There is, in fact, a considerable degree of host specificity, and some R factors have not so far been induced to enter certain hosts. Nevertheless, the host range of many R factors is very wide, and encompasses most of the enterobacteria.

R factors in S.typhimurium.

In the Enteric Reference Laboratory we have monitored the incidence of (among other serotypes) S.typhimurium for over 30 years. Our primary tool is phage-typing, but we supplement this with the identification of whatever genetic markers, including those for drug resistance, may be useful for strain identification. With these methods we have established that certain phage types of S.typhimurium are prevalent in particular animal hosts, often for long periods, and are communicated with roughly proportional frequency to man (Anderson, 1960, 1969a). Phage-typing and its ancillary methods thus indicate not only the relatedness of cases in a given outbreak, but the animal source from which the infection may have sprung.

In the early 1960s it was noted that a particular phage type of S.typhimurium, type 29, hitherto relatively rare, had become common in calves. Its increased incidence was associated with the appearance of drug resistance. Indeed, it was clear that resistance was a specific feature of the strain(s) concerned, which showed the resistance spectrum (R-type) SSu. By 1963 the resistant type had become established in calves, and human infections indicated that it was being communicated from calves to man (Anderson, 1965a, 1968a, b, 1971, 1973; Anderson & Lewis, 1965a, b). As the incidence of the type increased, so did its spectrum of drug resistance, with the appearance of T early in 1964, followed by resistances to ampicillin (A), chloramphenicol (C), furazolidone (Fu), and neomycin-kanamycin (K). The commonest R-types encountered were ASSuTFu and SSuTFu. All the resistances, with the exception of that to furazolidone, were transferable.

Investigations revealed the source of the organism, the reasons for its spread and those for the expanding range of drug resistance. The strain had been introduced into calves reared by the intensive farming method. A particular calf dealer was collecting animals very soon after birth, assembling them on a farm in Essex, and thereafter distributing them throughout Britain, using unsuitable transport, often over long journeys. The animals started off the journey in poor physical state, and were greatly enfeebled by the time they reached their destination: many indeed were moribund. They suffered from scours - infectious diarrhoea - and septicaemia, the organism concerned being drug-resistant S.typhimurium type 29. The calf dealer, who was passing 500 - 700 animals a week through his farm, was aware that his unit was acting as the source of infection, and was administering furazolidone and, it is suspected, ampicillin, to all his calves, irrespective of any signs of illness, to act as a prophylactic against the spread of infection to new stock. Moreover, he was distributing furazolidone with the animals he sent to other farms with a recommendation that it be used by his clients to prevent scours. As the animals were often already infected with type 29, and as the organism was already resistant to furazolidone, the results were the opposite of what was expected. The animals were if anything adversely affected by the drug, and spread of the infection was encouraged by its use. The result was not only that the animals already infected usually died, but that the infection rapidly spread to healthy animals, so that entire herds were affected, with very high mortality.

Naturally, veterinary help was sought, and antibiotics were again used in efforts to control the infection. They did not, but they did result in expansion of the R-type of 29; it was probably in this way that chloramphenicol and neomycin-kanamycin resistances were acquired. Fortunately, these proved to be rather unstable in this host and soon disappeared. On the other hand, the R-types ASSuTFu and SSuTFu are very stable.

Type 29 maintained a high incidence in bovines and man until 1968, but diminished thereafter, and disappeared by the end of 1970. The cause of its disappearance was the death of the calf dealer early in 1967. With the disappearance of the source, the network of infection resolved itself spontaneously, because there was negligible spread from the periphery. Nevertheless, it took over three years for type 29 to disappear, even when the central distribution had ceased.

The course of this outbreak is outlined in Fig. 1, which shows type 29 in man and animals as a percentage of total S.typhimurium in man and animals from 1960 to 1970 (Anderson, 1965a, 1968a, 1971, 1973; Anderson & Lewis, 1965a, b).

THE GENETICS OF DRUG RESISTANCE IN PHAGE TYPE 29

Studies of type 29 demonstrated that its pattern of resistance transfer differed materially from that of the R factors first observed in Japan and subsequently demonstrated in many other parts of the world (Anderson, 1968b, 1969b; Anderson & Lewis, 1965a, b). Primarily, the resistances in type 29 did not transfer as a single linkage group, but segregated in transfer, as shown in table 1. (The Su and Fu symbols will be omitted, the first because it always transferred with S, the second because it did not transfer: the original strain will thus be designated 29(AST).)

Table 2 shows the frequency of transfer of the segregated resistances from the various K12 progeny of this cross.

The crosses in table 2 show the same frequency of transfer of A and S, but a dramatic increase in the transfer frequency of T from about 10^{-6} in the initial 29(AST) x K12 cross to a figure approaching unity in the K12(T) x K12 cross. The explanation for this disparity was shown to be that the initial transfer of

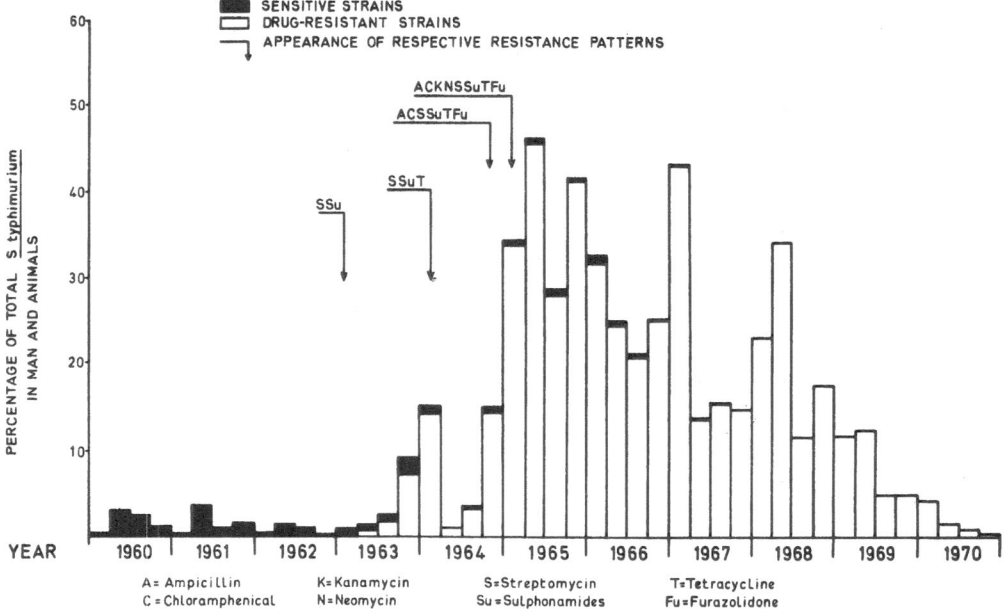

Fig. 1. Distribution of type 29 in man and animals 1960-1970

Table 1. Transfer of resistance markers from S.typhimurium phage type 29.

Cross	Selection	Progeny	Frequency
29(AST) x K12F⁻	A	K12(A)	10^{-2}
	S	K12(S)	10^{-2}
	T	K12(T)	c. 10^{-6}

T marked the occurrence of a very rare event - recombination between T and the
RTF. Thereafter, the transfer of T was equal to that of the RTF that carried it,
which approaches 10° in the overnight crosses routinely used in our laboratory
(Anderson & Lewis, 1965a, b). It was shown that the T-RTF resistance factor
caused heavy phage restriction in S.typhimurium.

The frequency of transfer of A and S remained constant at about 10^{-2} in
overnight crosses. If crosses from K12(A) and K12(S) to S.typhimurium were
interrupted at up to about 4 hours, most S.typhimurium(A) and S.typhimurium(S)
exconjugants were unable to transfer their resistance. These resistances could
be mobilised by the highly transferable tetracycline resistance resulting from
T transfer in the original 29(AST) x K12 cross (Anderson & Lewis, 1965b).

Table 2. <u>Transfer of resistance from K12 derivatives of type 29.</u>

Cross	Selection (including nalidixic acid)	Progeny	Frequency
K12(A) X K12Nal^r	ampicillin	K12(A)Nal^r	10^{-2}
K12(S) X K12Nal^r	streptomycin	K12(S)Nal^r	10^{-2}
K12(T) X K12Nal^r	tetracycline	K12(T)Nal^r	c. 10^{0}

K12Nal^r = K12 mutant resistant to nalidixic acid.

Further observations on transfer from K12(A) and K12(S) to <u>S.typhimurium</u> showed that in overnight crosses a factor with the following characters entered the <u>S.typhimurium</u> strain.

1) It did not carry resistance.

2) It caused heavy phage restriction in <u>S.typhimurium.</u>

3) It was transferred to almost 100% of the <u>S.typhimurium</u> recipient.

With the exception of the absence of drug resistance, these properties are identical with those of the highly transferable T. It was thus suspected that the transferable agent that did not carry drug resistance was in fact the RTF of the 29(AST) system, and that in its original state it was recombined with none of the resistances. This was confirmed by the triparental cross for determinant mobilisation, exemplified in table 3.

Strains 1 and 2 were mixed in equal amounts in late logarithmic growth in nutrient broth. After incubation for a few hours, strain 3 was added and the mixture incubated overnight. It was then plated in serial dilutions on medium containing streptomycin and nalidixic acid, the latter to eliminate strains 1 and 2, and incubated overnight. Transfer of S to K12Nal^r was then apparent. This was the result of transfer of the RTF from strain 1 to strain 2, mobilisation of S, and subsequent transfer of both S and the RTF to strain 3. The RTF concerned has been designated Δ (Anderson & Lewis, 1965b).

The genetics of the Δ transfer systems in 29(AST) can be summarised as follows. The A and S resistance determinants are independent plasmids. They are non auto-transferring but are mobilised by the Δ transfer factor. However, they remain independent of Δ in the new host. The state of the T determinant in the wild 29(AST) is unclear. It is certainly independent of A, S and Δ, but it is not known whether it is a plasmid in the same sense as the other three, or whether it is chromosomal in location. However, it is clear that once T is mobilised it has recombined with Δ in a relationship quite different from that between A or S and Δ. The T resistance factor is designated T-Δ, the hyphen indicating covalent linkage between the two; the A and S transfer systems are designated A,Δ and S,Δ respectively, the comma indicating the absence of covalent bonding. In fact the nature of the linkage, if any, between these determinants and the Δ transfer factor remains unknown.

Table 3. Triparental cross for determinant mobilisation

Parents	Selection	Progeny
1 2 3 S.typhimurium(RTF) X K12(S) X K12Nal^r	streptomycin + nalidixic acid	K12(S)(RTF)Nal^r

K12Nal^r = nalidixic acid-resistant mutant of K12.

The foregoing description indicates that the 29(ASTΔ) transfer systems are different from those first identified in Japan. In the first instance, there is no initial bonding between the Δ transfer factor and any of the determinants: secondly, the determinants are mobilised independently by Δ. Thirdly, A and S remain independent of each other and of Δ, but the T determinant recombines with Δ to form a single covalently-bonded R factor. There thus appears a point of similarity between these systems and those found in Japan, in that T-Δ, once formed, behaves in precisely the same way as the Japanese R factors: it is always transferred together with Δ and always remains transferable.

If these observations are correct, A and S should show independent transduction into K12 by phage P1, and should be non-transferring after transduction, even if Δ was present in the K12 donor strain. T-Δ, in contrast, should be transduced as a single plasmid and should remain transferable after transduction. All these postulates have been confirmed (Anderson & Natkin, 1972).

It has been shown that A and S are small plasmids, of 5.6 and 5.7×10^6 daltons molecular weight respectively. They are present in a multiplicity of between about 5 and 20 copies per cell (Smith et al., 1974), but only one carries out the function of master copy: probably that attached to the cell membrane and responsible for genetic continuity of the plasmid concerned. The A plasmid codes for β-lactamase synthesis, and the high level of ampicillin resistance it confers (minimal inhibitory concentration in K12 c. 3000μg/ml) is apparently related to the multiplicity of copies, each of which appears to function. Plasmids such as A and SSu can be mobilised by a wide range of transfer factors.

The Δ plasmid is present in an average of one copy per cell. It is a covalently closed circular element of about 59×10^6 daltons molecular weight (Humphreys et al., 1972). As would be expected from the genetic findings, T-Δ is similar in configuration to Δ and is also present as a single copy. However, the molecular weight of T-Δ is about 62×10^6 daltons, giving a possible weight of about 3×10^6 daltons for T.

It is evident from these findings that there are two types of resistance (or other plasmid) transfer system. We have designated these Class 1 and 2 (Anderson, 1968b, 1969b; Anderson & Natkin, 1972). Their properties are shown in table 4.

If the descriptions summarised in table 4 are generally applicable to enterobacterial transfer systems, both classes of transfer system should be found in nature, and since the components of Class 2 systems are independent plasmids, both the determinants and the transfer factors should be found separately. Moreover, since Class 1 R factors all possess transfer factors, such R factors should be found in nature transferring unlinked resistance (and other) determinants in a Class 2 relationship, as well as transferring their own resistances. These postulates have been confirmed. Class 1 and 2 transfer systems are commonly found in E.coli and salmonellae. The point of departure for the detection of transfer factors in drug-sensitive strains was the triparental cross summarised in table 3. The cross can be rewritten as in table 5.

The primary donor A is a wild drug-sensitive strain suspected of carrying the transfer factor x. The intermediate recipient B is a laboratory strain carrying a mobilisable resistance determinant r. The final recipient C is devoid of both transfer factor and R determinant, but is resistant to a drug to which both A and B are sensitive. The cross is performed as described earlier except that the time during which A and B, and then A, B and C are allowed to remain in contact may be extended for days if necessary, since some transfer factors may have a very low mobility into the bacterial strains we use as a routine. It has been shown by this technique that transfer factors devoid of any identifiable determinants are widespread in naturally-occurring E.coli and salmonellae (Anderson, 1965b).

Table 4. Enterobacterial plasmid transfer systems. Relationship
between transfer factor and resistance (or other genetic) determinants

Class 1	Class 2
Single covalently-bonded plasmid formed by recombination between determinant and transfer factor.	Resistance determinants are plasmids independent of transfer factors.
Transferred as a single linkage group.	Transferred separately or together with transfer factor.
One copy per cell.	Determinants, 5 - 20 copies per cell. Transfer factor, 1 copy per cell.
Transduced intact by phage P1.	Transduced separately by phage P1.
Examples	Examples
T-Δ 62 x 10^6 daltons	(SSu 5.7 x 10^6 daltons ((Δ 59 x 10^6 daltons
ColIb-P9 68 x 10^6 daltons	(ColE1 4.7 x 10^6 daltons ((F 59 x 10^6 daltons

Table 5

Parents		Progeny
A(x) X B(r)	X C $\longrightarrow$ C(xr)	
Primary donor Intermediate recipient	Final recipient	

If strain A is a laboratory line known to carry a transfer factor, and strain B is a wild drug-resistant strain unable to transfer its resistance, the triparental cross can be used to ascertain whether the resistance is coded by a mobilisable determinant. It has been found that many enterobacteria carry mobilisable R determinants but no transfer factor. The commonest "free" R determinants in our experience are those coding for streptomycin and sulphonamide resistance. Such determinants may be mobilisable only by particular groups of R factors. For example, in general, many SSu determinants are mobilisable only by I-like transfer factors (Anderson, 1968b).

The presence of a transfer factor in an enterobacterial strain will not only mobilise the resistance determinants in other strains. It will also operate to the advantage of the parent strain by potentiating the acquisition of drug resistance determinants by that strain. This process is illustrated in table 6.

Table 6. Acquisition of R determinant by transfer factor donor strain.

$$A(x) \times B(r) \longrightarrow A(x) + B(xr) \longrightarrow A(xr) + B(xr)$$

Although there may be exclusion of re-entry of the transfer factor into its parent strain, a Class 2 R determinant enters without difficulty and will protect the strain in the presence of antibiotics.

THE SOURCE OF R FACTORS AND R DETERMINANTS

R factors, and R determinants, are widespread in non-pathogenic enterobacteria throughout the world. Transfer factors are also widely distributed, though they have not been pursued on the same scale as R factors and R determinants, because they are technically more difficult to detect. Whatever the origin of determinants for drug resistance, they have become ubiquitous because of the pressure of the antibiotics against which they are active. The maintenance of this pressure by the indiscriminate use of antibiotics has resulted in the creation of an immense reservoir of R factors in the non-pathogenic enterobacteria of man and animals. If the phenomenon were limited to non-pathogens there would be little cause for alarm. However, as we have seen, it also affects pathogenic enterobacteria and has therefore been a source of much trouble. In many instances this trouble does not stem so much from the loss of specific treatability of the pathogens concerned, as from the survival advantage given to the pathogen in the face of drugs that will be used in the fight against it - an advantage that may have an adverse effect on the prognosis of the disease and may also help it to spread.

It may be thought that I am arguing that mass transfer of resistance to all bacterial pathogens is taking place. The operation of resistance transfer systems is certainly dynamic in non-pathogens and they constitute the reservoir that supplies transferable resistance to pathogens. But experience has shown that only a limited number of lines of a given enteric pathogen are ecologically important at a given time, and that individual lines of an organism such as S.typhimurium establish themselves in animals for periods which may extend into years. These lines are descendants of a single organism, that is, they are

clones. When they are transmitted from animals to man they retain the
distinctive features, including phage-type and drug resistance, they showed in
the animal host.

If we now return to the subject of type 29 of S.typhimurium, there is no
doubt that, from the beginning of 1964 at least, this constituted a single
strain, because it was in early 1964 that it acquired the T marker. This marker
had the peculiar property of being transferable initially at only a very low
frequency, but, once transferred, of becoming highly transferable. The reasons
for this phenomenon have been described earlier. The important point is that
all strains of 29 tested from 1964 until 1968 showed T with the same character
(Anderson, 1968a), which suggested that all the strains were isogenic. This
hypothesis was confirmed when Fu was acquired by 29 late in 1964. The Fu
marker is apparently chromosomal in origin and is non-transferable. It was present
in all strains of type 29 isolated from November 1964 onwards. This indicated
that at some time late in 1964 the parent line of 29 had become resistant to
furazolidone, and that from then on all strains disseminated from the central
source of the organism, that is, the dealer's farm in Essex, possessed the Fu
marker. In this respect it is significant to recall that the dealer was freely
using furazolidone and was distributing it with his animals, to be administered
after they had reached their destination.

It can thus be accepted that all of the thousands of bovine and human
infections with drug-resistant type 29, at least from 1964 to 1970, were caused
by the progeny of a single S.typhimurium organism.

These observations indicate that type 29 was not constantly acquiring
resistance over a period of years, but had acquired it in only a few events at
an early stage in the protracted epidemic: only four in the case of 29(ASSuTFu),
five when chloramphenicol resistance appeared, and six when neomycin-kanamycin
was added. The maintenance of resistances thereafter depended on their stability
in the strain and the pressure of antibiotics. In the event, the R type
29(ASSuTFu) proved to be stable; C and K were lost relatively easily. But this
is not the complete story, since the output from the Essex Farm was 29(ASSuTFu),
and there is evidence to support the suggestion that C and K were acquired at
the periphery of the chain of infection, where farmers were using chloramphenicol
and neomycin and related drugs in efforts to overcome calf infection caused by
29(ASSuTFu).

Type 29 may lose some of its resistance determinants, the frequency of
loss being usually in the order C, K, A, SSu. In the absence of antibiotics it
is thus ultimately reduced to 29(TFu); loss of these markers, or of the Δ
transfer factor, has not so far been observed.

When a bacterial strain carries a Class 1 R factor it has usually acquired
it in a single transfer event. Outbreaks caused by such strains are also clonal
in origin, as with type 29. It is thus evident that, although resistance transfer
is taking place continually in the non-pathogenic enterobacteria, and although
R factors are transferred to enterobacterial pathogens relatively frequently,
only a limited number of strains of resistant pathogens are ecologically important,
because the importance depends entirely on the organism being provided with the
opportunity to spread. However, given that opportunity they become of major
significance. It is worth noting at this point that, once dissemination has
occurred, the organism can be regarded as a resistant (or multiresistant)
mutant, because the transferable aspect of the resistance is no longer relevant
to the relationship between the infecting strain and its host. Indeed, some
drug-resistant S.typhimurium lines carry only a resistance determinant such as
SSu. They cannot transfer that determinant, but this in no way affects their
ability to cause infection or to manifest their drug resistance.

THE INCIDENCE OF TRANSFERABLE DRUG RESISTANCE IN SALMONELLAE

The very high incidence of transferable drug resistance in the non-pathogenic enterobacteria, the frequent appearance of transferable resistance in individual salmonellae, and the prevalence of resistant strains such as type 29 of S.typhimurium suggested that, if antibiotic pressure were sustained, it could lead to a situation in which resistant salmonellae were predominant and chronically hyperendemic. This would apply particularly to the commonest salmonellae such as S.typhimurium, because they would most frequently encounter an intestinal environment rich in non-pathogenic enterobacteria carrying R factors. The probability of resistance transfer into the pathogen would of course be augmented by the presence of antibiotics. Such a situation would be expected to arise most probably in developing countries where hygiene is poor, intestinal infection is common, and antibiotics are used indiscriminately by both doctors and the general public, to whom they are freely available.

Confirmation of these fears has occurred in many parts of the world, and I shall quote a few examples. One of the most striking is the upsurge in Central and South America of salmonellosis, due mainly to S.typhimurium, but also to other salmonella serotypes (Anderson, 1974a).

The countries involved, and the range of serotypes we have studied from each, are shown in Table 7.

Of the 472 cultures we examined, 431 (91.3%) were drug resistant. S.typhimurium predominated in all countries except Venezuela, where the predominant serotype was S.saintpaul.

Table 8 presents an analysis of the resistances involved.

Sixty-three different patterns of resistance occurred, but the commonest R-types were: ACKSSuTNal (26%); ACKSSuT (21.6%); and AK (7.6%).

Table 9 analyses the frequency of individual resistances and of resistance multiplicity.

Resistance to ampicillin is most frequent (92% of resistant strains). This is followed by resistances to neomycin-kanamycin (79%), sulphonamides (75%), streptomycin (74%), tetracyclines (69%), chloramphenicol (67%), and nalidixic acid (40%). Furazolidone (7%), trimethoprim (2%) and gentamicin (1%) resistances are uncommon. This frequency distribution of resistances probably indicates the frequency of use of the respective drugs.

Multiple resistance is of a high order, as shown in the right-hand section of table 9, where it is evident that 25% of strains were resistant to six antibiotics, and 32% to seven. Only 5% were resistant to one antibiotic.

All the Chilean strains of S.typhimurium belonged to phage type 12 of S.typhimurium, an indication of clonal origin. Most of the resistances were initially non-transferable, but could be mobilised with a suitable transfer factor. The resistance linkage groups in these strains were thus plasmid in nature but lacked a transfer factor, that is, they were R determinants.

The resistant S.typhimurium cultures isolated from countries east of the Andes mainly belonged to a group of recently identified types which are usually associated with drug resistance. Most of the resistance was transferable.

These salmonellae have caused troublesome infections, principally in paediatric units. The morbidity rate is up to 50%. Septicaemia and meningitis are common, and the case-mortality rate may be as high as 20 - 30%.

Table 7. Drug-resistant salmonellae from South and Central America

Country	No. of cultures	Serotypes
Chile	57	S.typhimurium
	2	S.newport
	2	S.newington
	2	S.anatum
	1	S.unidentified
	64	
Brazil	86	S.typhimurium
Uruguay	31	S.typhimurium
Paraguay	3	S.typhimurium
Argentina	85	S.typhimurium
	2	S.infantis
	87	
Venezuela	47	S.saintpaul
	11	S.typhimurium
	10	S.java
	29	Various serotypes
	97	
Mexico	100	S.typhimurium
	2	S.derby
	1	S.worthington
	1	S.saintpaul
	104	
Total	472	

Similar outbreaks of salmonellosis, principally S.typhimurium infection, have occurred in many other parts of the world.

CHLORAMPHENICOL-RESISTANT S.TYPHI

The appearance of chloramphenicol-resistant S.typhi has been feared almost since the discovery of transferable drug resistance. Although chloramphenicol

Table 8. R-types of salmonellae from South and Central America, 1971-1973.
(472 cultures examined, 431 (91.3%) drug-resistant; 63 R-types)

R-type	No.	R-type	No.	R-type	No.	R-type	No.	R-type	No.
ACKSSuTNal	114	ACKTFu	5	ACKSSu	3	AC	1	AKSuNal	1
ACKSSuT	93	ASSuT	5	AKSSu	3	ACKSSuTFuNal	1	AKSuFuNal	1
AK	33	ASu	5	AKSSuTNal	3	ACKSSuTTmNal	1	AS	1
ACKSSuTFu	15	Su	5	AKSTNal	3	ACKSuT	1	AT	1
ANal	13	ACKS	4	CKT	3	ACKSuTFuNal	1	ACKSTmNal	1
A	12	ACKST	4	ACK	2	ACKSuTNal	1	CSNal	1
ASSuNal	9	ACKT	4	ACSuT	2	ACS	1	CSSuTNal	1
AKSSuT	8	AKNal	4	ACSSuTNal	2	ACSSu	1	K	1
AKSu	7	CKSSuTTmNal	4	CKTFu	2	AKS	1	SNal	1
ACKSSuNal	6	SSuT	4	CKSSuTNal	2	AKSNal	1	SSu	1
ACKSSuTG	6			S	2	AKSSuFu	1	T	1
ACSSuT	6			SSuTFuNal	2	AKSSuTFu	1	Tm	1
ASSu	6			ST	2	AKST	1	Nal	1
				SuTm	2				

A = ampicillin; C = chloramphenicol; K = neomycin-kanamycin; S = streptomycin; Su = sulphonamides; T = tetracyclines;

G = gentamicin; Tm = trimethoprim; Fu = furazolidone; Nal = nalidixic acid.

Table 9. Drug-resistant salmonellae from South and Central America, 1971-1973.

Total number of strains	Drug-resistant	Number resistant to										Number resistant to (drugs)							
		A	K	Su	S	T	C	Nal	Fu	Tm	G	1	2	3	4	5	6	7	8
472	431 (91.3%)	395	342	324	321	299	288	174	29	9	6	23	60	29	33	35	109	140	2
	% of resistant salmonella	92	79	75	74	69	67	40	7	2	1	5	14	7	8	8	25	32	0.5
	% of total salmonella	84	72	69	68	63	61	37	6	2	1	5	13	6	7	7	23	30	0.4

resistance occurred in individual strains (Anderson & Smith, 1972), from some of which it was transferable, such resistance did not appear in epidemic typhoid until 1972. In that year a strain of the typhoid bacillus caused over 10,000 cases in Mexico, the largest outbreak on record. Infection was apparently waterborne, and a number of visitors, at least 52 American, two English and one Swiss, were infected (Anderson & Smith, 1972; Cohen, 1973; Waldvogel & Pitton, 1973). Ampicillin was substituted for chloramphenicol in treatment, but it is a second-line drug in this disease.

This outbreak was caused by a single degraded Vi-strain of S.typhi, that is, a clone, which carried an R factor coding for CSSuT resistances. This R factor belongs to compatibility group H_1.

Epidemic or hyperendemic chloramphenicol-resistant typhoid fever has also occurred in India (Paniker & Vimala, 1972), Vietnam (Butler et al., 1973; Anderson, 1974b, c) and Thailand (Anderson, 1974b, c; Lampe et al., 1974). In all cases the organism carried a group H_1 R factor. Most showed the R-type CSSuT, but in one phage type this had become ACSSuT, the ampicillin resistance having been added to the linkage group presumably as the result of ampicillin treatment. These findings are summarised in table 10.

Group H_1 R factors show the peculiarity of being difficult to transfer in vitro to sensitive S.typhi, and of being partially or totally lost from the organism with relative ease. Many R factors coding for chloramphenicol resistances transfer to the typhoid bacillus easily, and are stable in the serotype. It therefore seems paradoxical that group H_1 R factors should be those most commonly found in chloramphenicol-resistant S.typhi in different parts of the world. There are presumably some in vivo influences, of which we are unaware, which determine this predominance.

Group H_1 R factors are also common in S.typhimurium in animals and man in South East Asia, but in that serotype they code for AKT and AT resistances. There is an undoubted prevalence of these factors in salmonellae in South East Asia, and it can be postulated that they should occur frequently in the non-pathogenic enterobacteria, a point that is under investigation.

The upsurge in many parts of the world of epidemic salmonellae carrying R factors, of chloramphenicol-resistant S.typhi, of serious hospital outbreaks with drug-resistant gram-negative opportunist pathogens such as klebsiellae and pseudomonads (Price & Sleigh, 1970; Lowbury et al., 1972) are all the result of the indiscriminate use of antibiotics over a long period. It is important to remember that any drug represented in the resistance spectrum of a multiresistant bacterial strain will select for that strain and all its resistances. Moreover, the pressure of antibiotics in a mixed population of sensitive and resistant bacteria will offer a survival advantage to resistant organisms and will also promote the transfer of resistance to sensitive bacteria. The uncritical and increasing use of antibiotics throughout the world during the past three decades has created a gigantic reservoir of R factors in the non-pathogenic enterobacteria. From this reservoir have come the R factors that have declared their preference for particular hosts, such as H_1 factors for the typhoid bacillus and I-like factors for many salmonellae. The constant antibiotic pressure maintains the fullness of the reservoir, and pathogenic enterobacteria always find R factors in plentiful supply for their protection against antibiotics. It is doubtful whether anything short of complete withdrawal of antibiotics can repair this situation, and such withdrawal is a manifest impossibility. The only palliative is thus the exercise of much more prudence in the use of antibiotics, and perhaps their local withdrawal when an intractable problem exists - persistant epidemic or cross infection with resistant gram-negative bacilli. Antibiotics should be available to the public only on prescription from qualified practitioners. When an antibiotic exists that is specific for a particular infection, such as chloramphenicol for typhoid fever, it should be

Table 10. Group H$_1$ R factors in S.typhi.

Country of origin	Host	Phage types	Year of isolation	R-type	No. examined in ERL
Mexico	Human	Degraded Vi-strains	1972	CSSuT	8
India	Human	D1-N	1972	CSSuT	26
South Vietnam	Human	E7 (5)* D6 (8) 53 (1) 56 (32) Untypable Vi-strains** (25)	1972-1974	CSSuT***	71
Thailand	Human	D1 (5) 53 (12) Vi-negative variant (1)	1973-1974	ACSSuT (5) CSSuT (12) CSSuT	18

*   Number of cultures shown in parentheses.
**   Untypable with adapted Vi II phages.
*** One Vi-type 56 carries a CSSu group H$_1$ R factor.

reserved for treating that infection only. Chloramphenicol should be used in
man only for typhoid fever and perhaps haemophilus meningitis, and it should not
be used at all in animals.

Lastly, the recommendations of the Swann Committee (1969), that antibiotics
used for therapy in man and animals should be withdrawn from use as feed
additives, should be followed on a world-wide scale. These recommendations have
now been implemented in the United Kingdom. They have certainly had no
deleterious effect on protein production, and their implementation removes some
of the antibiotic pressure that has resulted in the present disquieting state
of resistance in the enterobacteria.

SUMMARY

The prevalence of R factors in the non-pathogenic enterobacteria of man and
animals is due to the world-wide use of antibiotics on an enormous scale. These
exert massive pressure on the intestinal bacteria, offering a survival advantage
to resistant lines and thereby promoting the transfer of R factors. In due course
the R factors are transferred to enterobacterial pathogens such as shigellae and
salmonellae. Continued pressure of drugs favours the emergence and maintenance
of resistant clones of these organisms. Transferable chloramphenicol resistance
has appeared in epidemic typhoid fever in Mexico and South East Asia. Many
countries, particularly those of South and Central America, have suffered from
lethal epidemics caused by salmonellae, especially S.typhimurium, carrying R
factors. The only way to diminish the high incidence of transferable drug
resistance is greatly to reduce the general use of antibiotics.

REFERENCES

Anderson, E. S.: Special methods used in the laboratory for the investigation
of salmonella food poisoning. Royal Soc. Health J. 80, 260-267 (1960).

Anderson, E. S.: Origin of transferable drug resistance factors in the
Enterobacteriaceae. Brit. Med. J. ii, 1289-1291 (1965a).

Anderson, E. S.: A rapid screening test for transfer factors in drug-sensitive
Enterobacteriaceae. Nature 208, 1016-1017 (1965b).

Anderson, E. S.: Transferable antibiotic resistance. Brit. Med. J. i, 574-575
(1968a).

Anderson, E. S.: The ecology of transferable drug resistance in the enterobacteria.
Ann. Rev. Microbiol. 22, 131-180 (1968b).

Anderson, E. S.: The use of bacteriophage typing in the investigation of
outbreaks of salmonella food poisoning. In: Bacterial Food Poisoning,
Royal Society of Health, London, 49-65 (1969a).

Anderson, E. S.: Ecology and epidemiology of transferable drug resistance. In:
Ciba Foundation Symposium on Bacterial Episomes and Plasmids (eds. G. E. W.
Wolstenholme and M. O'Connor) J. and A. Churchill Ltd. London, 102-119 (1969b).

Anderson, E. S.: The modern ecological study of Salmonella typhimurium infection.
In: Recent Advances in Microbiology (ed. A. Perez-Miravete & D. Pelaez).
Xth Int. Congr. Microbiol., Mexico City, 1970, 381-387 (1971).

Anderson, E. S.: The ecology of Salmonella typhimurium infection. Acta
Microbiol. Hellen. 18, 200-207 (1973).

Anderson, E. S.: Transferable drug resistance in salmonella in South and Central America. WHO Wkly. Epidem. Rec. No. 8, 65-69 (1974a).

Anderson, E. S.: Group H resistance factors in Southern Asia. WHO Wkly. Epidem. Rec. No. 29, 245-246 (1974b).

Anderson, E. S.: Chloramphenicol-resistant Salmonella typhi in Viet-Nam and Thailand. WHO Wkly. Epidem. Rec. In Press (1974c).

Anderson, E. S., and M. J. Lewis: Drug resistance and its transfer in Salmonella typhimurium. Nature 206, 579-583 (1965a).

Anderson, E. S., and M. J. Lewis: Characterisation of a transfer factor associated with drug resistance in Salmonella typhimurium. Nature 208, 843-849 (1965b).

Anderson, E. S., and E. Natkin: Transduction of resistance determinants and R factors of the Δ transfer systems by phage P1kc. Molec. gen. Genet. 114, 261-265 (1972).

Anderson, E. S. and H. R. Smith: Chloramphenicol resistance in the typhoid bacillus. Brit. Med. J. iii, 329-331 (1972).

Butler, T., N. N. Linh, K. Arnold and M. Pollack: Chloramphenicol-resistant typhoid fever in Vietnam associated with R factor. Lancet ii, 983-985 (1973).

Cohen, S. N.: Chloramphenicol-ampicillin resistant Salmonella typhi - California. Morbid. Mortal. 22, 183-184 (1973).

Humphreys, G. O., N. D. F. Grindley and E. S. Anderson: DNA-protein complexes of Δ-mediated transfer systems. Biochim. biophys. Acta 287, 355-360 (1972).

Joint Committee on the Use of Antibiotics in Animal Husbandry and Veterinary Medicine. Cmnd. 4190 H.M. Stationery Office 1969.

Lampe, R. M., P. Mansuwan and C. Duangmani: Chloramphenicol-resistant typhoid. Lancet i, 623-624 (1974).

Lowbury, E. J. L., J. R. Babb and E. Roe: Clearance from a hospital of gram-negative bacilli that transfer carbenicillin resistance to Pseudomonas aeruginosa. Lancet ii, 941-945 (1972).

Office of Health Economics: Antibiotics in Animal Husbandry, London (1969).

Paniker, C. K. J. and K. N. Vimala: Transferable chloramphenicol resistance in Salmonella typhi. Nature 239, 109-110 (1972).

Price, D. J. E. and J. D. Sleigh: Control of infection due to Klebsiella aerogenes in a neurosurgical unit by withdrawal of all antibiotics. Lancet ii, 1213-1215 (1970).

Smith, H. R., G. O. Humphreys and E. S. Anderson: Genetic and molecular characterisation of some non-transferring plasmids. Molec. gen. Genet. 129, 229-242 (1974).

Waldvogel, F. A. and J.-S. Pitton: Typhoid fever imported from Mexico to Switzerland: studies on R factor-mediated chloramphenicol resistance. J. Hyg. 71, 509-513 (1973).

Watanabe, T.: Infective heredity of multiple drug resistance in bacteria. Bact. Rev. 27, 87-115 (1963).

Structural Constraints in the Binding of Drugs to DNA

Michael Waring

INTRODUCTION

Drugs which interact with DNA so as to impair its function as a template for nucleic acid synthesis are used in the chemotherapy of so wide a range of infectious and malignant diseases that it is hard to over-estimate their importance in present-day medical practice. In the treatment of such conditions as malaria, trypanosomiasis, schistosomiasis and various forms of cancer they occupy a central place, in some instances providing virtually the only means of effective chemo-therapy. Even among the great number of compounds which are currently under active investigation as potentially useful antiviral agents there are many whose action derives from their ability to react with nucleic acids. Small wonder, then, that this topic has been the subject of numerous reviews in recent years (see, for example, Newton, 1970; Goldberg & Friedman, 1971; Waring, 1972; Corcoran & Hahn, 1974).

Yet there is a paradox surrounding the action of these drugs. No-one doubts the extreme specificity inherent in the structure of DNA, or more precisely in its sequence of nucleotides: indeed that sequence, for a DNA sample from any particular source, represents the very quintessence of specificity as regards its role in determining the form and function of a living cell or organism. Should one not therefore expect that drugs whose toxicity can be shown to result from their binding to DNA must be able to discriminate between DNAs from different sources, thus accounting for their selectivity? Far from it. Wherever investigations have been performed the results have been extremely disappointing. Even with drugs of proved therapeutic efficacy, such as acridines and ethidium (Waring, 1965,1972), the differences in their binding to DNAs from different sources have been found to be minimal if not actually non-existent. Where specificity has been demonstrated at all it is typically of a low order as in the case of actinomycin D which shows a requirement for G·C base-pairs in the DNA with a preference (far from absolute) for GpC sequences (Wells & Larson, 1970; Sobell et al., 1971). To be sure, the select-ive toxicity of drugs which bind to DNA is generally not impressive, certainly not compared with the selectivity of antibiotics which affect ribosomes or cell walls for instance, but it is nevertheless much greater than can be accounted for on the basis of their DNA-binding properties. Explanations for their selectivity in vivo have therefore generally had to invoke suggestions of differential permeability, uptake, or concentration by susceptible cells and organisms — a far cry from the site of toxic action of the drug once within the sensitive cell.

There is manifestly great need, and probably a bright future, for drugs endowed with better specificity for interaction with DNA. That specificity must ultimately involve the capacity to recognise distinct base-pair sequences, either by direct interaction between functional groupings on the base-pairs and the drug molecule or indirectly via recognition of a local conformational peculiarity of the

DNA associated with a particular sequence. As yet there are little more than encouraging signs that that goal will be attainable within the framework of existing expertise and our present understanding of drug-DNA interactions, but the issue is of sufficient importance to merit active pursuit.

In our laboratory during recent years we have increasingly turned our attention to questioning the nature of the forces and constraints which apply to the binding of drugs to DNA. The aim has been to determine the general character of the drug-DNA complex and then to delineate as precisely as possible the essential and non-essential features in the structure of the drug molecule which are involved in the binding reaction. These studies represent a first, essential step towards elucidating means and approaches likely to yield agents having improved binding specificity.

THE INTERCALATION MODEL

We are not concerned with substances which react with DNA by alkylation to yield a covalently bound product, such as the nitrogen mustards (Brookes, 1964) and the antibiotic mitomycin (Szybalski & Iyer, 1967), but rather with those drugs which interact with DNA to form a more or less tightly bound, reversible complex. This latter group comprises the majority of the clinically useful DNA-binding drugs, and most of them characteristically possess a polycyclic aromatic chromophore. Those which do contain such a chromophore fall immediately under suspicion as probable intercalating agents (Lerman, 1961; Fuller & Waring, 1964), though not all prove positive in this respect when subject to investigation (Waring, 1970,1972). Those which do not are considered likely to bind to DNA via some other mechanism, most probably involving some combination of electrostatic, hydrophobic, and/or hydrogen bonding interactions with the nucleic acid. In the intercalation model it is assumed that hydrophobic forces play a major part in stabilizing the complex, often reinforced by interactions of the other two types, but it is probably because the intercalation model is relatively well-defined that it has come to dominate thinking in this field. The intrinsic simplicity of its principal postulate, that the flat aromatic chromophore of the drug molecule becomes sandwiched between adjacent base-pairs stacked in the core of the double helix (Lerman, 1961,1964; Fuller & Waring, 1964) is very attractive and naturally lends itself to explain the binding of any agent which possesses a sufficiently large, flat substituent.

The stereochemical properties of the DNA helix are such that any simple process of intercalation demands a local unwinding of the helix at the point where the drug molecule binds, in order to permit the flat chromophore to slip between the base-pairs (Lerman, 1961,1964; Fuller & Waring, 1964). More complicated models can be envisaged in which the unwinding might be obviated or even reversed (Paoletti & LePecq, 1971) but as yet there are few grounds for making such postulates. At present the best estimate for the local unwinding associated with straightforward intercalation of a 3.4 Å thick aromatic chromophore is 12°, originally proposed for the ethidium intercalation model by Fuller & Waring (1964), but this value has not yet been unequivocally verified by experiment (for discussion on this point see Waring (1972,1974a); Pigram et al. (1973)). It remains, however, the best provisional estimate on which to base comparisons between the effects of different drugs.

More important for our present purposes is the qualitative assertion that some change in the winding of the DNA helix is to be expected for drugs which bind by intercalation but not necessarily for those which bind by other means (Waring, 1970). Indeed, failure to affect the winding of the helix provides sound prima facie evidence that intercalation does not take place. Based on this reasoning, and the experimental feasibility of detecting small changes in the winding of the DNA helix because of its consequences for the supercoiled state of closed circular duplex DNA (Crawford & Waring, 1967; Bauer & Vinograd, 1968), we have undertaken a survey of a wide variety of DNA-binding antibiotics and drugs to investigate whether intercalation plays any detectable part in their action (Waring, 1970,1972; Wakelin & Waring, 1974).

INTERACTION OF CHLOROQUINE, ADRIAMYCIN AND BERENIL WITH CIRCULAR DNA

To illustrate the sorts of conclusions which have been reached, experimental results for four drugs of diverse structure (Fig. 1) are presented in Figs. 2 - 4. In these plots the sedimentation coefficient of closed circular duplex DNA (and of the small proportion of nicked circular molecules present in the preparation) is determined as a function of the level of drug binding. The characteristic response for an intercalation process is a pronounced fall and rise in the S_{20} of

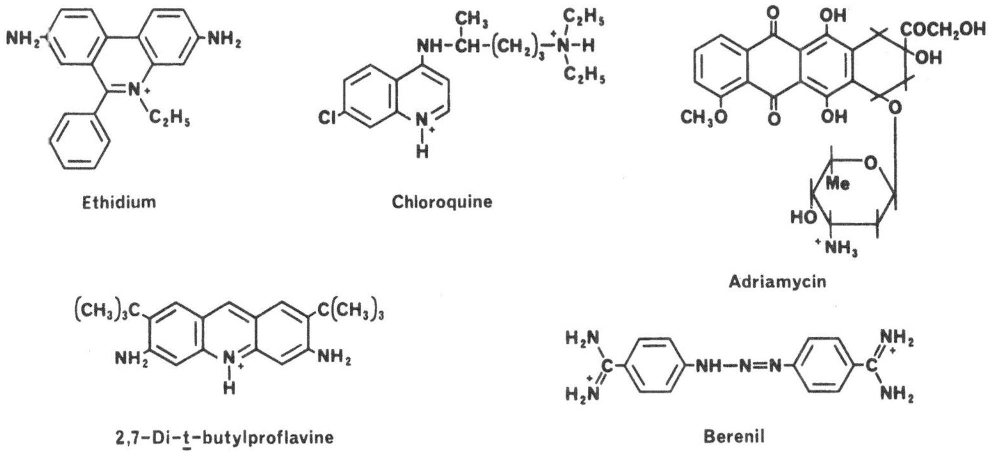

Ethidium Chloroquine Adriamycin

2,7-Di-t-butylproflavine   Berenil

Fig. 1. Structural formulae

the closed circular molecules, reflecting progressive removal and reversal of their supercoiling. [For full theoretical treatment and practical details see Crawford & Waring (1967), Bauer & Vinograd (1968) and Waring (1970)]. The position of the minimum in such a plot is termed the equivalence point, and by comparing the binding ratios at the equivalence point measured with two drugs under identical conditions it is a simple matter to calculate their relative helix-unwinding angles (Waring, 1970). If one of the two drugs is ethidium, an apparent unwinding angle for the second drug can be estimated by making the standard assumption that binding of each ethidium molecule unwinds the DNA helix by $12°$ (Fuller & Waring, 1964).

Fig. 2 shows that the antimalarial drug chloroquine yields the typical response expected for an intercalating agent, in agreement with conclusions drawn by earlier workers (see Hahn, 1971). With chloroquine the equivalence point appears unusually broad compared to the fairly sharp minimum observed with other intercalating drugs; indeed in this case it would be better to speak of an 'equivalence region' extending from 0.02 to 0.05 chloroquine molecules bound per nucleotide. At binding ratios within these limits the relaxed, closed circular DNA molecules co-sedimented with the nicked circles and could not be resolved from them. However, the equivalence region centres around 0.035 chloroquine molecules bound per nucleotide, which is practically the same as the equivalence point for ethidium (0.033 ± 0.009 drug molecules bound per nucleotide) under the same conditions. The conclusion is that binding of chloroquine leads to local unwinding of the helix by the same angle as binding of ethidium (taken to be $12°$), i.e. an apparent unwinding angle of $11.3° ± 5.8°$. The large limits of error are, of course, a consequence of the anomalously broad equivalence region seen with chloroquine, which might be due to its relatively weak binding compared to that of ethidium, though it is not obvious why this should be so.

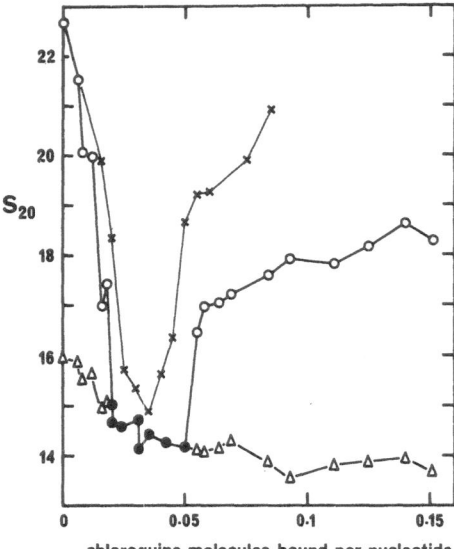

chloroquine molecules bound per nucleotide

Fig. 2. Effect of chloroquine on the sedimentation coefficient of bacteriophage
ØX174 replicative form DNA in 15 mM Na phosphate buffer (pH 5.9 at 20°).
The S_{20} of the closed circular duplex molecules is represented by O, that of
nicked circular molecules by Δ, and when the two forms of DNA co-sedimented as a
single unresolved boundary the symbol ● is used. For comparison, the effect of
ethidium on the S_{20} of closed circular molecules under the same conditions is shown
by X. Complexes were formed and subjected to analytical ultracentrifugation as
described by Waring (1970). Binding ratios of chloroquine-DNA complexes were
calculated using the parameters determined by Cohen & Yielding (1965) in this
buffer. The DNA preparation contained 65% closed circular molecules. Sedimentation coefficients are uncorrected values determined directly at 20°.

It is interesting that the unwinding angles associated with binding of these
two drugs should be the same, for the two-ring chromophore of chloroquine is substantially smaller in area than that of ethidium, though presumably the same thickness (approximately 3.4 Å). There seems, in fact, to be little or no correlation
among different intercalating drugs between the dimensions of the chromophore and
the helix unwinding angle. This point is further illustrated by results obtained
with the antitumour antibiotic adriamycin (Fig. 3). Here the equivalence point is
seen to lie at 0.115 ± 0.010 antibiotic molecules bound per nucleotide, whereas
with this DNA under the same conditions ethidium yields an equivalence point at a
binding ratio of 0.051 ± 0.006. The unwinding angle associated with binding of
adriamycin is therefore less than half the value of ethidium or chloroquine, i.e.
5.3° ± 0.8° based on the assumed 12° of ethidium. This value compares well with
the estimate of 5.2° ± 1.4° determined previously for daunomycin (Waring, 1970).
Daunomycin is another anthracycline antibiotic which differs from adriamycin only
in lacking the hydroxyl group of the -COCH$_2$OH substituent (Chandra et al., 1972);

it is an acknowledged intercalating agent (Pigram et al., 1972). The chromophores
of both these antibiotics are comparable in size to that of ethidium, containing
three fused six-membered aromatic rings in all cases. [The fourth ring of adriamycin and daunomycin is saturated and puckered; in the DNA complex it must
presumably project out, with its attached aminosugar, from the intercalated flat
aromatic portion and lie in one of the grooves of the helix — possibly the wide
groove (Pigram et al., 1972)].

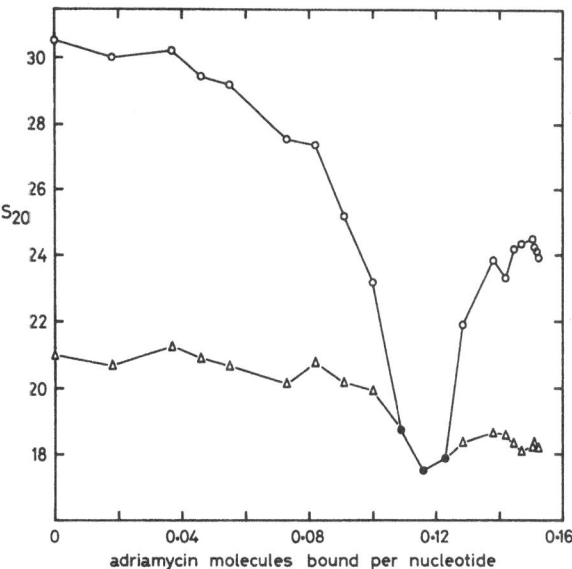

adriamycin molecules bound per nucleotide

Fig. 3. Removal and reversal of the supercoiling of bacteriophage PM2 DNA by adriamycin. The buffer was 50 mM tris-HCl (pH 7.9 at 20°). Symbols are as described in the legend to Fig. 2. The DNA preparation contained 90% closed circular duplex molecules. Binding ratios were determined from spectrophotometric measurements as previously described (Waring, 1970).

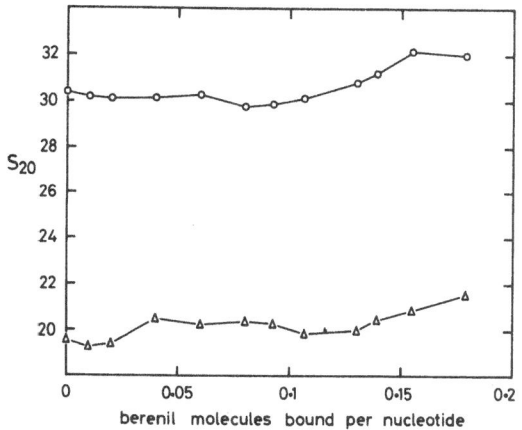

berenil molecules bound per nucleotide

Fig. 4. Effect of berenil on the sedimentation coefficient of PM2 DNA in 50 mM tris-HCl (pH 7.9 at 20°). Symbols and conditions are as described in the legends to Figs. 2 and 3. The binding was measured by spectrophotometry.

Fig. 4 provides a clear example of a negative result, in which the binding of the trypanocidal drug berenil (Newton, 1974) is shown to produce no detectable change in the supercoiling of circular DNA. This experiment is an improved version of one reported earlier (Waring, 1970) in which an impure commercial sample of the drug was employed. The results in Fig. 4 were obtained with a pure, homogeneous sample free from the antipyrine stabilizer present in the commercial material (55.5% stabilizer by weight). The characteristic dip in the S_{20} of the closed circular molecules seen with intercalating drugs is totally lacking; in fact up to a binding ratio of 0.18, approaching saturation of the binding sites available to berenil, there is barely any detectable effect on the sedimentation behaviour of either closed or nicked circular molecules. The very slight increase in S_{20} of the closed circles (no more than about 2S) is mirrored in the behaviour of the nicked circles. We can conclude that there is no detectable unwinding of the DNA helix associated with binding of berenil, and therefore that any simple intercalation-type model for its binding is eliminated. Based on the observation that binding of 0.18 molecules of berenil per nucleotide has no detectable effect on the supercoiling, whereas binding of 0.04 molecules of ethidium produces almost complete loss of the supercoils, we can calculate that berenil does not alter the winding of the DNA helix by any angle greater than $2.7°$ per bound drug molecule (cf. the analogous calculations for a non-intercalating dibutylproflavine derivative presented by Müller et al., 1973).

STUDIES WITH HOMOLOGOUS SERIES OF DRUGS

Experiments such as those illustrated above have been performed with a great variety of antibiotics and drugs which form reversible complexes with DNA. For a compilation of results see Waring (1972,1973a). The technique, which we can refer to as the circular DNA-binding test, is now firmly established as a prime criterion for sorting drugs into intercalating and non-intercalating categories. From the accumulated information it has been possible to build up a general impression of what structural features are likely to endow a molecule with the capacity to bind to DNA by intercalation, and conversely what features can be expected to militate against an intercalation mechanism, but precise conclusions are rendered difficult because of the very diversity in structure of the drugs tested. Most were chosen for study because of their importance in clinical and experimental medical practice, not for their potential as probes of a molecular interaction process. Since, as indicated earlier, we have grown increasingly concerned to define the structural constraints and forces involved in drug-DNA interaction it became clear that studies with homologous series of closely-related compounds would be necessary, so that individual substituents might be varied independently and in a controlled fashion, enabling their specific influence upon the parameters of the interaction to be investigated. Accordingly, four lines of approach have been pursued as outlined below. The first two sets of studies are essentially complete, at least so far as equilibrium measurements go, while the latter two are at a preliminary stage though sufficiently informative to be worth mentioning despite their present incompleteness.

(1) Di-tertiary-butyl-proflavine

This compound (Fig. 1) was synthesised with the explicit intention of applying bulky groups to the proflavine chromophore which should prevent it from intercalating in the straightforward fashion required by Lerman's model (1961, 1964). Such proved to be the case. The circular DNA-binding test revealed no significant effect on the supercoiling of PM2 DNA, which, together with other evidence on the optical, hydrodynamic and kinetic properties of the binding reaction, established that the remaining interaction was of a non-intercalative type (Müller et al., 1973). The chief surprise was the discovery that this derivative, unlike the parent compound proflavine, displayed marked specificity for binding to sites rich in A·T base-pairs — an unexpected bonus which may lead to considerable practical application.

(2) <u>Phenanthridinium analogues of ethidium bromide</u>

In a more extensive series of experiments the effect of systematically removing, modifying, or substituting the various functional groupings on the ethidium chromophore was investigated (Wakelin & Waring, 1974). Table 1 summarises the principal findings, beginning with variations in the quaternising group at position 5 (R_4), then modifications to the phenyl substituent at position 6 (R_3), and finally blockage, removal or substitution of the amino groups at positions 8 and 3 $(R_1$ and $R_2)$. A complete description of the results is given in Wakelin & Waring (1974); only a brief outline of the main conclusions need be re-stated here.

The nature of the quaternising group seems to be practically immaterial: intercalation, as evidenced by removal and reversal of the supercoiling of the circular DNA, is not measurably affected by the change from methyl to ethyl to trialkylaminopropyl, nor by the additional positive charge of the latter substituent.

The phenyl group at position 6 is, by contrast, more important. While its presence does not seem to contribute significantly to the binding energy (witness the relative association constant of the des-phenyl derivative M&B 2421) it strongly influences the distribution of bound drug molecules between outside-bound and intercalated states. When it is missing the drug molecule as a whole is practically planar so that stacked aggregates are readily formed which cause precipitation of the DNA. When such precipitation is suppressed by raising the ionic strength, the soluble complex which forms has a substantially lowered unwinding angle, pointing to the persistence of a significant proportion of bound, non-intercalated drug — very likely attached externally to the backbones of the helix.

Introduction of a <u>para</u>-carboxylate grouping on the phenyl ring imparts an extra negative charge to the molecule, yielding a zwitterion. As a result the binding constant falls five-fold but the nature of the intercalated complex is not affected, at least in respect of the unwinding angle. The change in binding energy provides an indication of the contribution of electrostatic forces to the stabilization of the intercalated complex.

It seems, then, that steric effects resulting from alterations in the quaternising group or substitution on the phenyl ring are slight. This is not unexpected, for these substituents should project out from the intercalated chromophore into one of the grooves of the helix. They therefore provide sites at which further substitutions might be made to improve the biological properties of the drug without affecting its fundamental mechanism of action as a DNA-intercalating agent.

When the amino groups at positions 3 and 8 are interfered with the consequences are more severe, though intercalation, perhaps in a modified form, is not abolished. Blockage of both amino groups has clearly more drastic consequences than blockage or removal of only one. The most interesting results were obtained with derivatives lacking both amino groups or having them replaced by bromine atoms. With these compounds the association constant was lowered by a factor of 10 - 30, from which it may be calculated that the presence of the two amino groups contributes some 1.7 Kcal/mole to the stability of the intercalated ethidium complex. This would be consistent with the suggestion of Fuller & Waring (1964) that hydrogen bonds may be formed from these amino groups to phosphate oxygens in the complementary DNA strands, though other interpretations (Wakelin & Waring, 1974) are not excluded. The dibromo analogue, whose unwinding angle of 12° speaks for the formation of an intercalation complex geometrically identical to that formed by ethidium, promises to be of much interest in future studies of the intercalation process.

Finally, the large measure of coincidence between structure-activity relations for phenanthridines in the intercalation reaction and for their biological activity (Seaman & Woodbine, 1954; Woolfe, 1956) suggests that the present study may not be without direct relevance to the chemotherapeutic action of these drugs and means for its possible improvement.

TABLE 1

INTERACTION BETWEEN PHENANTHRIDINES AND CLOSED CIRCULAR DUPLEX DNA

The data are compiled from Wakelin & Waring (1974). With one exception (propidium; Waring, 1970) they refer to experiments with bacteriophage PM2 DNA performed in aqueous buffers of neutral pH and ionic strength in the range 0.01 – 0.5. Values of the apparent helix unwinding angle per bound drug molecule were calculated from measurements of sedimentation coefficients determined by boundary sedimentation in the analytical ultracentrifuge; the estimates of error should be regarded as limits rather than statistical standard errors. Equilibrium constants were determined from Scatchard plots based on spectrophotometric measurements of binding, except for the two derivatives bearing blocked amino groups where equilibrium dialysis was employed. Association constants are expressed relative to that of ethidium in the same buffer. The sign ~ indicates an approximate estimate derived from a curved Scatchard plot. Where the value is given as ~1? the binding was too tight to determine an accurate association constant and it is presumed that the strength of interaction was little, if any, different from that of ethidium.

Drug	R_1	R_2	R_3	R_4	Relative association constant	Apparent unwinding angle
Ethidium	NH_2	NH_2	C_6H_5	C_2H_5	[1]	[12^0]
Dimidium	NH_2	NH_2	C_6H_5	CH_3	~1?	$11.5^0 \pm 2.2^0$
Propidium	NH_2	NH_2	C_6H_5	$(CH_2)_3-\overset{+}{N}(MeEt_2)$	~1?	$12.0^0 \pm 3.4^0$
M&B 2421	NH_2	NH_2	H	CH_3	0.96	$8.3^0 \pm 0.7^0$
M&B 3492	NH_2	NH_2	$C_6H_4-COOH(p)$	CH_3	~0.2	$11.8^0 \pm 1.4^0$
M&B 4594	$NHCOCH_3$	NH_2	C_6H_5	CH_3	~0.5	$8.1^0 \pm 0.8^0$
RD 16101	NHCOOEt	NHCOOEt	C_6H_5	C_2H_5	0.07	$5.1^0 \pm 0.6^0$
Phenidium	NH_2	H	$C_6H_4-NH_2(p)$	CH_3	~1?	$8.6^0 \pm 0.7^0$
M&B 3016	NH_2	H	$C_6H_4-NH_2(p)$	C_2H_5	~1?	$10.6^0 \pm 1.5^0$
M&B 3427	H	H	C_6H_5	CH_3	0.1 / 0.05	$7.7^0 \pm 1.3^0$ / $\not> 4.6^0$
M&B 1765	Br	Br	C_6H_5	CH_3	– / 0.03	$12.0^0 \pm 2.2^0$ / $\not> 7.2^0$

(3) <u>Thiaxanthenone schistosomicides</u>

     As part of a broadly-based programme to improve the therapeutic efficacy of schistosomicidal drugs and to eliminate possible toxic and mutagenic side-effects we have studied a series of newly-synthesised thiaxanthenone compounds related to the established schistosomicides Miracil D (lucanthone) and hycanthone. Earlier work has established hycanthone as a DNA-intercalating agent (Waring, 1970) and the mechanism of action of the thiaxanthenones has recently been reviewed (Weinstein & Hirschberg, 1971; Hirschberg, 1974). The availability of this series of homologous compounds provided a third opportunity to examine the relation between chemical structure and DNA-binding among a group of potentially intercalating drugs. Preliminary results on four indazole analogues of lucanthone and hycanthone have been published (Waring, 1973b). Comparable data for six more thiaxanthenones are presented in Fig. 5. As with the four previous drugs, the interchange of methyl

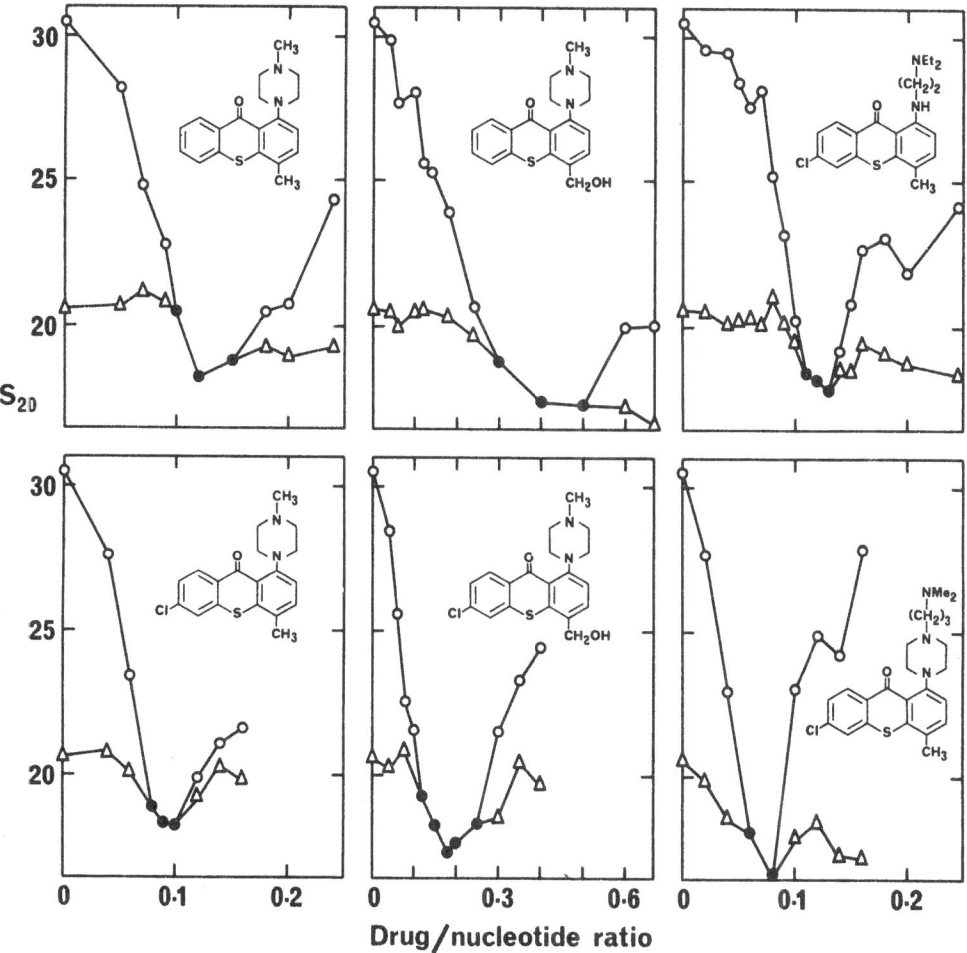

Fig. 5. Interaction between thiaxanthenone compounds and PM2 DNA. The solvent was 50 mM tris-HCl (pH 7.9 at 20°) and the DNA preparations contained 85-95% closed circular molecules. Symbols and conditions of measurement of sedimentation coefficients are as described in the legend to Fig. 2. The abscissa shows the molar ratio of <u>added</u> drug to DNA nucleotides.

and hydroxymethyl groups at position 4 of the ring system, and substitution of chlorine at position 6, does not prevent the intercalation reaction occurring but may influence the drug/nucleotide ratio at which equivalence (removal of the super-coiling) is achieved. From the data in Fig. 5 it appears that compounds bearing a 4-hydroxymethyl group are less effective in removing and reversing the supercoiling than equivalent compounds having the 4-methyl group, and that the presence of a 6-chloro substituent shifts the equivalence ratio to slightly lower values. These observations are not consonant with the earlier findings on the indazole analogues, however (Waring, 1973b). When the nature of the side-chain at position 1 is varied there are also significant changes; the observations suggest that the methyl-piperazinyl substituent yields a lower equivalence ratio than the dialkylaminoalkyl substituent, but that the lowest equivalence ratio of all is attained with a 1-substituent possessing both functional moieties. Until accurate measurements of binding are available it is not possible to attribute the differences evident in the plots in Fig. 5 to variations in the unwinding angles, the binding constants, or both. Previous attempts to determine binding parameters were unsuccessful (Waring, 1973b) but further experimentation is desirable.

(4) <u>Steroidal diamines</u>

The three studies described above have all concerned structural constraints and forces operating in the intercalation reaction. However, the usefulness of the circular DNA-binding test is not restricted to probing the phenomenon of intercala-tion since it can in principle yield precise information about any mode of inter-action with DNA which results in unwinding of the helix. Some years ago it was discovered that binding of irehdiamine A, a steroidal diamine, results in removal and reversal of the supercoiling of circular DNA (Waring, 1970). The unwinding angle per bound steroid molecule was subsequently determined to be approximately 5^{0} (Waring & Chisholm, 1972) which, bearing in mind the non-aromatic character of the steroid nucleus and its much greater thickness (5.9 Å) compared with the chromo-phores of intercalating drugs (3.4 Å), argues strongly against any intercalation-type mechanism as an explanation for the source of the unwinding. To investigate the nature of the interaction further, and to attempt to elucidate the structural features of the steroid molecule responsible for the unwinding effect, we have made detailed measurements with a complete series of isomeric diaminoandrostane compounds (Table 2). All are bisquaternary 3,17-dipyrrolidin-1'-yl-androstane bismethiodides (Davis <u>et al</u>., 1967) differing in their stereochemistry at the 3, 5 and 17 positions as shown. The 5α, 3β, 17β isomer is known as dipyrandium, a potent, non-depolarizing neuromuscular blocking agent (Bamford <u>et al</u>., 1967). These compounds have the advantage over other steroidal diamines that the androst-ane nucleus is relatively rigid, so that the precise conformation of each isomer can be predicted with some certainty, allowing estimation for example of the 'interonium' distance separating the charged centres.

The results, summarised in Table 2, allow the following conclusions.
(a) The preferred stereochemistry for the amino substituents at positions 3 and 17 is β in both cases, and the orientation of the 17-substituent is the more critical of the two. (b) Although all the rings are saturated and puckered into a 'chair' conformation the flatter 5α androstane nucleus is preferred over the more folded 5β nucleus. (c) The unwinding angles associated with binding of the three 17β isomers which removed and reversed the supercoiling of PM2 DNA lie within the range 4.3^{0} – 6.1^{0}, not very different from the values of 5.1^{0} and 4.7^{0} previously deter-mined for irehdiamine A (Waring & Chisholm, 1972). By contrast, the unwinding angle of the only positive 17α isomer is 2.7^{0} and its binding is relatively weak, as evidenced by the high free drug concentration in equilibrium with the relaxed circular DNA complex at equivalence.

We interpret these findings as identifying the preferred site for interact-ion with DNA to be the C – D ring end of the molecule with a 17β substituent. Intermolecular contacts with the DNA probably occur on the α-face beneath the C and

TABLE 2

INTERACTION BETWEEN STEREOISOMERIC ANDROSTANE-3,17-BISQUATERNARY AMMONIUM SALTS AND CLOSED CIRCULAR DUPLEX PM2 DNA

The data are compiled from unpublished experiments of M.J. Waring and S.M. Henley; for a preliminary account see Waring (1974). Measurements were made at 20° using the viscometric technique described by Revet et al. (1971) in a buffer containing 4 mM NaCl, 20 mM HEPES and 0.1 mM EDTA (pH 7.0 at room temperature). The DNA samples contained >95% closed circular duplex molecules. Where a blank is recorded the isomer in question failed to relax the supercoiling of the DNA (303 μM with respect to nucleotides) at a drug/nucleotide input ratio of 1:1. Estimates of error are standard deviations of least-squares fitted lines from a plot of the critical diamine concentration required to relax the supercoiling as a function of DNA concentration; in these plots the DNA concentration was varied between 80 and 800 μM in nucleotides. Interonium distances (measured on Dreiding models) and estimates of biological potency are taken from Bamford et al. (1967).

Isomer			Binding ratio at equivalence	Free drug (μM) at equivalence	Apparent unwinding angle	Interonium distance (Å)	Relative potency in vivo	
							Cat	Monkey
5α	3β	17β	0.102 ± 0.003	8 ± 2	6.1° ± 0.2°	11.0	— 1.00 —	
5α	3α	17β	0.143 ± 0.002	21 ± 1	4.3° ± 0.1°	10.4	0.56	0.86
5α	3β	17α	0.233 ± 0.016	88 ± 10	2.7° ± 0.2°	10.6	1.00	0.92
5α	3α	17α	-	-	-	9.6	0.43	0.76
5β	3β	17β	0.136 ± 0.005	49 ± 3	4.6° ± 0.2°	10.0	0.91	1.25
5β	3α	17β	-	-	-	9.9	0.09	0.08
5β	3β	17α	-	-	-	9.3	0.67	0.79
5β	3α	17α	-	-	-	8.7	0.09	0.07

D rings since this would be sterically obstructed by the large quaternary substituent in a 17α isomer. However, the anomalous positive response given by the 5α, 3β, 17α isomer points to the existence of a secondary, less favourable, site of interaction on the α-face beneath the A and B rings.

These conclusions are in good agreement with results of earlier workers on weak interactions between hormonal steroids and nucleic acid-related materials (Munck et al., 1957; Molinari & Lata, 1962; Cohen et al., 1969). They have been checked by measuring the effects of a number of mono-amino steroids, which confirmed the over-riding importance of a 17β-substituent rather than a 3β-substituent and also revealed that the second quaternary centre in a diamine, even if unfavourably oriented in the α-configuration, nevertheless helps to stabilise the complex (Waring, 1974b).

It is probably significant that the interonium distance of isomers which yielded a positive response is 10 Å or greater, whereas for those isomers which failed to remove the supercoiling of the DNA it is <10 Å (Table 2). However, it is clear that this is by no means the only constraint on the nature of the interaction. It is also clear that structure-activity relations for the DNA-binding reaction are not well correlated with those for neuromuscular blocking potency, which appears to depend more critically upon a 3β-substituent than a 17β-substituent (Bamford et al. 1967). That is hardly surprising; there is no reason to expect that the structural constraints governing drug-receptor interaction at the neuromuscular junction resulting in rapid, reversible paralysis should be mimicked when the same drugs interact with DNA. We incline to the view that these two biological properties of steroidal diamines are quite separate and distinct; indeed it appears simply fortuitous that they are combined within the pharmacology of a single molecule. Nevertheless, it is important that the DNA-binding characteristics of steroidal diamines be properly understood if they are to be employed clinically, for their capacity to bind to DNA should caution against indiscriminate use.

CONCLUDING REMARKS

The experiments described here serve to emphasise the value of the circular DNA-binding test as a means of discriminating between intercalating and non-intercalating drugs. Moreover, by providing a precise parameter relating to conformational changes associated with the binding reaction, i.e. the helix unwinding angle per bound drug molecule, they yield uniquely valuable information for the construction of acceptable molecular models. Any consideration of a recognition process involving binding of a small molecule to a macromolecule is like a kind of jigsaw puzzle in which the detailed interaction of complementary groups and surfaces on the interacting species must be deduced. However, unlike a jigsaw puzzle the interlocking elements cannot be treated as static entities since allowance must be made for their conformational flexibility. Indeed conformational adjustments — 'induced fit', adoption of strained transition states, and the like — are probably widespread features of drug-receptor interaction leading to a biological response. It is in this context that the availability of some measure of the conformational change realises its full importance.

So far as the field of drug-DNA interaction is concerned the interpretation of the unwinding angle associated with an intercalation process is of obvious significance. It is particularly gratifying that we have been able to extend the same sort of measurement to probe the nature of a different mode of binding, that of steroidal diamines, especially since so much less is known in general about non-intercalative interactions. We are all the more convinced that the binding of steroidal diamines involves a process fundamentally different from intercalation by our discovery of the positive unwinding action of a 5β-diaminoandrostane isomer, whose structural resemblance to any known intercalating agent is quite remote and whose unwinding angle is the lowest yet determined for any DNA-binding drug. It is too early to say whether the information gained about structural constraints operating in this novel mode of binding will prove of practical value in the design of better, more specific DNA-binding agents, but it will certainly contribute significantly to our understanding of recognition processes involving nucleic acids.

ACKNOWLEDGMENTS

It is a pleasure to record my appreciation to those workers and drug companies who so generously supplied antibiotics and drugs: Dr S. Archer (Sterling-Winthrop Research Institute) for chloroquine; Dr B. Camerino (Farmitalia) for adriamycin; Dr H. Loewe (Hoechst) for berenil; Dr W. Müller (Stöckheim) for di-t-butyl-proflavine; Dr G. Woolfe (Boots) for phenanthridines; Drs R. Slack, S.S. Berg, M. Davis and K. Wooldridge (May & Baker) for phenanthridines and steroidal diamines; Dr E. Bueding (Johns Hopkins University) for thiaxanthenones. Many colleagues, particularly Messrs L.P.G. Wakelin and S.M. Henley, Dr E. Cundliffe, Professor E.F. Gale, and my wife Dr A.J. Waring provided invaluable advice and criticism. The technical assistance of Mr N.F. Totty is recorded with appreciation. Financial support was made available by the Royal Society and the Medical Research Council.

REFERENCES

BAMFORD, D.G., D.F. BIGGS, M. DAVIS & E.W. PARNELL: Neuromuscular blocking properties of stereoisomeric androstane-3,17-bisquaternary ammonium salts. Brit. J. Pharmacol. Chemother. 30, 194-202 (1967)

BAUER, W. & J. VINOGRAD: The interaction of closed circular DNA with intercalative dyes. I. The superhelix density of SV40 DNA in the presence and absence of dye. J. Mol. Biol. 33, 141-171 (1968)

BROOKES, P.: Reaction of alkylating agents with nucleic acids. In 'Chemotherapy of Cancer' (ed. P.A. PLATTNER), Elsevier, Amsterdam, pp 32-43 (1964)

CHANDRA, P., A. DI MARCO, F. ZUNINO, A.M. CASAZZA, D. GERICKE, F. GIULIANI, C. SORANZO, R. THORBECK, A. GÖTZ, F. ARCAMONE & M. GHIONE: Influence of some anti-tumor antibiotics on viral neoplasia. Naturwissenschaften 59, 448-455 (1972)

COHEN, P., R.C. CHIN & C. KIDSON: Interactions of hormonal steroids with nucleic acids. II. Structural and thermodynamic aspects of binding. Biochemistry 8, 3603-3609 (1969)

COHEN, S.N. & K.L. YIELDING: Spectrophotometric studies of the interaction of chloroquine with DNA. J. Biol. Chem. 240, 3123-3131 (1965)

CORCORAN, J.W. & F.E. HAHN (eds.): Antibiotics. III. Mechanism of Action of Antimicrobial and Antitumor Agents. Springer-Verlag, Berlin-Heidelberg-New York (1974).

CRAWFORD, L.V. & M.J. WARING: Supercoiling of polyoma virus DNA measured by its interaction with ethidium bromide. J. Mol. Biol. 25, 23-30 (1967)

DAVIS, M., E.W. PARNELL & J. ROSENBAUM: Steroid amines. Part IV. 3,17-Diamino-androstane derivatives. J. Chem. Soc. (C) 1967, 1045-1052

FULLER, W. & M.J. WARING: A molecular model for the interaction of ethidium bromide with DNA. Ber. Bunsenges. Physik. Chem. 68, 805-808 (1964)

GOLDBERG, I.H. & P.A. FRIEDMAN: Antibiotics and nucleic acids. Ann. Rev. Biochem. 40, 775-810 (1971)

HAHN, F.E. (ed.): Antimalarials and nucleic acids. Progress in Molecular and Sub-Cellular Biology 2, 69-133 (1971)

HIRSCHBERG, E.: Thiaxanthenones: Miracil D and hycanthone. In 'Antibiotics. III. Mechanism of Action of Antimicrobial and Antitumor Agents' (eds. J.W. CORCORAN & F.E. HAHN), Springer-Verlag, Berlin-Heidelberg-New York (1974).

LERMAN, L.S.: Structural considerations in the interaction of DNA and acridines. J. Mol. Biol. 3, 18-30 (1961)

LERMAN, L.S.: Acridine mutagens and DNA structure. J. Cell. and Comp. Physiol. 64, Suppl. 1, 1-18 (1964)

MOLINARI, G. & G.F. LATA: Interaction of steroids with some pyrimidine and purine derivatives. Arch. Biochem. Biophys. 96, 486-490 (1962)

MÜLLER, W., D.M. CROTHERS & M.J. WARING: A non-intercalating proflavine derivative. Eur. J. Biochem. 39, 223-234 (1973)

MUNCK, A., J.F. SCOTT & L.L. ENGEL: The interaction of steroid hormones and coenzyme components. Biochim. Biophys. Acta 26, 397-407 (1957)

NEWTON, B.A.: Chemotherapeutic compounds affecting DNA structure and function. Adv. Pharmacol. Chemother. 8, 149-184 (1970)

NEWTON, B.A.: Berenil. In 'Antibiotics. III. Mechanism of Action of Antimicrobial and Antitumor Agents' (eds. J.W. CORCORAN & F.E. HAHN), Springer-Verlag, Berlin-Heidelberg-New York (1974).

PAOLETTI, J. & J.B. LE PECQ: The change of the torsion of the DNA helix caused by intercalation. I. A discussion of the two different possibilities, winding or unwinding. Biochimie 53, 969-972 (1971)

PIGRAM, W.J., W. FULLER & M.E. DAVIES: Unwinding the DNA helix by intercalation. J. Mol. Biol. 80, 361-365 (1973)

PIGRAM, W.J., W. FULLER & L.D. HAMILTON: Stereochemistry of intercalation: interaction of daunomycin with DNA. Nature New Biol. 235, 17-19 (1972)

REVET, B.M.J., M. SCHMIR & J. VINOGRAD: Direct determination of the superhelix density of closed circular DNA by viscometric titration. Nature New Biol. 229, 10-13 (1971)

SEAMAN, A. & M. WOODBINE: The antibacterial activity of phenanthridine compounds. Brit. J. Pharmacol. 9, 265-270 (1954)

SOBELL, H.M., S.C. JAIN, T.D. SAKORE & C.E. NORDMAN: Stereochemistry of actinomycin-DNA binding. Nature New Biol. 231, 200-205 (1971)

SZYBALSKI, W. & V.N. IYER: The mitomycins and porfiromycins. In 'Antibiotics. I. Mechanism of Action' (eds. D. GOTTLIEB & P.D. SHAW), Springer-Verlag, Berlin-Heidelberg-New York, pp 211-245 (1967).

WAKELIN, L.P.G. & M.J. WARING: The unwinding of circular DNA by phenanthridinium drugs: Structure-activity relations for the intercalation reaction. Mol. Pharmacol. 10, 544-561 (1974)

WARING, M.J.: Complex formation between ethidium bromide and nucleic acids. J. Mol. Biol. 13, 269-282 (1965)

WARING, M.J.: Variation of the supercoils in closed circular DNA by binding of antibiotics and drugs: Evidence for molecular models involving intercalation. J. Mol. Biol. 54, 247-279 (1970)

WARING, M.J.: Inhibitors of nucleic acid synthesis. In 'The Molecular Basis of Antibiotic Action' (E.F. GALE, E. CUNDLIFFE, P.E. REYNOLDS, M.H. RICHMOND & M.J. WARING), Wiley, London, pp 173-277 (1972)

WARING, M.J.: Studies with closed circular duplex DNA as a probe for conformational alterations. Studia Biophysica (Berlin) 40, 151-157 (1973a)

WARING, M.J.: Interaction of indazole analogs of lucanthone and hycanthone with closed circular duplex DNA. J. Pharm. Exp. Ther. 186, 385-389 (1973b)

WARING, M.J.: Ethidium and propidium. In 'Antibiotics. III. Mechanism of Action of Antimicrobial and Antitumor Agents' (eds. J.W. CORCORAN & F.E. HAHN), Springer-Verlag, Berlin-Heidelberg-New York (1974a).

WARING, M.J.: Stacking interactions. Chemistry and Industry, in press (1974b)

WARING, M.J. & J.W. CHISHOLM: Uncoiling of bacteriophage PM2 DNA by binding of steroidal diamines. Biochim. Biophys. Acta 262, 18-23 (1972)

WEINSTEIN, I.B. & E. HIRSCHBERG: Mode of action of Miracil D. Progress in Molecular and Subcellular Biology 2, 232-246 (1971)

WELLS, R.D. & J.E. LARSON: Studies on the binding of actinomycin D to DNA and DNA model polymers. J. Mol. Biol. 49, 319-342 (1970)

WOOLFE, G.: Trypanocidal action of phenanthridine compounds: Effect of changing the quaternary groups of known trypanocides. Brit. J. Pharmacol. 11, 330-333 (1956). Trypanocidal action of phenanthridine compounds: Further 2,7-diamino phenanthridinium compounds. Brit. J. Pharmacol. 11, 334-338 (1956)

Molecular Aspects of the Biosynthesis of R Factor DNA

Royston Clowes, Toshihiko Arai, and Gerry Anderson

As we have heard from DR.ANDERSON'S presentation, infectious antibiotic resistance determined by plasmids is now a major clinical and economic problem. The ideal measure to reduce the prevalence of such resistant bacteria would clearly be one resulting in the loss of resistance (R) plasmids from the bacterium. Procedures leading to elimination of the R plasmid so far reported are, as we shall hear later, rather arbitrary and not too satisfactory. Clearly, if the control of replication of chromosomal and plasmid DNA were better understood, more suitable elimination regimes could be devised. The experiments reported below investigate the replication of certain plasmids under conditions inhibiting chromosomal replication, as a basis for further experiments exploring the mechanisms controlling replication.

Previous experiments in our laboratory and in those of other workers have shown that plasmids are extrachromosomal genetic elements (for reviews, see NOVICK, 1969; MEYNELL et al., 1969), and are present in the bacterium in the form of "circular" duplex DNA molecules (see Fig. 1). These circular molecules probably contain genes which permit them to replicate, as well as other genes determining resistance to one or more antibiotics. They may also contain genes leading the host cell to conjugate with other cells lacking the plasmid, and resulting in the transfer of one of the two strands of the DNA duplex. The consequent synthesis of the complementary DNA strands in both donor and recipient cells results in the effective transfer of the plasmid (VAPNEK and RUPP, 1971) (plasmids with this property are called conjugative plasmids). The genes determining transfer, and those determining antibiotic resistance may be on the same circular DNA molecule (in a plasmid cointegrate), or on separate molecules (in a plasmid aggregate — in this case, co-transfer of the antibiotic-resistance plasmid, together with the transfer-gene plasmid is often found), so that in both cases, the genes for antibiotic resistance are spread throughout a bacterial population (CLOWES, 1972). When the DNA of plasmid(s) is isolated, a major proportion of the circular molecules have both DNA strands intact and are therefore covalently-closed circular (CCC) molecules (Fig. 1). Since chromosomal DNA is usually sheared into linear segments under the conditions of cell lysis used, it can be separated from the CCC plasmid DNA by use of the dye ethidium bromide, which intercalates as described by DR. WARING, and leads to its separation as a less dense band to the heavier plasmid DNA, when the cell lysate is centrifuged in cesium chloride in the presence of ethidium bromide (RADLOFF et al., 1967) (see Fig. 2).

Fractionation of the tube contents permits the separation of the heavier satellite band and visualization of the plasmid DNA by electron microscopy. If some of the CCC molecules undergo one nick in one of their strands, these molecules adopt an open configuration, which permits measurement of their contour length

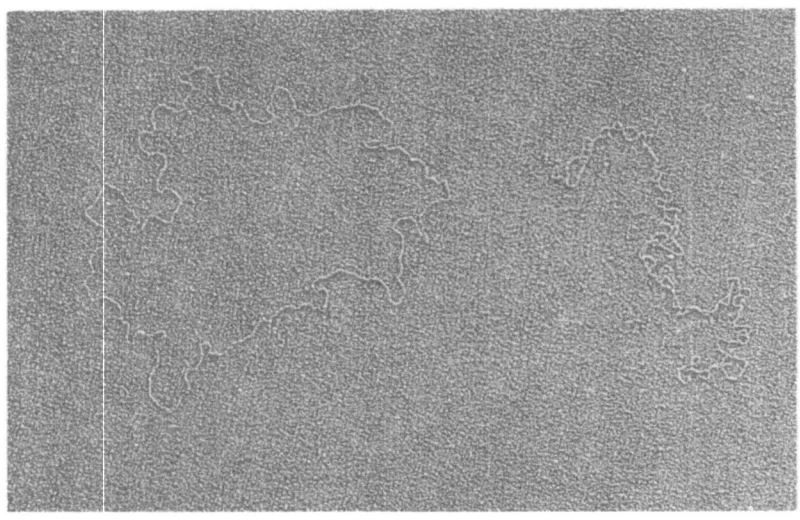

Fig. 1. *Electron micrograph of R factor molecules.* The DNA of the plasmid, R6K, was obtained from a heavy satellite band after centrifugation procedure as shown in Fig. 2. The *open circular* (OC) molecule on the left is produced by a single nick in one of the two strands of the supercoiled molecule (which is a *covalently-closed circular* [CCC] structure) shown on the right (Magnification x 27,500).

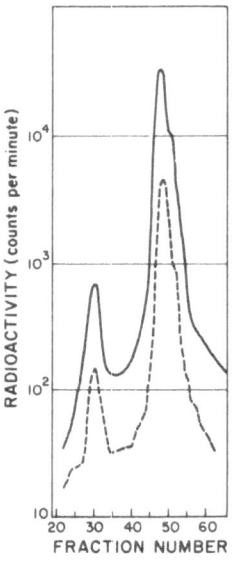

Fig. 2. *Typical profile of uptake of radioactivity into DNA of fractions isolated after lysis and centrifugation in cesium chloride-ethidium bromide of a labelled culture of a bacterial strain containing a plasmid.* The broken line shows the counts of radioactivity of ^{14}C-thymidine present in the culture before the change in cultural conditions. The solid line similarly shows counts of ^{3}H-thymidine added after the change of conditions. (Control experiments, from a host strain which did *not* contain a plasmid, gave rise to only one peak, corresponding in position and radioactivity to the main peak on the right, the smaller (satellite) peak being absent. The satellite band is therefore taken to be plasmid DNA.) The replication of plasmid DNA after the change of growth conditions is therefore given by the ratio of ^{3}H:^{14}C counts in the two satellite peaks, and replication of the chromosome by a similar ratio of counts in the main peaks. (In both cases, the ratio equivalent to one replication is derived from a control experiment where the initial conditions remained unchanged with the change in isotope, and replication was continued for one generation before lysis.)

and hence calculation of the molecular weight of the plasmid. (Such calculations show that the size of plasmids range from about one megadalton [Md] to more than 100 Md). Moreover, if the *amount* of DNA in the plasmid and chromosomal bands is measured, then from a knowledge of the molecular weight of each, the numbers of plasmid molecules for every chromosome (termed the plasmid *copy number*) can be calculated. When such calculations are made, they lead to the remarkable finding that for many plasmids, the copy number is about one. This implies some form of coordinate control of chromosome and plasmid replication *and* segregation. The replication of such plasmids has been termed *stringently regulated*. In other plasmids, a multiple copy number, usually greater than 10 is found, and the replication of these plasmids is sometimes termed *relaxedly regulated* (see CLOWES, 1972).

Our experiments have focused on two R plasmids, R6K and R28K. Both are conjugative plasmid cointegrates and are 28 Md and 44 Md respectively. However R28K is stringently regulated, whereas R6K is relaxed in its replication (KONTOMICHALOU *et al.*, 1970). We have also used two other plasmids that have been extensively investigated by others. As the prototype stringent plasmid, we have used the *E. coli* F sex factor (62 Md), and as another relaxed plasmid we have used the colicin E1 factor (ColE1) which is about 5 Md in size (BAZARAL and HELINSKI, 1968) (see Table 1).

It is now generally accepted that replication of the bacterial chromosome occurs by initiation of new cycles of replication starting at a fixed site on the DNA molecule. The rate of the extension of the two daughter duplexes is however constant in a particular organism, even though the overall rate of DNA replication can vary considerably — the rate of replication being controlled through the control of the frequency with which new cycles are initiated. (For example, in rapidly growing cells, the initiation of one or more further cycles of replication occurs before previous cycles have been terminated [see COOPER and HELMSTETTER, 1968]). Moreover it has been tacitly assumed that replication of plasmid DNA occurs through a similar control of initiation and that the rate of growth of plasmid DNA chains is the same as those of the chromosomes.

By use of a double labelling method, we have investigated the replication of plasmid DNA under a number of conditions in which replication of chromosomal DNA is inhibited. Host cells harboring a specific plasmid are grown for several generations under normal conditions with a DNA precursor, usually ^{14}C-thymidine, so that the DNA of plasmid and chromosome is uniformly labelled in both DNA strands with ^{14}C-thymidine. The cells are then rapidly washed and incubation continued under conditions where chromosomal replication is inhibited, the ^{14}C label being replaced with ^{3}H. Thus, newly synthesized DNA strands would be labelled with ^{3}H-thymidine. A control experiment maintains a portion of the culture with the ^{3}H label at the normal growth conditions for one generation, the ratio of ^{3}H label to ^{14}C label in this control culture being equivalent to one round of replication of both plasmid and chromosomal DNA. At various times at the new growth conditions, samples are removed, the cells are lysed and the lysate is centrifuged in the presence of ethidium bromide in a cesium chloride solution for about 60 h at 100,000 g, separating the chromosomal and plasmid DNA into two bands. The contents of the centrifuge tube are fractionated, and the ^{3}H and ^{14}C isotopes in each fraction are counted. The ratio of ^{3}H/^{14}C in the chromosomal and plasmid DNA bands then gives a measure of the replication of plasmid and chromosome under the growth conditions used (see Fig. 2).

The conditions chosen are of two major kinds. Firstly, growth is investigated in the presence of 150 µg/ml of chloramphenicol (CAP). This has been shown to inhibit bacterial chromosomal replication, with kinetics consistent with the idea that CAP inhibits the initiation of new rounds of replication, but does not interfere with the completion of rounds already initiated (see SMITH, 1973). The second method uses a series of mutants of the host cell in which chromosomal DNA replication is inhibited at a temperature of 42°C but not at 32°C. These temperature-sensitive mutations have been mapped by crosses and by complementation tests to lie in seven genes termed *dnaA*, *B*, *C*, *E*, *F*, *G*, and *H*, and we have used mutant hosts from the groups *dnaA*, *B*, *C*, and *E*. The mutants *dnaA* and *dnaC* have been shown to be defective in initiation, whereas *dnaB* and *E* mutants are defective in chain elongation (WECHSLER and GROSS, 1971). Only one of these functions has been further specified; the *dnaE* gene apparently controls the synthesis of the enzyme, DNA polymerase III (GEFTER *et al.*, 1971).

The plasmids R6K, R28K, F and ColEl were independently transferred to each of these mutant host strains and replication of each plasmid-containing strain was studied. Three general types of response have been found, summarised in Fig. 3. The first, found in a wild-type cell carrying ColEl, replicating in CAP, is referred to as type I. As previously demonstrated by CLEWELL (1972), ColEl continues to replicate under these conditions where initiation of new rounds of chromosomal replication is inhibited. However under these same conditions, the replication of R28K, F or R6K followed that of the chromosome, and is shown as type II replication. In a *dnaA* mutant at 42°C, the replication of F and R28K was inhibited, also with type II responses, whereas that of R6K showed an unusual biphasic growth pattern, shown as type III. (Preliminary experiments with ColEl in a *dnaA* host also showed a type II response.) In *dnaB* and *dnaC* mutants, all four plasmids showed a type II response. In *dnaE* mutants however, R6K showed a type I response, whereas R28K and F showed a type II response. (Preliminary experiments with ColEl in the *dnaE* host showed a response intermediate between types I and II.) These results are summarized below in Table 1.

Table 1. Characteristics of four plasmids R6K, R28K, F, and ColEl

Plasmid	Size(Md)[1]	Phenotype[2]	Copy No.[3]	C/NC[4]	Growth in[5]					
					CAP	*dnaA*	*dnaB*	*dnaC*	*dnaE*	*polI*
R6K	26	ApSm	15	C	II	III	II	II	I	+
R28K	44	Ap	1	C	II	II	II	II	II	+
F	62	–	1	C	II	II	II	II	II	+
ColEl	5	Col	15	NC	I	(II)	II	II	(II)	–

(1) Md = megadaltons
(2) Ap,Sm = resistance to ampicillin and streptomycin respectively, Col = colicinogeny for ColEl
(3) Copy No. = number of copies of each plasmid molecule per copy of chromosome
(4) C = conjugative; NC = non-conjugative
(5) Roman numerals refer to growth response as shown in Fig. 3 *polI* indicates plasmid replication in cells temperature-sensitive for the enzyme, DNA polymerase I

Table 1 also shows the growth response of plasmids in host cells defective for the enzyme, DNA polymerase I. It has previously been shown that ColEl does not replicate in such cells (KINGSBURY and HELINSKI, 1971) whereas our experiments show no dependence of F, R6K or R28K replication on this enzyme.

Certain patterns are apparent from the data summarised in Table 1. The most obvious is that the replication of the two stringent plasmids F and R28K is closely co-ordinated with that of the chromosome, and all conditions which result in inhibition of chromosomal replication results in similar inhibition of these plasmids. (Similarly, a deficiency of the *polI* enzyme which does not inhibit chromosomal replication, does not inhibit stringent plasmid replication.) Nevertheless, when initiation of the chromosomal replication is inhibited, one further round of plasmid replication seems always to be possible. (If plasmid DNA initiation were immediately inhibited, and if we assume a plasmid chain-growth rate equivalent to that of the chromosome [of size 2500 Md] then, under

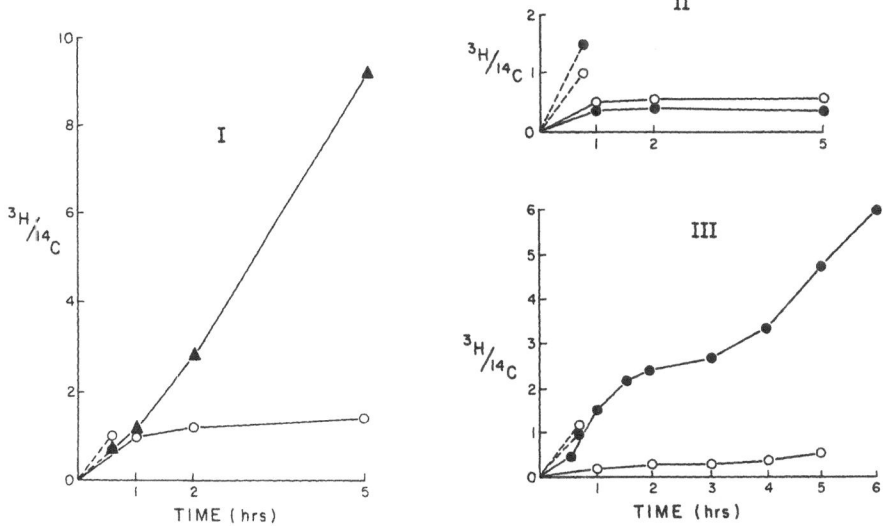

Fig. 3. *Plasmid and chromosomal replication under different cultural conditions.*
At each time, samples were taken, lysed and centrifuged as shown in Fig. 2 and
the ^{3}H and ^{14}C counts in the satellite and main peaks were calculated. The
broken lines represent relative ^{3}H:^{14}C counts in the control culture maintained
at normal growth conditions for one generation after isotope change, the ratio
being taken as 1. The solid lines represent similar samples taken after the
change to conditions inhibiting chromosomal replication. The open circles (O)
represent ratios of counts in the main band (taken as chromosomal DNA), and the
closed symbols (● or ▲), the corresponding ratios in the satellite band (taken
as plasmid DNA). The symbols I, II and III are representative of the responses
referred to as type I, type II and type III, respectively. For further explanation see the text and Table 1.

the conditions used, with a mean cell generation time of about 40 min, it would
take only about 5s, 25s, 45s, and 1 min for replication of the ColE1, R6K, R28K
and F molecules, respectively. Thus, there should be no further plasmid replication shortly after the imposition of the initiation inhibiting conditions.)
Furthermore, based on the observations that, when the F factor is integrated
within the chromosome it can provide a new site for initiation of chromosomal
replication in *dnaA* and *dnaC* mutants under non-permissive conditions, it has been
concluded that F is independent of the *dnaA* and C products (NISHIMURA *et al.*,
1971). (Similar data have been found with R28K in a *dnaA* mutant — T. ARAI,
personal communication.) Nevertheless F (and R28K) in the extrachromosomal state
does not undergo more than one round of replication in *dnaA* and *dnaC* mutants. It
may thus be concluded that the initiation of stringent plasmid replication is
dependent upon the same event (possibly the elongation of the cell envelope
[HELMSTETTER, 1974]) that initiates chromosomal replication, but that this event
permits one further round of initiation of plasmid replication at any time
during the subsequent cell cycle.

In contrast, extensive replication of the relaxed plasmids ColE1 and R6K
can occur in the absence of chromosomal replication. The conditions for this
vary according to the plasmid. Thus, ColE1 replicates in high concentrations
of CAP but does not replicate in the absence of polymerase I. R6K replicates
in the absence of polymerase III but is not dependent on polymerase I and is
inhibited in CAP. It can also replicate in a limited way in *dnaA* mutants.

Our more recent work makes use of these differences in the replication control of plasmids determined above, by investigating the interactions of two or more different plasmid replication systems when coupled on the same molecule. Usually, when two unit plasmid replicons replicate in the same cell, independent control is maintained, whereas when two plasmid replicons are co-integrated, the replication characteristics of only one of the replicons is expressed. Thus, when the F sex factor (whose independent replication is hypersensitive to acridine orange) is integrated into the chromosome, replication of the co-integrated circular (Hfr) structure appears to be determined by the chromosomal replicon (BIRD *et al.*, 1972). If however, this replication is defective, as in temperature-sensitive initiator-defective mutants (such as the *dnaA* mutants at 42°C), then replication of the cointegrate appears to be initiated at the F replicon, and exhibits the acridine orange replication-sensitivity of F initiation (NISHIMURA *et al.*, 1971). As a second example, certain plasmid cointegrates such as R222, comprised of a cointegrated transfer-factor replicon and one or more drug-resistance replicons, separate in *Proteus* hosts into their component replicons. Under these conditions, the drug-resistance replicon appears to be relaxed, whereas the transfer replicon is stringently controlled, as is the control of the replication of the cointegrate (NISIOKA *et al.*, 1969, 1970). Finally, when F and ColE1 are harbored in the same cell, the multi-copy nature of ColE1 is maintained, whereas F retains its 1:1 relationship with the chromosome. Moreover, ColE1 is still dependent upon the DNA polymerase I enzyme under these conditions (CLOWES, unpublished). Thus when two replicons are cointegrated, it seems likely that one or other of the replicons controls replication of the whole (CIS-relationship) although such dominance is not expressed when the plasmids are independent (TRANS-relationship). Such CIS-TRANS effects could help in clarifying the mechanisms of replication.

We are now constructing plasmid hybrids between R28K, R6K and ColE1, and we have also made use of the small plasmid pSC101 (derived from a stringently replicating plasmid [COHEN and CHANG, 1973], so that its replication may be expected to be stringently controlled). The hybrids are assembled through the use of the restriction endonuclease, EcoR1. In brief, this endonuclease recognizes a specific sequence of six bases present on DNA of plasmids and phage at intervals of about 2 to 15 Md. The endonuclease makes a break in both strands between the outside pair of bases at the 5'-3' end of the sequence. In this way, when the strands are separated, they have single-stranded, four-base termini which are complementary (BOYER, 1974). Thus, the end of any fragment can pair with either end of any other fragment and, if these fragments originate from distinct molecules, then hybrid molecules can be produced if the single-strand nicks are sealed with the joining enzyme, E. *coli* ligase (COHEN *et al.*, 1973). The DNA of intact plasmids and of EcoR1-generated fragments is conveniently separated by agarose-gel electrophoresis (SHARP *et al.*, 1973), and the biological activity of the circular molecules, either intact plasmid DNA, or ligated EcoR1-generated DNA, can be tested in a transformation system with an E. *coli* recipient (COHEN *et al.*, 1972).

pSC101 and ColE1 have been shown to have only one EcoR1-sensitive sequence (COHEN *et al.*, 1973; HERSCHFIELD *et al.*, 1974). Our preliminary data is that R6K has two sequences, recognized by the EcoR1 enzyme to produce two fragments of approximately 10 and 15 Md, as shown by separation on agarose-gel electrophoresis (see Fig. 4). If pSC101 is cut with EcoR1, then ligated, the DNA can be used to transform E. *coli* , selection being made for tetracycline resistance carried by this plasmid (COHEN *et al.*, 1973). Neither the 10 Md or the 15 Md R6K fragments, when ligated separately produce either ampicillin or streptomycin transformants, although when the mixture is ligated, numerous transformants for both characters can be found. A simple explanation for this result would be if the Ap and Sm genes were located on one fragment and the replication locus on the other. Such appears to be the case, for when the 15 Md fragment was ligated in the presence of EcoR1-treated pSC101, then transformants for Ap, Sm and Tc resistance could be selected (whereas no transformants were found when the 10 Md fragment was

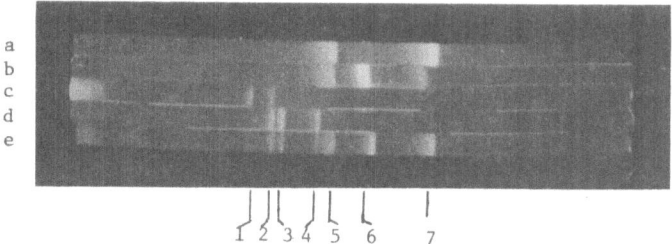

Fig. 4. *Agarose-gel electrophoresis of plasmid DNAs.* DNA samples were layered on top of the gel (shown on the left). After electrophoresis and staining, they were photographed by UV light of long wavelength. The gels contained (a) pSC101 (b) pSC101(+ *EcoR1*) (c) R6K (d) R6K(+ *EcoR1*) (e) R6K, R6K(+ *EcoR1*), pSC101 and pSC101(+ *EcoR1*). The bands are taken to be those of (1) R6K(OC) (2) R6K(CCC) (3) R6K(linear ∿ 15 Md) (4) R6K(linear ∿ 10 Md) (5) pSC101(OC) (6) pSC101(linear) (7) pSC101(CCC).

similarly treated). The DNA of several of these transformants contained a single species of DNA molecule of about 20 Md molecular weight, which when treated with *EcoR1* produced fragments equivalent in size to the 15 Md R6K fragment and linear pSC101.

Hybrids between the 10 Md fragment of R6K and pSC101 (or ColE1) have been constructed and experiments are now in progress to investigate the replication of these hybrid molecules under conditions non-permissive for one or other of the component replicons.

These experiments, together with others planned to locate the physical origin of DNA initiation on the parental plasmids and on the hybrids, should permit an insight into the regulatory mechanisms of plasmid replication.

Acknowledgements

This work was carried out with support from Public Health Service grant from the National Institute of Allergy and Infectious Diseases (AI-10468). We are grateful to DR. JAMES A. WECHSLER for the temperature sensitive *dna* mutants, to DR. STANLEY N. COHEN for plasmid pSC101 and our initial samples of the *EcoR1* endonuclease, to DR. D. JAMES McCORQUODALE for advice on agarose-gel electrophoresis and to DR. DIMITRIJ LANG for electron microscopy.

References

BAZARAL, M., and D. R. HELINSKI: Circular DNA forms of colicinogenic factors E1, E2 and E3 from *Escherichia coli. J. molec. Biol.* **36**, 185-194 (1968).

BIRD, R. E., J. LOUARN, J. MARTUSCELLI, AND L. G. CARO: The origin and sequence of chromosome replication in *Escherichia coli. J. molec. Biol.* **70**, 549-566 (1972).

BOYER, H. W.: R factor controlled restriction and modification of DNA. *Microbiology 1974* (in press) (ASM, Baltimore, 1974).

CLEWELL, D. B.: The nature of *Col* E1 plasmid replication in *Escherichia coli* in the presence of chloramphenicol. *J. Bact.* **110**, 667-676 (1972).

CLOWES, R. C.: Molecular structure of bacterial plasmids. *Bact. Rev.* **36**, 361-405 (1972).

COHEN, S. N., A. C. Y. CHANG, and L. HSU: Nonchromosomal antibiotic resistance in bacteria: genetic transformation of *Escherichia coli* by R-factor. *Proc. nat. Acad. Sci. Wash.* **69**, 2110-2114 (1972).

COHEN, S. N., and A. C. Y. CHANG: Recircularization and autonomous replication of a sheared R-factor DNA segment in *Escherichia coli* transformants. *Proc. nat. Acad. Sci. Wash.* 70, 1293-1297 (1973).

COHEN, S. N., A. C. Y. CHANG, H. W. BOYER, and R. B. HELLING: Construction of biologically functional bacterial plasmids *in vitro*. *Proc. nat. Acad. Sci. Wash.* 40, 3240-3244 (1973).

COOPER, S., and C. E. HELMSTETTER: Chromosomal replication and the division cycle of *Escherichia coli* B/r. *J. molec. Biol.* 31, 519-540 (1968).

GEFTER, M. L., Y. HIROTA, T. KORNBERG, J. A. WECHSLER, and C. BARNOUX: Analysis of DNA polymerases II and III in mutants of *Escherichia coli* thermosensitive for DNA synthesis. *Proc. nat. Acad. Sci. Wash.* 68, 3150-3153 (1971).

HELMSTETTER, C. E.: Initiation of chromosome replication in *Escherichia coli*. II. Analysis of the control mechanism. *J. molec. Biol.* 84, 21-36 (1974).

HERSCHFIELD, V., H. W. BOYER, C. YANOFSKY, M. A. LOVETT and D. HELINSKI: Plasmid ColE1 as a molecular vehicle for cloning and amplification of DNA. *Proc. nat. Acad. Sci. Wash.* 71, in press (1974).

KINGSBURY, D. T. and D. R. HELINSKI: Temperature-sensitive mutants for the replication of plasmids in *Escherichia coli*: Requirement for deoxyribonucleic acid polymerase I in the replication of the plasmid ColE1. *J. Bact.* 114, 1116-1124 (1973).

KONTOMICHALOU, P., M. MITANI, and R. C. CLOWES: Circular R-factor molecules controlling penicillinase synthesis, replicating in *Escherichia coli* under either relaxed or stringent control. *J. Bact.* 104, 34-44 (1970).

MEYNELL, E., G. G. MEYNELL and N. DATTA: Phylogenetic relationships of drug-resistance factors and other transmissible bacterial plasmids. *Bact. Rev.* 32, 55-83 (1968).

NISHIMURA, Y., L. CARO, C. B. BERG, and Y. HIROTA: Chromosome replication in *Escherichia coli*. IV. Control of chromosome replication and cell division by an integrated episome. *J. molec. Biol.* 55, 441-456 (1971).

NISIOKA, T., M. MITANI, and R. C. CLOWES: Composite circular forms of R-factor deoxyribonucleic acid molecules. *J. Bact.* 97, 376-385 (1969).

NISIOKA, T., M. MITANI, and R. C. CLOWES: Molecular recombination between R-factor deoxyribonucleic acid molecules in *Escherichia coli* host cells. *J. Bact.* 103, 166-177 (1970).

NOVICK, R. P.: Extrachromosomal inheritance in bacteria. *Bact. Rev.* 33, 210-257 (1969).

RADLOFF, R., W. BAUER, and J. VINOGRAD: A dye-buoyant-density method for the detection and isolation of closed circular duplex DNA: the closed circular DNA in HeLa cells. *Proc. nat. Acad. Sci. Wash.* 57, 1514-1520 (1967).

SHARP, P. A., B. SUGDEN, and J. SAMBROOK: Detection of two restriction endo-nuclease activities in *Haemophilus parainfluenzae* using analytical agarose-ethidium bromide electrophoresis. *Biochemistry* 12, 3055-3063 (1973).

SMITH, D. W.: DNA synthesis in Prokaryotes: Replication. *Progr. Biophysics* 26, 321-408 (1973).

VAPNEK, D., and W. D. RUPP: Identification of individual sex-factor DNA strands and their replication during conjugation in thermosensitive DNA mutants of *Escherichia coli*. *J. molec. Biol.* 60, 413-424 (1971).

WECHSLER, J. A., and J. D. GROSS: *Escherichia coli* mutants temperature sensitive for DNA synthesis. *Molec. gen. Genet.* 113, 273-284 (1971).

Elimination of Plasmidic Determinants by DNA-Complexing Compounds

Fred E. Hahn and Jennie Ciak

I. INTRODUCTION

Solutions to problems posed by R-factor determined multiresistance of pathogenic bacteria to chemotherapeutic drugs might be approached by several avenues. Firstly, one might search for new chemotherapeutic drugs. Secondly, one could think of interfering with the formation of R-factor gene products through inhibition of the transcription of messenger RNA or of its translation into proteins. In instances in which new drugs had these modes of action, the two first approaches would become unitary. Thirdly, one might hope to forestall the recombinatorial formation of new R-factors. Fourthly, one could think of inhibiting the transmission of R-factors, and, lastly, one might attempt to eliminate R-factors by selective inhibition of R-factor DNA replication. To the extent to which this replication is required for recombination of plasmidic genes into new R-factors or for transmission, the last three approaches would be served jointly by effective inhibition of plasmidic DNA replication. This is the approach which we have taken.

The discovery that extrachromosomal genetic elements in bacteria can be eliminated by intercalating chemicals was made in 1957 by Hirota and Iijima who grew Escherichia coli K12 in the presence of acriflavine and determined by genetic analysis that the bacteria lost their F-factor. Later, Hirota (1960) extended these observations to acridine orange and proflavine and referred to known effects of acridines on yeast mitochondria and on trypanosomal kinetoplasts as precedents of elimination of extrachromosomal genetic entities in micro-organisms other than bacteria.

On the basis of these results, Watanabe and Fukasawa (1960, 1961) and Mitsuhashi and his associates (1961) obtained the first eliminations of drug resistance determinants from bacterial R-factors by acriflavine and acridine orange. At the same time, Lerman developed the DNA intercalation theory for aminoacridines (1961). However, these two bodies of knowledge remained unconnected. Five years later it was shown by Falkow, Citarella, Wohlhieter and Watanabe (1966) that R-factors which had been transferred from several gram-negative enteropathogenic bacteria into Proteus mirabilis were DNA in nature. Shortly thereafter, Rownd, Nakaya and Nakamura (1966) grew several R-factor containing bacterial strains in the presence of acriflavine and isolated those bacteria which had lost all drug resistance determinants of their plasmids. When these organisms were then analyzed for DNA, no remaining plasmid DNA was detected. That was the first critical study of chemical elimination of plasmidic determinants and showed that this effect was the result of a physical elimination of R-factor DNA from bacteria.

But in these precise and detailed studies of Rownd and his associates (1966), no thought was given to the possible binding of acriflavine to R-factor DNA and no reference was made to Lerman's studies on intercalation which had been concluded and summarized two years earlier (Lerman, 1964).

The next step in the development of a theory of chemical elimination of plasmidic determinants came from the work of Michael Waring (Crawford and Waring, 1967) and of Bauer and Vinograd (1968) who studied the conformational changes in circular supercoiled DNA upon intercalation binding of ethidium bromide; this was followed by Waring's survey of a number of DNA-complexing substances as concerns their systematic influence on the conformation of the supercoiled replicative form of ϕX 174 DNA as a test for intercalation binding (Waring, 1970).

These findings became critically important to the consideration of chemical elimination of plasmidic determinants when it was shown first for the F' lac factor (Freifelder, 1968) and subsequently for R-factors from Proteus (Nisioka, Mitani and Clowes, 1969) that these extrachromosomal entities could be isolated in the form of circular supercoiled DNA.

At that point in time, we began our own work with studies on the elimination of the lac determinant from E. coli harboring the F' lac episome. Our first preliminary communication in 1969 (Ciak, Wormley and Hahn) was entitled Elimination of the F lac episome from E. coli by substances which intercalate into DNA, and closed with the sentence, "We propose that elimination of the F lac episome is a group property of intercalative substances and consider it significant that the F'lac DNA molecule has been found to be circular." To our knowledge, this was the first time that intercalation binding was regarded as a property of plasmid-eliminating compounds. Shortly thereafter, Chabbert, Baudens and Bouanchaud (1969) mentioned intercalative substances in a tabulation of several classes of R-factor eliminating chemicals.

One year later, we presented our first results on elimination of resistance determinants from an R-factor in E. coli before the New York Academy of Sciences (Hahn and Ciak, 1971) and introduced our work with the following sentence, "We propose the hypothesis that chemical substances which bind to double-helical DNA by intercalation will eliminate bacterial episomes through a molecular mechanism by which closed circular episomal DNA is converted into unnatural left-handed supercoils and cannot be replicated in this conformation."

Before going on to our experimental results, it is necessary to discuss this hypothesis. A major criticism emerges from the fact that the molecular conformation of R-factors inside the bacterial cell in vivo has not been determined; neither have conformational changes which may accompany R-factor DNA replication. Our hypothesis tacitly assumed that the closed circular form in which many R-factor DNAs have been isolated also exists prominently inside the bacterial cell. We still do not know if such is the case.

On the positive side, there exist several lines of evidence which indicate that ethidium affects selectively extrachromosomal DNAs in vivo in eucaryotic cells such as yeast, trypanosomes, mammalian cells in culture and Tetrahymena (rev. Borst, 1972; Upholt and Borst, 1974; Steinert, 1969). In vitro, super-coiled DNA preferentially binds ethidium (Bauer and Vinograd, 1971), and the drug is about one order of magnitude more active as a DNA template poison when the template is circular supercoiled in structure as compared to unconstrained DNA (Richardson and Parker, 1973). Our results show that intercalating compounds do, indeed, have the group property of eliminating plasmidic determinants. The exact mechanism of this action remains hypothetical but most likely is based on template toxicity in plasmidic DNA replication.

II.   ELIMINATION OF THE LAC MARKER FROM THE F' LAC EPISOME IN E. COLI

The first major drug for which intercalation binding into DNA had been demonstrated was quinacrine (Lerman, 1963). We had found, subsequently, that quinacrine was bacteriostatic for Escherichia coli B at 2×10^{-4} M (Ciak and Hahn, 1967), and now grew strain 3876 of the K12 group overnight in the presence of graded sub-inhibitory concentrations of this drug. These cultures were plated on MacConkey agar which contains lactose as a major source of carbon and neutral red as an acid indicator. The total numbers of colonies and the numbers of lac⁻ colonies were counted and the extent of elimination of the lac marker was expressed as the percentage of lac⁻ colonies. From these data, the probit transformation of the dosage response correlation was drawn which is shown in Fig. 1. According to principles summarized earlier in this Symposium (Hahn), this correlation results from reversible occupancy of receptors by a drug according to the mass action law.

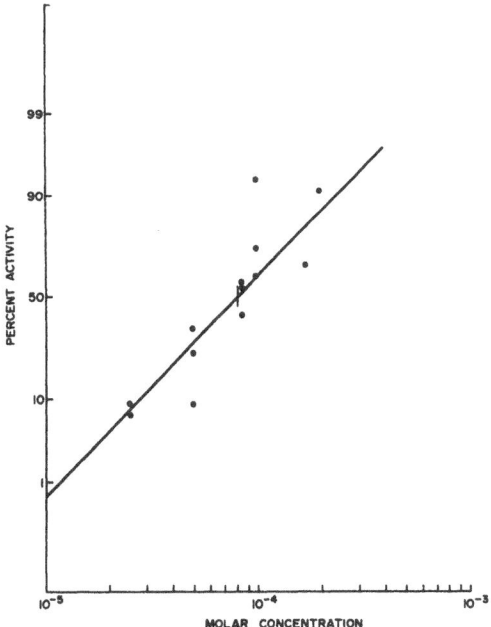

Fig. 1.   Dosage-response correlation for the elimination of the lac[+] marker from E. coli 3876 by quinacrine.

The best straight line was fitted by the method of least squares. This was also done for the dosage-response lines in Fig. 2 which compares the relative potencies of acridine orange, ethidium bromide and chloroquine to that of quinacrine. From such lines, the ED_{50}s, i.e. the fifty per cent eliminating concentrations were interpolated, and these values are listed in Table 1 for the series of compounds studied (Ciak, Wormley and Hahn, 1969). Independently, Bouanchaud, Scavizzy and Chabbert (1969) obtained 20 per cent elimination of the lac marker in E. coli K12 by "subinhibitory concentrations" of ethidium bromide, and Hohn and Korn (1969) studied the kinetics of lac elimination in a strain of the K12 group by acridine orange. In that last work, it was shown that elimination was the result of a dilution of the original lac[+] cell population with the lac⁻ progeny owing to a blockade of episome replication by acridine orange.

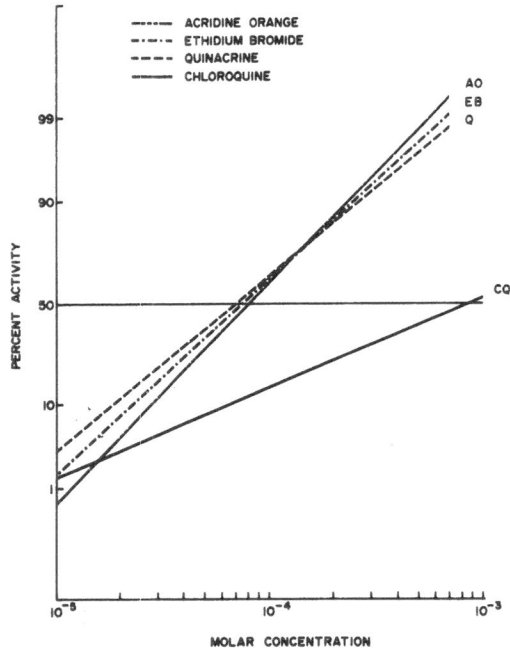

Fig. 2. Dosage response correlations for the elimination of the lac[+] marker from E. coli 3876 by acridine orange, ethidium bromide, quinacrine and chloroquine.

TABLE 1

FIFTY PERCENT EFFECTIVE DOSES, $ED_{50}S$, OF COMPOUNDS ELIMINATING THE Lac[+] MARKER FROM E. COLI 3876

Compound	ED_{50}
Quinacrine	7.2×10^{-5} M
Ethidium bromide	7.5×10^{-5} M
Acridine orange	8.2×10^{-5} M
Chloroquine	9.0×10^{-4} M
Miracil D	3.3×10^{-3} M*
Quinine	**
Methylene blue	**
p-Rosaniline	**

* Extrapolated
** No 50 percent activity attained

These various observations on the elimination of the lac determinant from F' lac by intercalating compounds raised the question of the physical fate of the F-factor. Hirota (1960) had determined the loss of mating ability in E. coli K12 grown in the presence of aminoacridines but no molecular studies of the fate of the episomal DNA had been carried out which could compare to the demonstration of Rownd and his associates (1966) that the DNA of an R-factor was no longer present in bacteria after all resistance determinants had been eliminated by acriflavine. We labeled the global DNA of lac⁺ and lac⁻ E. coli K12 with ¹⁴C-thymidine, extracted the DNA and subjected it to cesium chloride density gradient centrifugation in the presence of ethidium bromide which renders circular supercoiled DNA heavy followed by fractionation (Bazarel and Helinski, 1968). The results are shown in Fig. 3. The DNA of untreated cells contained a large fraction of heavy DNA at left; the rise of the curve toward lower densities signaled the presence of chromosomal DNA. At right, for cells from which lac had been eliminated by quinacrine, the satellite peak was grossly diminished; the area under this peak is about 20 per cent of that under the large satellite DNA peak at left. We inferred that the elimination of the lac determinant had not caused a complete loss of episomal DNA (Hahn and Ciak, 1971).

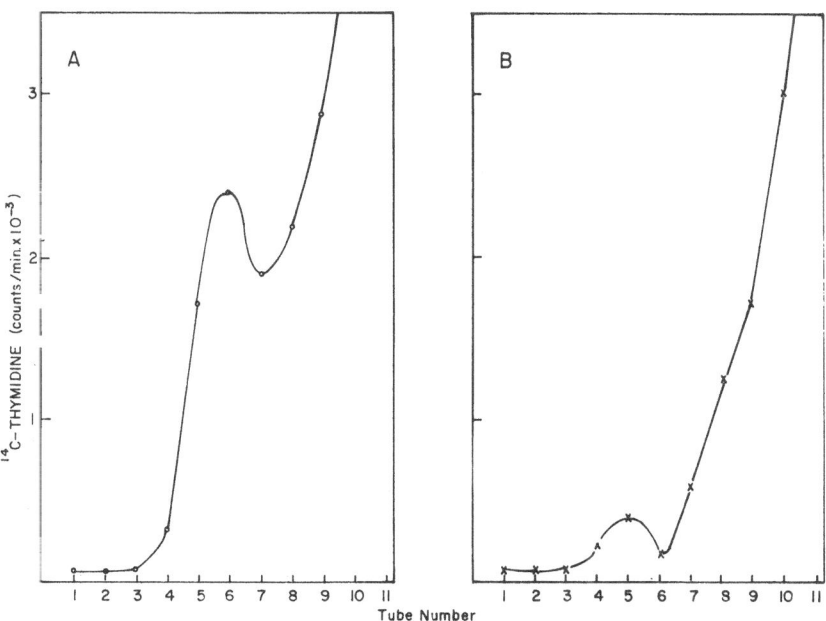

Fig. 3. Isopycnic centrifugation profiles of A: global DNA of E. coli 3876, and B: DNA of the same organism after elimination of lac⁺ by quinacrine.

III. ELIMINATION OF RESISTANCE DETERMINANTS FROM AN R-FACTOR IN E. COLI

After these preliminary studies, we began to investigate the elimination of resistance determinants in E. coli. Our test strain was RS-2 of the K12 group which had been genetically constructed by Silver and Falkow (1970) and contained an R-factor with resistance determinants to kanamycin, chloramphenicol, ampicillin, streptomycin and sulfonamide which had been transferred into RS-2 from an original isolate of Datta. These bacteria were grown overnight in the presence of a 10^{-4} M concentration of test compounds, the cultures plated on drug-free agar and on plates containing singly each of the five chemotherapeutic drugs, and all colonies counted. The differences between the numbers of colonies on drug-containing plates and those on drug-free control plates were expressed as percentages of total colonies on the latter and were considered percentages of elimination of determinants which had been accomplished. In order to prevent the carry-over of small amounts of eliminating compounds onto the drug-containing test plates which might have produced synergistic growth suppression and faulty numbers of excessive eliminations, we passed the original experimental cultures once over drug-free plates, suspended the organisms from such plates and then carried out differential plating. The results from both procedures were not significantly different.

TABLE 2

FREQUENCIES OF ELIMINATION OF DETERMINANTS IN E. COLI RS-2

Compound 10^{-4} M	Kanamycin	Percent Curing of R Factors for: Chlor-amphenicol	Ampicillin	Streptomycin	Sulfadiazine
Ethidium bromide	59 ± 4	61 ± 4	15 ± 8	0	0
Quinacrine	25 ± 3	22 ± 8	4 ± 2	0	0
Acridine orange	21 ± 5	22 ± 3	0	0	0
Berberine	9 ± 4	9 ± 4	0	0	0
Quinine	10 ± 3	0	0	0	0
Chloroquine	10 ± 6	0	0	0	0
Spermine	11 ± 2	0	9 ± 4	0	0
p-Rosaniline	0	0	0	0	0
Methylene blue	0	0	0	0	0

Table 2 lists the results of elimination of resistance determinants from E. coli RS-2. It is immediately apparent that the active compounds produced marked segregation of the individual determinants. The kanamycin determinant was eliminated by 7 out of 9 compounds, the chloramphenicol determinant by 4, the ampicillin determinant by 2 or perhaps 3, and the determinants of resistance to streptomycin and sulfadiazine were not eliminated by any of our test compounds. In the original work of Watanabe and Fukasawa (1960, 1961) no segregation had been observed. Our results do confirm, however, that elimination frequencies in E. coli are low (Watanabe, 1963; Bouanchaud et al., 1969).

For the most active compound, ethidium bromide, we carried out dosage-response determinations for the elimination of the kanamycin and chloramphenicol determinants. The results are shown in Fig. 4. Both lines have similar slopes and the 50 per cent eliminating concentrations for both determinants interpolate to 7.5 x 10^{-5} M.

The outcome of this study, 12 eliminations out of numerically possible 35 such observations with intercalating drugs and 2 out of 5 possible eliminations by the non-intercalating spermine, could not be considered a conclusive test of our hypothesis that the ability of eliminating determinants from plasmids is a group property of intercalating substances.

IV. ELIMINATION OF RESISTANCE DETERMINANTS FROM AN R-FACTOR IN SALMONELLA TYPHIMURIUM

For such a more conclusive test, we made use of the well-known fact that elimination frequencies are much higher in strains of Salmonellae (Bouanchaud et al., 1969; Lebek, 1969) than in E. coli and that various Salmonella species

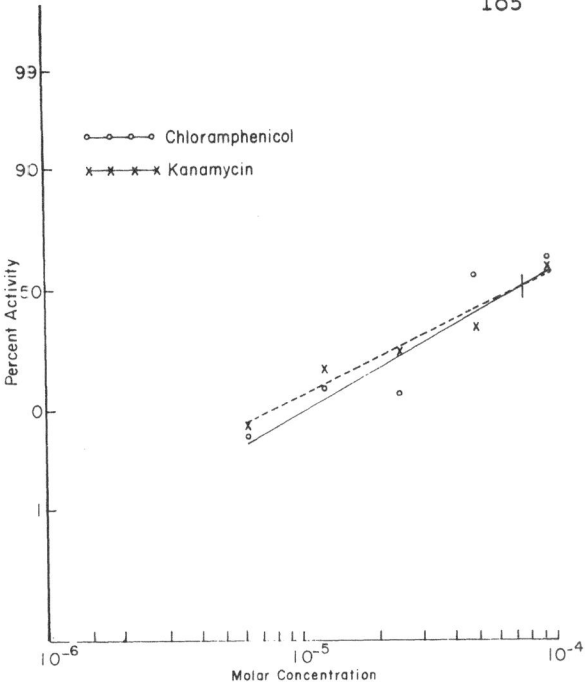

Fig. 4. Dosage-response correlations for the elimination of the kanamycin and chloramphenicol resistance determinants from E. coli RS-2 by ethidium bromide.

can also exhibit considerable spontaneous segregation of plasmidic resistance determinants (Watanabe and Lyang, 1962; Anderson, 1968). The R-factor from E. coli RS-2 was transferred into Salmonella typhimurium LT-2. Since this strain was, before the transfer, resistant to >25 mg/ml of sulfadiazine, the elimination of the sulfonamide determinant could not be measured and our studies were therefore restricted to eliminations of the determinants of resistance to kanamycin, chloramphenicol, ampicillin and streptomycin. Experimental procedures and data handling were the same as used previously with E. coli.

TABLE 3

PER CENTS ELIMINATION OF RESISTANCE DETERMINANTS IN S. TYPHIMURIUM

Compounds	Kana	Chloramph	Strepto	Ampicill
6.25×10^{-6} M Nalidixic acid	70	56	60	64
2.5×10^{-5} M Nitroacridine II	99	96	96	97
Daunomycin	86	80	77	81
Proflavine	86	79	64	68
5×10^{-5} M Nitroakridin 3582	82	69	70	69
8×10^{-4} M Coumadine	70	56	60	64

The growth inhibitory properties of several of our test compounds were such that the substances could not be used at the standard concentration of 10^{-4} M. Results with these compounds are shown in Table 3. The two nitroacridines were gifts from Farbwerke Hoechst, and the compound designated as nitroacridine II is a derivative of the well-known compound 3582 in which the two methoxy groups have been deleted from the acridine ring system. This was the most active substance which at 2.5×10^{-5} M eliminated all four resistance determinants completely within the limits of statistical significance. Nalidixic acid could be used only over a very narrow concentration range without causing its typical bactericidal effect. A slight elimination of determinants from R-factors in Shigella flexneri and E. coli by nalidixic acid had been tabulated earlier by Chabbert and his associates (1969). Coumadine does not intercalate into DNA and exhibited low activity at a high concentration of 8×10^{-4} M.

TABLE 4

PER CENTS ELIMINATION OF RESISTANCE DETERMINANTS IN S. TYPHIMURIUM

Compounds at 10^{-4} M	Kana	Chloramph	Strepto	Ampicill
Ethidium	96	82	84	82
Miracil D	91	82	81	82
Quinacrine	92	79	81	71
Propidium	89	78	71	71
Tilorone	85	80	74	78*
p-Rosaniline	87	71	73	66
Acridine orange	85	71	69	68
Berberine	83	68	70	62
Quinine	81	60	66	57
Spermine	81	56*	71	58
Chlorpromazine	78	63	67	72*
Hoechst 33258	72	64	64	67*
Chloroquine	80*	58	52	53
Methylene blue	68	50	48	41

*Significant inversions in activity sequence

Table 4 lists results for all compounds which could be employed at 10^{-4} M which can, therefore, be directly compared. All listed substances are known to form complexes with DNA; intercalation binding of Hoechst 33258 can be assumed but has not yet been determined. It is probably excluded for p-rosaniline (Neville and Davies, 1966) and is, of course, impossible for spermine. All others are known intercalators.

The first fact which emerges from an examination of the Table is that all resistance determinants were eliminated in contrast to the incomplete effects of intercalants on the determinants of the same R-factor when it had been carried by E. coli (Table 2). On the other hand, segregation was not so drastic as in E. coli although the kanamycin determinant was consistently eliminated at higher frequencies than the other three.

The second fact which can be recognized is that the eliminating potencies of the studied compounds fell into a fairly consistent sequence. The compounds have been listed in their order of decreasing potency which shows only a few inversions in the activity sequence which may not all be statistically significant. We have interpreted the occurrence of this systematic sequence as an expression of the greater or lesser tendency of these substances to complex with DNA.

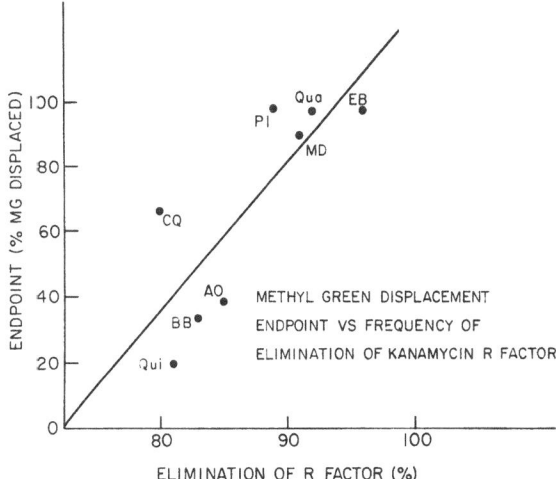

Fig. 5. Correlation between the endpoints of methyl green displacement from
calf-thymus DNA and the elimination frequencies for the kanamycin
determinant in S. typhimurium LT-2 by eight intercalating compounds.
Qua: quinacrine; EB: ethidium bromide; PI: propidium iodide;
MD: miracil D; CQ: chloroquine; AO: acridine orange; BB: berberine;
Qui: quinine.

This rests on a correlation between the endpoints of displacement of methyl
green from DNA which Anne Krey and I have studied extensively (Krey and Hahn,
1971) and of the potencies of the same compounds in eliminating the kanamycin
determinant. This correlation is shown in Fig. 5. The only point which falls
somewhat far from the straight line is that for chloroquine, CQ, and this was one
of the instances in which an inversion in the activity sequence was quite
apparent. If we consider endpoints of the displacement of methyl green by these
intercalants a relative measure of their total binding to DNA, it follows that
the ability to eliminate resistance determinants was a function of this
stoichiometry.

The significant activities of p-rosaniline and of spermine may, perhaps,
require a broadening of our original working hypothesis. Both substances bind to
DNA but not by intercalation. We may infer, from this, that there exist
instances in which DNA complexing compounds eliminate plasmidic resistance
determinants even when they do not intercalate. Hirota (1960) has shown this for
the F-factor with propamidine at low frequency.

V. STERILIZATION OF S. TYPHIMURIUM BY COMBINATIONS OF AMPICILLIN AND
ELIMINATING COMPOUNDS

Based upon the kinetics of elimination of the lac determinant from F' lac
by acriflavine which in the study of Hohn and Korn (1969) was the reflection of a
progressive dilution of preexisting lac$^+$ population with the lac$^-$ progeny, we
expected that a complete inhibition of the replication of the ampicillin
determinant in S. typhimurium, for example, by ethidium, would result in the
destruction of all progeny cells when ampicillin also was present so that the
bacterial titer of such cultures should remain constant, at least for a time.

Our R-factor containing test strain is resistant to 2,500 μg/ml of ampicillin in conventional serial dilution test tube assays with incubation overnight. When we added ethidium to 10^{-4} M plus 60 μg/ml of ampicillin to an exponentially growing culture which contained at that point in time 2 x 10^4 bacteria per ml and removed samples at two hour intervals for plating and colony counting, we obtained results of which a typical example is shown in Fig. 6. The control culture without any additions grew exponentially to a final concentration of 4 x 10^9 organism per ml. Another culture to which only ethidium had been added, showed an initial decline in the number of colony-forming bacteria by a factor of 20, after which it resumed exponential growth with increasing rates which, beyond the 14 hr experimental period shown here, approached the rate of the control. A third culture to which only ampicillin had been added showed an initial decline in the number of colony-forming bacteria by a factor of 40 but then resumed exponential growth at a rate which between hours 6 and 8 equalled the growth rate of the control. The experimental culture to which ethidium plus ampicillin had been added declined in viability until by the sixth hour there were one or no viable cells left per ml. Further incubation for several days did not produce a resumption of growth, and bacteriologically the culture remained sterile.

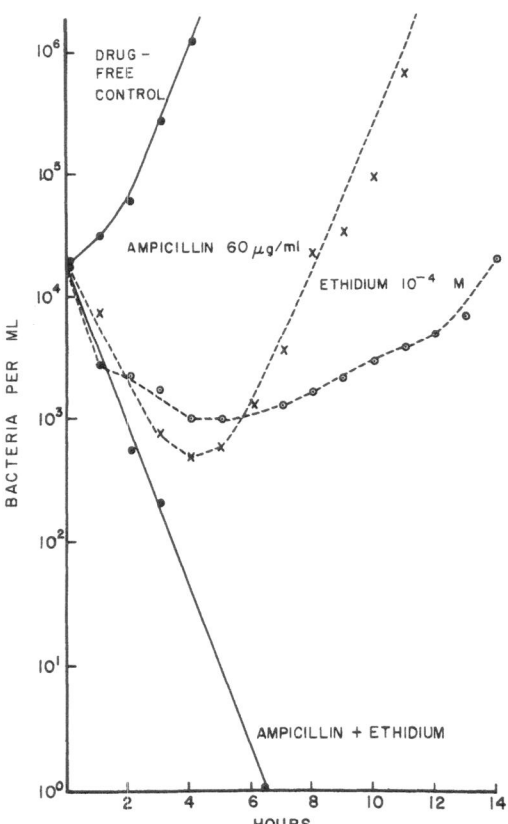

Fig. 6. Numbers of viable cells of S. typhimurium in cultures exposed to 60 μg/ml ampicillin, 10^{-4} M ethidium bromide or to a combination of both drugs.

Such results could be obtained over a pH range of from 7.4 to 8.0 when the pH was adjusted by the addition of potassium hydroxide. Cultures which were exposed to ethidium alone and had resumed growth by the sixth hour were sterilized when ampicillin was added at that point in time. In contrast, cultures which had received ampicillin alone and had resumed growth by the sixth hour were not sterilized by the addition of ethidium.

We have obtained analogous results with combinations of ampicillin and tilorone at 10^{-4} M or with quinacrine at 4×10^{-4} M. Most important, such results were also seen with a combination of ampicillin and Nitroakridin 3582 at a low concentration of 5×10^{-6} M, i.e. 2.5 µg/ml.

VI. DISCUSSION

In the aggregate, our results support the hypothesis that the ability to eliminate plasmidic determinants is a group property of chemicals which bind to DNA, foremost, of those which are intercalated. The relatively low activity of chloroquine is probably explained by the low affinity of the drug for DNA for which association constants of 10^3 to 10^4 M^{-1} have been determined (Stollar and Levine, 1963; Cohen and Yielding, 1965). Methylene blue, our least potent compound, has been shown by Hirota (1960) actually to antagonize the elimination of the F-factor from E. coli by aminoacridines; he has made reference to the classical phenomenon of therapeutic interference (Browning and Gulbranson, 1922) between substances of similar chemical structure.

Preferential inhibition of R-factor DNA replication is not restricted to substances which form complexes with DNA. Ultraviolet irradiation (Rownd et al., 1956), mitomycin C (Kawakami and Landman, 1965), nalidixic acid (Table 3), phenethyl alcohol (Unowsky and Bontempo, 1967), trimethoprim which converts prototrophic bacteria into phenocopies of thymine auxotrophs (Pinney and Smith, 1972), or thymine starvation of genuine auxotrophs (Pinney and Smith, 1971), all have a selective effect on the biosynthesis of plasmid DNA. In the absence of knowledge on the mechanism of plasmid DNA replication, we do not wish to speculate on reasons why this process is more susceptible to inhibitions than is the biosynthesis of chromosomal DNA.

DNA intercalators also inhibit the transfer of R-factors between bacteria. This was shown by Levy and Watanabe (1966) for quinacrine and investigated in some detail by Hayashi and his associates (Hayashi, Kodaira, Ogawa, Baba, Kikuchi, Tada and Iwasaki, 1965). Among 17 compounds tested, 12 were derivatives of acridine. Unsubstituted acridine and acridine N-oxide were inactive. In contrast, aminoacridines inhibited R-factor transfer and this activity was maintained when the amino groups were methylated or acetylated; larger amino substituents such as propionyl or benzoyl abolished activity. It is not difficult to read into these results the structural rules for intercalation binding which have been discussed earlier in this Symposium. Since Fenwick and Curtiss (1973a) have recently shown that transmission of plasmids requires active conjugal DNA biosynthesis and can, for this reason, be inhibited by nalidixic acid (Fenwick and Curtiss, 1973b), it follows that an inhibition of R-factor replication by intercalative drugs will result also in non-occurrence of R-factor transfer: DNA which is not synthesized can not be transferred.

Our results on sterilization of S. typhimurium with combinations of ampicillin and four different DNA-intercalating compounds require comment. We had hoped to restrict test cultures to the original R-factor containing populations and merely to preclude the proliferation of an R⁻ progeny. The complete sterilization of cultures within 6 hours was unexpected.

A first explanation would be the occurrence of synergistic growth inhibition. This does not appear likely because we carried out analogous experiments with combinations of kanamycin and ethidium and saw no growth inhibition or bactericidal effect. The presence of kanamycin has been reported to protect Salmonellae against spontaneous as well as chemically induced loss of the kanamycin resistance determinant (Lebek, 1969). A second explanation would be that ethidium caused selective inhibition of RNA transcription, resulting in a failure of the formation of the plasmid-determined β-lactamase enzyme. However, quinacrine with which similar results were obtained, inhibits bacterial RNA synthesis not at all and protein synthesis only partly at the concentration levels employed (Ciak and Hahn, 1967) and Nitroakridin 3582 at 5×10^{-6} M has no effect on bacterial RNA or protein biosyntheses (Wolfe, Cook and Hahn, 1971). We do not think, therefore, that the result of our drug combination experiments was produced by inhibitions of the phenotypic expression of the ampicillin determinant.

The exponential loss of viability of S. typhimurium in the ampicillin combination experiments is, however, difficult to explain on the basis of the assumption that the four R-factor eliminating drugs caused only a blockade of R-factor replication. The mitochondrial DNA in yeast undergoes rapid degradation upon exposure to ethidium (Goldring, Grossman, Krupnick, Cryer and Marmur, 1970; Perlman and Mahler, 1971). If a similar dissimilation of bacterial plasmid DNA were stimulated by ethidium or the other drugs which we tested, this would explain the rapid loss of viability which was observed. However, tests for such a contact effect have been carried out for the F-episome with acridine orange by Hirota (1960) and for our R-factor in E. coli RS-2 with ethidium (Hahn and Ciak, 1973) in our laboratory, both with negative results. At this point we feel that further study is required in order to explain the bactericidal effect which is produced by ampicillin combinations with R-factor eliminating drugs.

SUMMARY

Originally, we proposed the hypothesis that the ability to eliminate genetic determinants from bacterial plasmids is a group property of compounds which bind to DNA by intercalation and act as template poisons in the replication of plasmid DNA. This was tested for the lac determinant of F' lac in E. coli, for five resistance determinants of the R-factor in E. coli RS-2 and for four resistance determinants of the same R-factor after it had been transferred into S. typhimurium LT-2. The results were in accord with the hypothesis. Spermine and p-rosaniline which bind to DNA but do not intercalate, also showed activity. Populations of S. typhimurium with R-factor determined resistance to 2500 µg/ml of ampicillin were rapidly sterilized by combinations of 60 µg/ml of this antibiotic with quinacrine (4×10^{-4} M), ethidium bromide (10^{-4} M), tilorone (10^{-4} M) or Nitroakridin 3582 (5×10^{-6} M).

REFERENCES

Anderson, E.S.: The ecology of the transferable drug resistance in the enterobacteria. Ann. Rev. Microbiol. 22, 131 (1968).

Bauer, W. and J. Vinograd: The interaction of closed circular DNA with intercalative dyes. I. The superhelix density of SV40 DNA in the presence and absence of dye. J. Mol. Biol. 33, 141 (1968).

Bauer, W. and J. Vinograd: The use of intercalative dyes in the study of closed circular DNA. In Progr. Mol. Subcell. Biol. 2, 181 (1971). F.E. Hahn edt. Springer, Berlin-Heidelberg-New York.

Bazaral, M. and D.R. Helinski: Circular form of colicinogenic factors E1, E2 and E3 from Escherichia coli. J. Mol. Biol. 36, 185 (1968).

Borst, P.: Mitochondrial nucleic acids. Ann. Rev. Biochem. 41, 333 (1972).

Bouanchaud, D.H., M.R. Scavizzi and Y.A. Chabbert: Elimination by ethidium bromide of antibiotic resistance in Enterobacteria and Staphylococci. J. Gen. Microbiol. 54, 417 (1969).

Browning, C.H. and R. Gulbranson: An interference phenomenon in the action of chemotherapeutic substances in experimental trypanosome infections. J. Path. Bact. 25, 395 (1922).

Chabbert, Y.A., J.G. Baudens and D.H. Bouanchaud: Medical aspects of transferable drug resistance. In Bacterial Episomes and Plasmids, Ciba Foundation Symp. Churchill, London, 1969, p 227.

Ciak, J. and F.E. Hahn: Quinacrine (Atebrin): Mode of action. Science 156, 655 (1967).

Ciak, J., S. Wormley and F.E. Hahn: Elimination of the F lac episome from Escherichia coli 3876 by substances which intercalate into DNA. Bact. Proc. 1969, 67 (1969).

Cohen, S.N. and K.L. Yielding: Spectrophotometric studies of the interaction of chloroquine with deoxyribonucleic acid. J. Biol. Chem. 240, 3123 (1965).

Crawford, L.V. and M. Waring: Supercoiling of polyoma virus DNA measured by its interaction with ethidium bromide. J. Mol. Biol. 25, 23 (1967).

Falkow, S., R.V. Citarella, J.A. Wohlhieter and T. Watanabe: The molecular nature of R-factors. J. Mol. Biol. 17, 102 (1966).

Fenwick, R.G. and R. Curtiss: Conjugal deoxyribonucleic acid replication by Escherichia coli K12: Stimulation in dnaB(ts) donors by minicells. J. Bact. 116, 1212 (1973a).

Fenwick, R.G. and R. Curtiss: Conjugal deoxyribonucleic acid replication by Escherichia coli K12: Effect of nalidixic acid. J. Bact. 116, 1236 (1973b).

Freifelder, D.: Studies on Escherichia coli sex factors. III. Covalently closed F' lac DNA molecules. J. Mol. Biol. 34, 31 (1968).

Go'dring, E.S., L.I. Grossman, D. Krupnick, D.R. Cryer and J. Marmur: The petite mutation in yeast: Loss of mitochondrial DNA during induction of petites with ethidium bromide. J. Mol. Biol. 52, 323 (1970).

Hahn, F.E. and J. Ciak: Elimination of bacterial episomes by DNA-complexing compounds. Ann. New York Acad. Sci. 182, 295 (1971).

Hahn, F.E. and J. Ciak: Restoration of drug-resistant bacteria to sensitivity to chemotherapeutic drugs. Proc. 1972 Army Sci. Conf. 2, 1 (1973).

Hayashi, K., T. Kodaira, Y. Ogawa, K. Baba, K. Kikuchi, K. Tada and K. Iwasaki: Studies on substances which act on episomal infective transfer systems. Jap. J. Bact. [In Japanese] 20, 498 (1965).

Hirota, Y.: The effect of acridine dyes on mating type in Escherichia coli. Proc. Natl. Acad. Sci. USA 46, 57 (1960).

Hirota, Y. and T. Iijima: Acriflavine as an effective agent for eliminating F factor in Escherichia coli. Nature 180, 655 (1957).

Hohn, B. and D. Korn: Cosegregation of a sex factor with the Escherichia coli chromosome during curing by acridine orange. J. Mol. Biol. 45, 385 (1969).

Kawakami, M. and O.E. Landman: Experiments concerning the curing and intra-cellular site of episomes. Biochem. Biophys. Res. Comm. 18, 716 (1965).

Krey, A.K. and F.E. Hahn: Methyl green-DNA complex: Displacement of dye by DNA-binding substances. Proc. First Eur. Congr. Biophys. 1, 223 (1971).

Lebek, G.: Die infektiöse bakterielle Antibiotika-Resistenz. Hans Huber, Bern and Stuttgart, 1969.

Lerman, L.S.: Structural considerations in the interaction of DNA and acridines. J. Mol. Biol. 3, 18 (1961).

Lerman, L.S.: The structure of the DNA-acridine complex. Proc. Nat. Acad. Sci. USA 49, 94 (1963).

Lerman, L.S.: Acridine mutagens and DNA structure. J. Cell. Comp. Physiol. 64, Suppl. 1, 1 (1964).

Levy, S.B. and T. Watanabe: Mepacrine and transfer of R-factors. Lancet 2, 1138 (1966).

Mitsuhashi, S., K. Harada and M. Kameda: Elimination of transmissible drug-resistance by treatment with acriflavine. Nature 189, 947 (1961).

Neville, D.M. and D.R. Davies: The interaction of acridine dyes with DNA: An x-ray diffraction and optical investigation. J. Mol. Biol. 17, 57 (1966).

Nisioka, T., M. Mitani and R. Clowes: Composite circular forms of R factor deoxyribonucleic acid molecules. J. Bact. 97, 376 (1969).

Perlman, P.S. and H.R. Mahler: Effect of ethidium bromide on yeast cells. Nature New Biol. 231, 12 (1971).

Pinney, R.J. and J.T. Smith: R-factor elimination by thymine starvation. Genet. Res. Camb. 18, 173 (1971).

Pinney, R.J. and J.T. Smith: Elimination of an R-factor by trimethoprim. J. Pharm. Pharmacol. 24, Suppl. 126 p (1972).

Richardson, J.P. and S.R. Parker: Effect of ethidium bromide on transcription of linear and circular DNA templates. J. Mol. Biol. 78, 715 (1973).

Rownd, R., R. Nakaya and A. Nakamura: Molecular nature of the drug-resistance factors of the Enterbacteriaceae. J. Mol. Biol. 17, 376 (1966).

Silver, R.P. and S. Falkow: Specific labeling and physical characterization of R-factor deoxyribonucleic acid in Escherichia coli. J. Bact. 104, 331 (1970).

Steinert, M.: Specific loss of kinetoplastic DNA in trypanosomatidae treated with ethidium bromide. Exptl. Cell Res. 55, 248 (1969).

Stollar, D. and L. Levine: Antibodies to denatured deoxyribonucleic acid in lupus erythematosus serum. V. Mechanism of DNA-ant-DNA inhibition by chloroquine. Arch. Biochem. Biophys. 101, 335 (1963).

Unowsky, J. and J. Bontempo: The elimination of R-factor-mediated drug resistance by phenethyl alcohol and acriflavine. Abstr. Seventh Intersci. Conf. Antimicr. Agents & Chemoth. 57 (1967).

Upholt, W.B. and P. Borst: Accumulation of replicative intermediates of mitochondrial DNA in Tetrahymena pyriformis grown in ethidium bromide. J. Cell Biol. 61, 383 (1974).

Waring, M.: Variations of the supercoils in closed circular DNA by binding of antibiotics and drugs: Evidence for molecular models involving intercalation. J. Mol. Biol. 54, 247 (1970).

Watanabe, T.: Infective heredity of multiple drug resistance in bacteria. Bact. Rev. 27, 87 (1963).

Watanabe, T. and T. Fukasawa: Episomic resistance factors in Enterobacteriaceae. III. Elimination of resistance factors by treatment with acridine dyes. [In Japanese] Med. Biol. (Tokyo) 56, 71 (1960).

Watanabe, T. and T. Fukasawa: Episome-mediated transfer of drug resistance in Enterobacteriaceae. II. Elimination of resistance factors with acridine dyes. J. Bact. 81, 679 (1961).

Watanabe, T. and K.W. Lyang: Episome-mediated transfer of drug resistance in Enterobacteriaceae. V. Spontaneous segregation and recombination of resistance factors in Salmonella typhimurium. J. Bact. 84, 422 (1962).

Wolfe, A.D., T.M. Cook and F.E. Hahn: Antibacterial nitroacridine, Nitroakridin 3582: Effects on bacterial growth and macromolecular biosynthesis in vivo. J. Bact. 108, 320 (1971).

III. Ribosomes as Drug-Receptors

Antibiotic Receptor-Sites in Escherichia coli Ribosomes

Georg Stöffler and Gilbert W. Tischendorf

INTRODUCTION

The translation of mRNA into protein at the ribosomal level can be divided into three phases: initiation, elongation and termination. The initiation phase can be divided into: (a) Recognition of initiation factors and mRNA by the 30S subunit, (b) binding of f-Met-tRNA$_F^{Met}$ and (c) combination of this initiation complex with a 50S subunit. The elongation phase follows initiation of protein biosynthesis and is composed of repeated cycles. Each cycle can be divided into: (a) EF-Tu dependent aminoacyl-tRNA-binding, (b) peptide bond formation and (c) translocation. The translocation step requires the elongation factor G and GTP. The elongation cycle occurs repeatedly until the termination codon of the mRNA is reached. In response to this codon, release factors are bound and promote release of a newly synthesized protein from the tRNA moiety in a reaction catalyzed by the ribosomal peptidyltransferase (Haselkorn and Rothman-Denes, 1973; Porgs et al., 1974).

Specific inhibition of bacterial protein synthesis was first described almost 25 years ago (Hahn and Wisseman, 1951). Studies on the mechanism of antibiotic action have been so widely developed that now specific antibiotic inhibitors are known for all steps of protein synthesis (Weisblum and Davies, 1968; Pestka, 1971; Pestka and Bodley, 1974; Vazquez, 1974).

A number of mutants with altered response to antibiotics that block protein synthesis by affecting the ribosomes were isolated: such mutants were in general more resistant than the parental strain but sometimes also more sensitive or even dependent on the drug. The fact that mutational alteration of the ribosomes is the primary resistance mechanism has proved of great utility. Resistance to antibiotics in bacteria has been shown to produce specific alterations in components of the 30S or 50S ribosomal subunits and allowed genetic mapping of the loci responsible for the synthesis of these components, e.g. a given ribosomal protein (review by Osawa et al., 1972).

The finding that ribosomal subunits can be reconstituted from RNA and proteins offered a further test system to trace the site of action of an antibiotic (Staehelin et al., 1969; Traub and Nomura, 1968; Nomura and Erdmann, 1970). To date mutational alterations have been found in several different ribosomal proteins (for refs. see Wittmann and Wittmann-Liebold, 1974).

Inhibitors of ribosomal function will be divided in this review in two major classes: 30S and 50S inhibitors of bacterial ribosomal functions. We shall discuss almost exclusively antibiotics whose mode of action could be correlated to individual ribosomal components, predominantly to proteins. Thus, mutational alterations in ribosomal proteins, conferring drug-sensitivity or dependence, are discussed. The mode of action of streptomycin is particularly emphasized. Reconstitution of antibiotic binding sites or of active centers of particular ribosomal functions, as well as affinity labeling techniques, were useful to elucidate the identity of a ribosomal protein (see Pongs *et al*. and Nierhaus, this volume).

The localization of these proteins on the surface of ribosomal subunits was determined by immune electron microscopy. An attempt was made to establish the three-dimensional arrangement of the proteins involved in hypothetical antibiotic binding sites.

A complete survey of the literature could not be given due to limited space; instead, a number of very recent reviews are cited to provide sources for original research contributions.

RIBOSOME STRUCTURE AND FUNCTION

In order to correlate ribosomal structure and function it is essential to first have information on the properties of the individual components. This problem has received the attention of several laboratories. There is now general agreement that the 30S subunit of *E.coli* contains 21 proteins and one 16S rRNA molecule. The larger 50S subunit contains two rRNA species (5S and 23S rRNA) and 34 proteins. The ribosomal proteins have been purified and characterized with respect to their chemical, physical and immunological properties. More recently, the complete amino acid sequences of a few, and partial sequences of a number of ribosomal proteins were determined. Moreover, the amino acid alterations leading to some altered responses towards antibiotics have been elucitated. In addition, work on the primary structure of 5S rRNA is completed, the sequence of 16S rRNA is almost completely known and sequence studies of the 23S rRNA are progressing rapidly (for refs. see: Fellner, 1974; Wittmann, 1974; Wittmann and Wittmann-Liebold, 1974).

IDENTIFICATION OF RIBOSOMAL COMPONENTS INVOLVED IN DRUG BINDING SITES.

Various methods have been used to characterize the binding of antibiotics which inhibit protein synthesis at the ribosomal level. (1) Radioactive antibiotics have been and still are of great value to localize the site of action of a given antibiotic (Vazquez, 1974; see also Nierhaus, this volume). (2) Affinity labeling uses chemically modified antibiotics that are capable of covalent linkage to ribosomal components to identify individual ribosomal proteins involved in antibiotic binding sites. This method has recently been very useful (for refs. see Pongs *et al*., this volume). (3) Production of specific antibodies to each of the 55 ribosomal proteins of *E.coli* provided another means to investigate which proteins are involved in the binding of drugs. The rationale of this method is to test whether a prebound specific antibody (IgG or Fab) blocks drug binding (Lelong *et al*., 1974; Stöffler, 1974). (4) The examination of molecular alterations of ribosomal components from cells with an altered response towards an antibiotic has led to exciting progress during the last years (Wittmann and Wittmann-Liebold, 1974).

30S INHIBITORS

The identification of protein S12 as the *strA* gene product.
The development of research which finally led to the molecular localization of streptomycin resistance is an interesting story. Streptomycin was found very early to be an inhibitor of protein synthesis
(Fitzgerald *et al.*, 1948; Hahn and Ciak, 1959). The development of
cell-free protein synthesizing systems allowed the conclusion that
streptomycin inhibits protein synthesis *in vitro* (Erdös and Ullmann,
1959). Mutants of *E. coli* were isolated which were resistant to
streptomycin both *in vivo* and *in vitro* (Newcombe and Nyholm, 1950;
Hashimoto, 1960; Davies *et al.*, 1964). Poly(U) translation by ribosomes from streptomycin-resistant cells is not inhibited by streptomycin, regardless of whether the supernatant enzyme fraction is derived from extracts of sensitive cells or from extracts of resistant
cells (Flaks *et al.*, 1962; Speyer *et al.*, 1962). Other experiments
with hybrid ribosomes reconstituted from one subunit of the wild type
strain and the complementary subunit of a streptomycin resistant
mutant showed that the mutational alteration conferring streptomycin
resistance is on the 30S subunit (Cox *et al.*, 1964; Davies, 1964).
Partial *in vitro* reconstitution experiments of 30S subunits then
indicated that the critical alteration was localized in proteins and
not in RNA (Staehelin and Meselson, 1966; Traub *et al.*, 1966). By reconstitution studies in which each wild type protein was replaced
with its homologous protein from the streptomycin resistant mutant,
it was finally possible to establish that the alteration is in one
ribosomal protein, namely S12 (Ozaki *et al.*, 1969).

All 55 ribosomal proteins of *E. coli* can be separated by two-dimensional electrophoresis (Kaltschmidt and Wittmann, 1971). This
method has greatly facilitated the search for altered proteins in
various mutant strains (Deusser *et al.*, 1970; Stöffler *et al.*, 1971;
Hasenbank *et al.*, 1973). Comparative CM-cellulose chromatography of
ribosomal proteins from the mutant and from the parental strain proved
equally useful in the detection of mutationally altered proteins
(Otaka *et al.*, 1968). With both methods, however, only alterations
due to a change in the net charge or the size of a protein are detectable. The final proof whether an electrophoretically altered protein
is in fact responsible for the altered response towards the antibiotic is still possible only by reconstitution experiments.

LOCATION OF THE AMINO ACID REPLACEMENTS IN PROTEIN S 12

Streptomycin resistance. Several mutants (Sm[R]) of *Escherichia coli*
resistant to high levels of streptomycin were isolated (Hashimoto,
1960; Gorini and Kataja, 1964). All appear to map within the *strA*
gene but on two different chromosomal sites which are separated by
0.3 map units (Breckenridge and Gorini, 1970). Mutants A1, A2 and
A60 were located together on one of the sites, mutant A40 on the other.
The four mutants differ in their restriction of genotypic and phenotypic suppression.

Protein S12, the product of the *strA* gene, from the wild type
strain and from the four mutants was investigated (Funatsu *et al.*,
1972a; Funatsu and Wittmann, 1972). The polypeptide chain of S12
consists of 120 amino acids. The amino acid replacement in protein
S12 from streptomycin resistant mutants occurs at only two amino
acid positions: a lysine residue at position 42 and another lysine
at position 87 (Fig. 1). The lysine at position 42 is replaced by
asparagine, threonine and arginine in the mutant A1, A2 and A60 re-

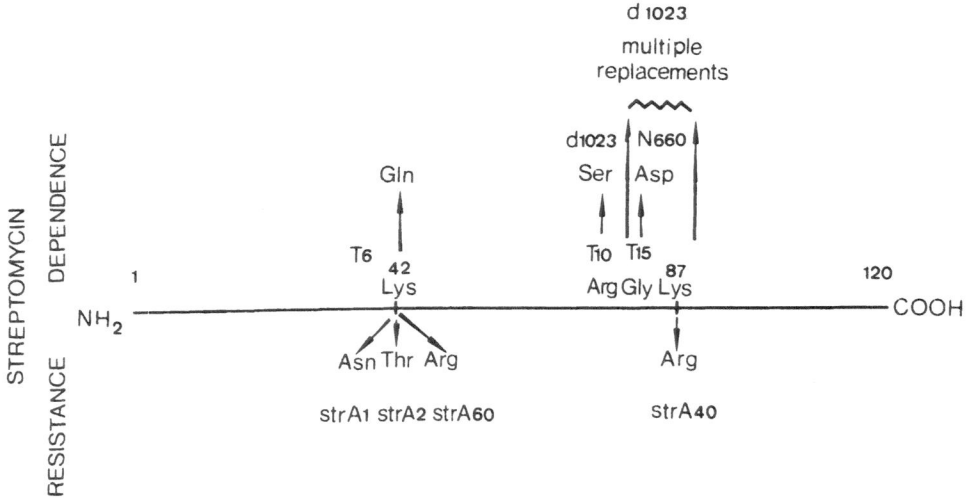

Fig. 1. Mutational alterations in ribosomal protein S12 of *Escherichia coli*, conferring streptomycin resistance or dependence. For references see text.

spectively (Fig. 1). In mutant A40 the lysine residue at position 87 is exchanged for arginine (Funatsu and Wittmann, 1972; Funatsu *et al*., 1972a).

Streptomycin dependence. Many of the mutants surviving streptomycin treatment are not resistant but are dependent on the drug (Hashimoto, 1960). It has been demonstrated by *in vitro* reconstitution that again an alteration in protein S12 is responsible for streptomycin dependence (Birge and Kurland, 1969). Genetic fine structure analysis revealed that streptomycin dependent mutants, most of which are also dependent on other drugs, map at three sites within the S12 gene locus (Momose and Gorini, 1971). Polypeptide analysis has revealed a replacement of the lysine residue at position 42 by glutamine in S12 of one of the mutants (Funatsu and Wittmann, 1972; Fig. 1). Amino acid replacements close to the lysine in position 87 were found in other mutants. It appears, however, that amino acid exchanges are not restricted to the lysine in position 87. Other amino acids in the close neighborhood of this region were found to be substituted; aspartic acid for glycine (in tryptic peptide T15 of mutant N660) as well as serine for arginine in the third position of tryptic peptide T10 from mutant d1023. T10 is an adjacent peptide of T15 (Itoh and Wittmann, 1973). Besides the single amino acid replacement in T10, rather drastic differences in the amino acid compositions between peptides T15 of proteins S12 from wild type (A19) and from the mutant d1023 have been detected (Itoh and Wittmann, 1973). Alterations leading to streptomycin dependence are, therefore, not restricted to only two positions in the polypeptide chain as it was found for resistant mutants (Fig. 1).

Phenotypic reversion from streptomycin dependence to independence. Phenotypic revertants from streptomycin dependence to independence are the results of a second mutation which maps outside the locus for protein S12 (Hashimoto, 1960). This second mutation maps, however, still in the ribosomal cluster and mutants of this type have altered ribosomes. It has been shown that the altered protein is either S5 or S4 (Deusser *et al*., 1970; Birge and Kurland, 1970; Stöffler *et al*.,

1971; Kreider and Brownstein, 1971, 1972; Hasenbank *et al.*, 1973). Among 100 revertants, the two-dimensional polyacrylamide gel electrophoresis of ribosomal proteins from 100 revertants revealed that 16 mutants had an electrophoretically altered S5 protein whereas 24 showed alteration in protein S4 (Hasenbank *et al.*, 1973). Serological investigations, however, yielded a larger number of alterations in S4. The proteins probably had a replacement of neutral amino acids. Alterations in proteins other than S5 and S4 were not found.

The alterations in the S5 proteins are single amino acid replacements, as found by sequence analysis of the proteins from two mutants. The following amino acid replacements were found: Arginine was replaced by leucine in S5 from mutant d1023, and glycine was replaced by arginine in S5 from mutant N660 (Fig. 2). Both alterations were found in one and the same tryptic peptide, namely T2 (Itoh and Wittmann, 1973).

The mutational alterations in protein S4 are, in contrast to those found in S5, rather drastic (Funatsu *et al.*, 1972b; Donner and Kurland, 1972). In several mutants a shortening of the S4 molecule was found; in a few mutants S4 was found to be considerably longer than the wild type protein. These variable sizes of the mutant S4 protein chain reflect drastic changes at the C-terminal region of protein S4 (Funatsu *et al.*, 1972b; Schiltz, unpublished results; Reinbolt and Schiltz, 1973; Wittmann and Wittmann-Liebold, 1974). A combination of a deletion with a frameshift could lead to a new termination codon. Such a mutational event would account for the alterations observed (Schiltz, unpublished results; Wittmann and Wittmann-Liebold, 1974).

The *ram* (ribosomal ambiguity) gene leads to the streptomycin independent phenotype when introduced into streptomycin dependent mu-

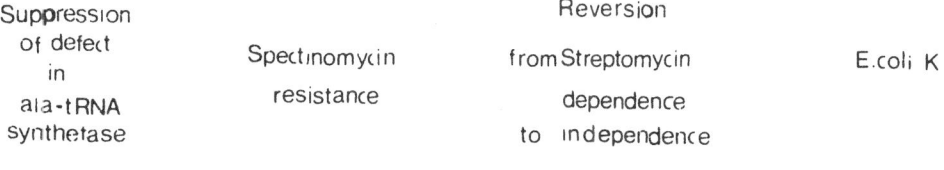

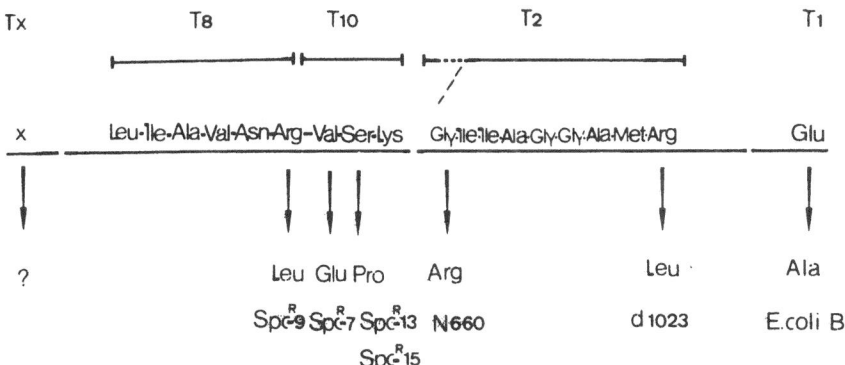

Fig. 2. Summary of the various mutational alterations in ribosomal protein S5 (The order of tryptic peptides in the diagram is arbitrary).

tants (Bjare and Gorini, 1971). *Ram* mutants showed an increased level of ambiguity and misreading (Rosset and Gorini, 1969). It has been demonstrated that protein S4 is the *ram* gene product (Zimmermann *et al.*, 1971; Hasenbank *et al.*, 1973). It is likely, although not yet proved, that the molecular mechanism for the *ram* alteration is similar to the one described for the revertants.

The complexity of the site of action of streptomycin. Spotts and Stanier (1961) postulated that the ribosome is not only the site of action of streptomycin but also is the entity in which sensitivity, resistance or dependence are phenotypically expressed. Ribosomes from streptomycin sensitive bacteria exhibit a high affinity for the drug, whereas ribosomes from resistant bacteria show a lower affinity probably because the alteration modifies the binding site. This hypothesis has been proved with one exception (see above). There is no evidence that streptomycin inhibits the binding of mRNA to the ribosome.

Mutational alterations in three different proteins of the 30S subunit (S12, S4, S5) were clearly shown to exert an influence on streptomycin action and therefore on the fidelity of translation. The amino acid exchanges in protein S12 occur at two unique positions. The kind of amino acid substitution in one and the same position (lysine 42) affects the phenotype of the ribosomes from the mutants differently (Fig. 1). A1, A2 and A60 differ strongly from each other in translational misreading. The conservative amino acid exchange of one or the other lysine in position 42 or 87 of the wild type protein by another basic amino acid (arginine), as was found in mutants A40 and A60, does not lead to such a drastic alteration in translational misreading as does the replacement of the lysine in position 42 by asparagine and threonine (Fig. 1). However, the two mutants A40 and A60 also differ in their ability to restrict phenotypic and genotypic suppression in translation. The four classes of Sm[R] mutations which have been distinguished on the basis of quantitative differences in the restriction they impose on nonsense suppression are, therefore, caused by a specific single amino acid exchange. This is an exciting result and sustains the view of the importance of the many cooperative interactions of the individual components in the ribosome. It is more than astonishing that functionally active hybrid ribosomes can be reconstituted with ribosomal proteins from two unrelated bacteria as *B. stearothermophilus* and *E. coli*, but that a single specific amino acid exchange of one out of a total number of 8.000 amino acids per ribosome exerts such severe functional alterations.

The heterogeneity in the streptomycin dependent class of mutants is even more striking (Momose and Gorini, 1971). Although it is necessary to study the amino acid exchanges in protein S12 of a larger number of mutants, the data so far available support the genetic results (see Fig. 1). The mutational alterations in protein S4 start at different amino acid positions, whereas the alterations in protein S5 seem to be restricted to a small portion of the molecule. The notion that S12 is the specific site of streptomycin action is at least highly unlikely, since all these complex alterations can be hardly reduced to a common denominator.

Several other independent results support this view and provide strong indication for a more complex binding site: (1) Biswas and Gorini (1972) provided evidence that streptomycin interacts with the 16S ribosomal RNA. They confirmed earlier data, indicating that two streptomycin molecules are bound per 30S subunit (Kaji and Tanaka, 1968). In a reinvestigation of the conditions of *in vitro* streptomycin binding, Schreiner and Nierhaus (1973) reported that there is one binding site per 30S subunit, and it is not 16S rRNA. (2) The same authors presented evidence that proteins S3 and S5 but not S12 are required for reconstitution of the binding site from 30S core particles (Schreiner and Nierhaus, 1973). (3) Protein S11 opposes the function of protein S12: Reconstituted 30S particles completely deficient in protein S11 showed an increase in translational error frequency (Nomura *et al.*, 1969). (4) A streptomycin analogue used as an affinity label was attached to protein S4; hence, this protein should be close to the site where the streptose moiety of streptomycin is bound (Pongs and Erdmann, 1973). (5) Specific monovalent antibodies to seven ribosomal proteins of the 30S subunit (anti-S1, -S10, -S11, -S18, -S19, -S20 and -S21) inhibited streptomycin binding (Lelong *et al.*, 1974). Of these, only S11 belongs to the group of proteins that were so far shown to be involved in translational fidelity. However, four of the proteins whose antibodies inhibited streptomycin binding were shown to be close to the binding site of either IF-2 or IF-3 (Bollen et al., personal communication). Since it has been shown that initiation factors also prevent the binding of streptomycin (Lelong *et al.*, 1972) the blocking effect of some antibodies could mimic such an effect. (6) Protein S6 could be also included into the proteins involved in the fidelity group since neomycin and kanamycin also cause misreading (see below).

Although a tremendous amount of information on the mode of action of streptomycin has been accumulated, a molecular localization of the drug binding site is still not possible. Additional information concerning the complexity of the drug receptor, the ribosome, and the numerous interactions among the many components is required before the problem can be solved.

Resistance to kanamycin and neomycin. The aminoglycoside antibiotics kanamycin and neomycin cause misreading in cell-free systems (Davies *et al.*, 1965; Tanaka *et al.*, 1967). A mechanism of action similar to that of streptomycin has been proposed (Masukawa, 1969). Mutants of *E. coli*, resistant to neo- and kanamycin, however, showed an altered S6 protein by two dimensional polyacrylamide gel electrophoresis (Wittmann and Apirion, unpublished results; Wittmann and Wittmann-Liebold, 1974).

Kasugamycin resistance. Kasugamycin, another member of the group of aminoglycoside antibiotics, lacks the streptamine moiety and does not cause misreading. It has been shown that resistance to kasugamycin in *E. coli* is due to two different mechanisms: (1) The lack of methylation of two adjacent adenine residues in the 16S rRNA was found to cause kasugamycin resistance (Helser *et al.*, 1971, 1972). (2) An alteration in protein S4 was also observed (Zimmermann *et al.*, 1973). This mutation was mapped apart from the structural gene for protein S4, outside of the *strA* region. It is, therefore, likely that the alteration in protein S4 is due to a secondary modification of the protein.

Spectinomycin resistance. Spectinomycin is an aminoglycoside which contains the sugar residue actinamine. Although an effective inhibitor of protein synthesis in cells and in cell-free systems, the antibiotic does not induce translational errors. Spectinomycin acts on the 30S subunit, and it appears to affect translocation (Burns and Cundliffe, 1973). Spectinomycin resistant mutants are easily isolated. In fact, rapid development of resistance has been inhibitory to the therapeutic use of this drug. Very recently, spectinomycin gained therapeutic value in the treatment of gonorrhoea. Drug dependence has not been found and phenotypic suppression was thought to be not allowed until recently (P.E. Berg and S.S. Kang, personal communication).

Spectinomycin resistance is conferred by an alteration in protein S5 (Bollen *et al.*, 1969; Dekio and Takata, 1969). Proteins S5 from several spectinomycin resistant mutants were investigated for their amino acid replacements (Funatsu *et al.*, 1971, 1972c; De Wilde and Wittmann-Liebold, 1973). It was shown that amino acid replacements conferring spectinomycin resistance are located within three adjacent amino acids of the S5 polypeptide (tryptic peptide T10). The region is clearly separated from the locus which is altered in revertants from streptomycin dependence (Fig. 2).

Another spectinomycin-resistant mutant (spc-49-1) was found to have also the "sad" phenotype. A mutation in protein S5 of this mutant confers not only spectinomycin resistance but leads also to cold-sensitivity and to the accumulation of 30S and 50S subunits (Guthrie *et al.*, 1969; Nashimoto and Nomura, 1970; Nashimoto *et al.*, 1971). The amino acid exchange in protein S5 of this mutant has not yet been investigated.

It is worth mentioning that altered S5 proteins have also been detected in two other classes of mutants: (a) A mutation in S5 was isolated as a suppressor of a defect in alanyl-tRNA synthetase (Buckel *et al.*, 1972). The alteration in S5 differs from all other alterations so far known in S5 mutant proteins (Fig. 2; Wittmann *et al.*, 1974). (b) An alanine residue in peptide T1 of protein S5 from *E. coli* B is exchanged for glutamic acid at the corresponding position in S5 from *E. coli* strain K12 (Fig. 2; Wittmann-Liebold and Wittmann, 1971).

Specific antibodies to six 30S ribosomal proteins inhibited binding of spectinomycin and streptomycin to ribosomes almost identically (Lelong *et al.*, 1974; Bollen, Maschler and Stöffler, unpublished results; see above). Spectinomycin-binding was not inhibited by an antibody to the "fidelity protein" S11. Anti-S11 interfered, however, with the binding of streptomycin. This result is compatible with the finding that spectinomycin does, in contrast to streptomycin, not cause misreading.

THE THREE-DIMENSIONAL ARRANGEMENT OF EIGHT RIBOSOMAL PROTEINS ON THE SURFACE OF THE 30S SUBUNIT

To localize antibiotic action to a precise physical site on the ribosome and to precise temporal positions during the various steps of protein synthesis, the three-dimensional structure of the ribosome must ultimately be known. However, information on the spatial arrangement of the proteins and the RNA within the ribosome *in situ* has lagged behind progress on chemical and physical characterization. At present there is relatively little information available on the topography and conformations of the ribosomal proteins in intact ribosomes. The necessity for such information is of intrinsic importance for an understanding of ribosome structure and function and the mechanism of protein synthesis. Such knowledge would also provide indispensable information for the physical characterization of a drug binding site.

In the last few years some information on the arrangement of ribosomal components within the ribosome emerged. These results can be briefly summarized as follows: (1) Each of the 55 ribosomal proteins is at least in part on the ribosome surface (Stöffler *et al.*, 1973; for literature see Stöffler, 1974). (2) A group of proteins is located at or near the interface of the two ribosomal subunits. This group comprises the 30S proteins S9, S11, S12 and S20 as well as the 50S proteins L14, L19, L23 and L27 (Morrison *et al.*, 1973; Highland *et al.*, 1974; Stöffler, 1974). (3) Other proteins bind specifically and independently to 16S rRNA, 5S rRNA or 23S rRNA. These sites of protein binding on the RNA have also been identified (for reviews see: Garrett and Wittmann, 1973; Zimmermann and Fellner, 1974). The characterization of ribonucleoprotein particles obtained by mild RNase digestion of ribosomes and ribosomal subunits has proven useful to establish both protein-RNA and protein-protein interactions (Morgan and Brimacombe, 1973; Székely *et al.*, 1973). (4) Cross-linking of protein pairs by bifunctional reagents has provided substantial evidence for protein neighborhoods (Lutter *et al.*, 1972; for refs. see Kurland, 1974 and Traut, 1974). (5) An alternative method for measuring the distance between close and remote pairs of proteins is the fluorescent dye-marker technique (Huang and Cantor, 1972; Cantor, 1974). The interpretation of these results is limited by our lack of knowledge about the shape of the proteins (see above) but even more important, these data do not provide any information on the absolute location of a protein.

Determination of the location of ribosomal proteins on the surface of the 30S ribosomal subunit by immune electron microscopy. The immunological finding that antigenic determinants for each protein are on the surface of the ribosome can be applied to determine the spatial arrangement of the proteins. Bivalent IgGs specific to single ribosomal proteins can be bound to ribosomal subunits. After being incubated with bivalent antibody molecules the subunits were subjected to sucrose density gradient centrifugation and 30S-IgG-30S or 50S-IgG-50S complexes ("dimers") were collected and investigated by the negative staining technique in the electron microscope (Tischendorf *et al.*, 1974a). The antibody that links two subunits can be seen directly and the binding site which is the location of the protein antigen can then be determined and related to structural features on the surface of the subunits. Orientation points found on the surfaces of the ribosomal subunits allow physical localization of the attachment sites of various antibodies. This method has previously been used for the location of several proteins of the 30S and the 50S subunit (Tischendorf *et al.*, 1974a,b; Wabl, 1974). It was employed here to localize ribosomal proteins that are involved in the reaction of an antibiotic with the ribosome.

The structure of the 30S subunit as studied by electron microscopy. The 30S subunits are elongated and asymmetric in shape and consist of two unequal globular parts. Some particles revealed a compact triangular body, others showed a hollow between the two globules. A few negatively stained 30S subunits from controls and typical views of small subunits are shown schematically (Figs.3 and 5). The 30S subunit structure therefore provides sufficient distinct points of orientation to allow localization of the exposed portions of proteins on the ribosomal surface by antibody labeling.

Proteins S13, S14 and S19 occupy a confined area on the surface of the 30S subunit. Proteins S13 and S14 were previously located on the top of the small head of the 30S subunit (Tischendorf *et al.*, 1974a; Fig. 3). The subunits are linked together by the antibody which shows a Y- or T-like structure (Fig. 3). There is no evidence so far that these proteins are involved in the interaction with antibiotics which act on the 30S subunit.

The attachment point of anti-S19 was located in the vicinity of S13 and S14 (Tischendorf, Zeichhardt and Stöffler, unpublished results). It should be noted that S19 and S13 were cross-linked to a ribosome bound initiation factor IF-2 (Bollen, personal communi-

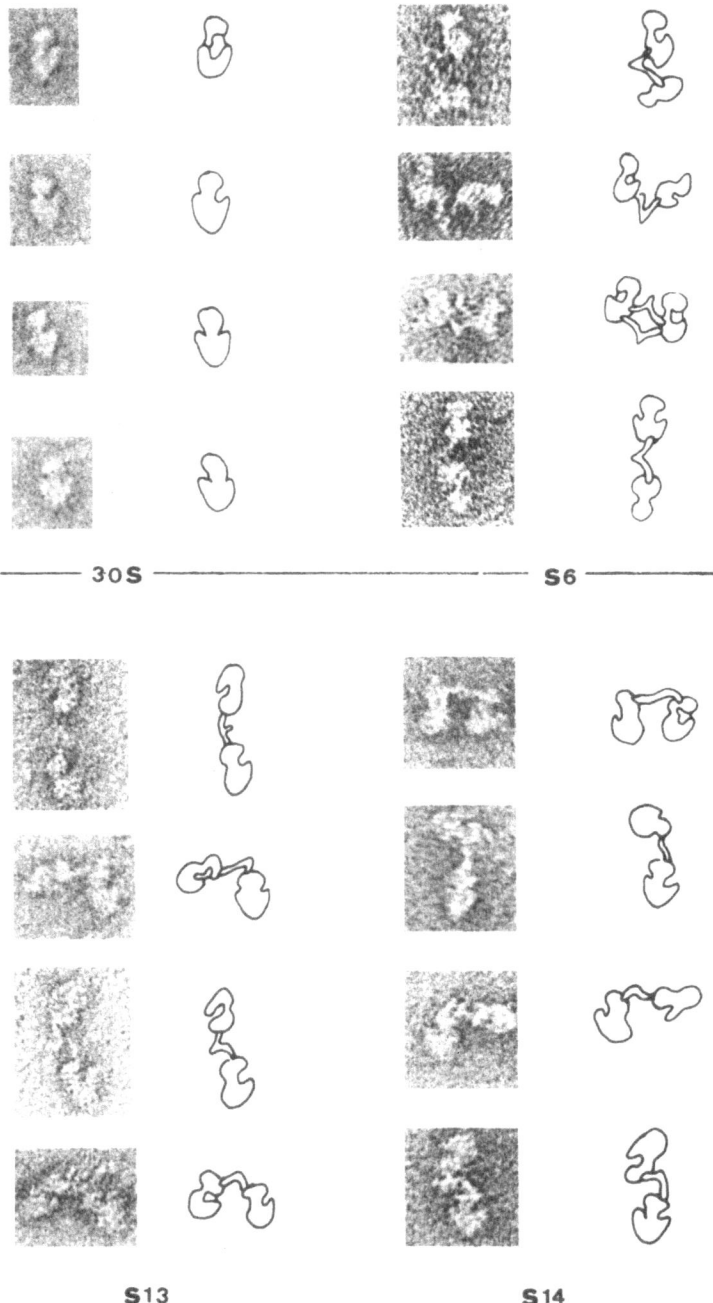

Fig. 3. Selected images and their interpretive drawings of 30S subunits and 30S-IgG-30S complexes obtained with anti-S6, -S13 and -S14.
X 300.000.

cation; Traut, 1974). Anti-S19 also strongly inhibited streptomycin binding to 30S subunits (Lelong et al., 1974 and above). S13, S14 and S19 should be close neighbors in the 30S subunits. S19 has been identified in two cross-linked protein-pairs: S13-S19 and S14-S19 (Lutter et al., 1974; Bode et al., 1974). This result is supported by the finding that S13, S14 and S19 were also found associated with a common region of 16S rRNA (Morgan and Brimacombe, 1973; Székely et al., 1973).

S5 is located at three separate sites in the neck region. We have previously shown that S5 is located at multiple sites in the neck region of the bipartite 30S particle (Tischendorf et al., 1974a; Fig. 4). The three sites of S5 are in close vicinity to each other but they are clearly discernible. The maximum distance between them is about 50 Å. These results indicate that S5 is not a globular protein but has an elongated structure within the 30S subunit.

Mutational alterations in S5 at separate sites within the polypeptide chain leads to spectinomycin resistance or to reversion of streptomycin dependence. Four different mutational events have been shown to occur in separate portions of the gene coding for S5 (see above and Fig. 2). Antigenic determinants of proteins with defined sequences can be associated with certain parts of the protein sequence (Benjamini, 1972). Antisera specific for protein S5 contain a mixture of antibody populations which are specific for six different antigenic determinants randomly distributed on the polypeptide chain (Stöffler and Wittmann, 1971). An antigenic determinant has a minimal size of four amino acids. Some antisera elicited against the polypeptide chain of wild type S5 contain fractions of specific antibodies which no longer react with the mutationally altered S5 proteins isolated from spectinomycin resistant cells (Spc^R-9; see Fig. 2). Similarly, the mutations conferring reversion of streptomycin dependence or suppression of the defect in the alanyl-tRNA synthetase, revealed a quantitatively reduced cross reactivity with antisera raised against the wild type S5-protein. 30S subunits from these mutants are presently being investigated by immune electron microscopy. Possible disappearance of one of the three antibody binding sites would provide a tool to physically localize the various mutated portions of protein S5 on the ribosomal surface (Figs. 2 and 5).

The location of the proteins of the fidelity group. A group of at least five proteins, namely S3, S4, S5, S11 and S12 were shown to be somehow involved in translational fidelity (see above). Parts of these proteins were located on the surface of the 30S ribosome.

Protein S4 has an extended conformation. Anti-S4 IgG was found to bind to three separate regions on the ribosomal surface (Fig. 5). Our interpretation of these data is that each of the sites is an antigenic determinant of S4, indicating that this protein has an elongated conformation in situ. The polypeptide chain seems to go from the small head through the neck region to the lower and larger globular section and seems to continue to one of the edges which is elongated and protruded like an earlobe. The sites are separated by approximately 120 Å with a maximal distance of 150 Å. Protein S4 contains 203 amino acids (Reinbolt and Schiltz, 1973). Assuming the entire polypeptide to be an alpha-helix, it would be sufficiently large to extend to almost 300 Å. The expected diameter for an assumed spherical conformation would not exceed 35 to 40 Å. Work is in progress to correlate the three binding sites to specific parts of the polypeptide sequence. This is facilitated by the availability of mutationally altered S4 proteins with drastic changes at their C-terminal ends.

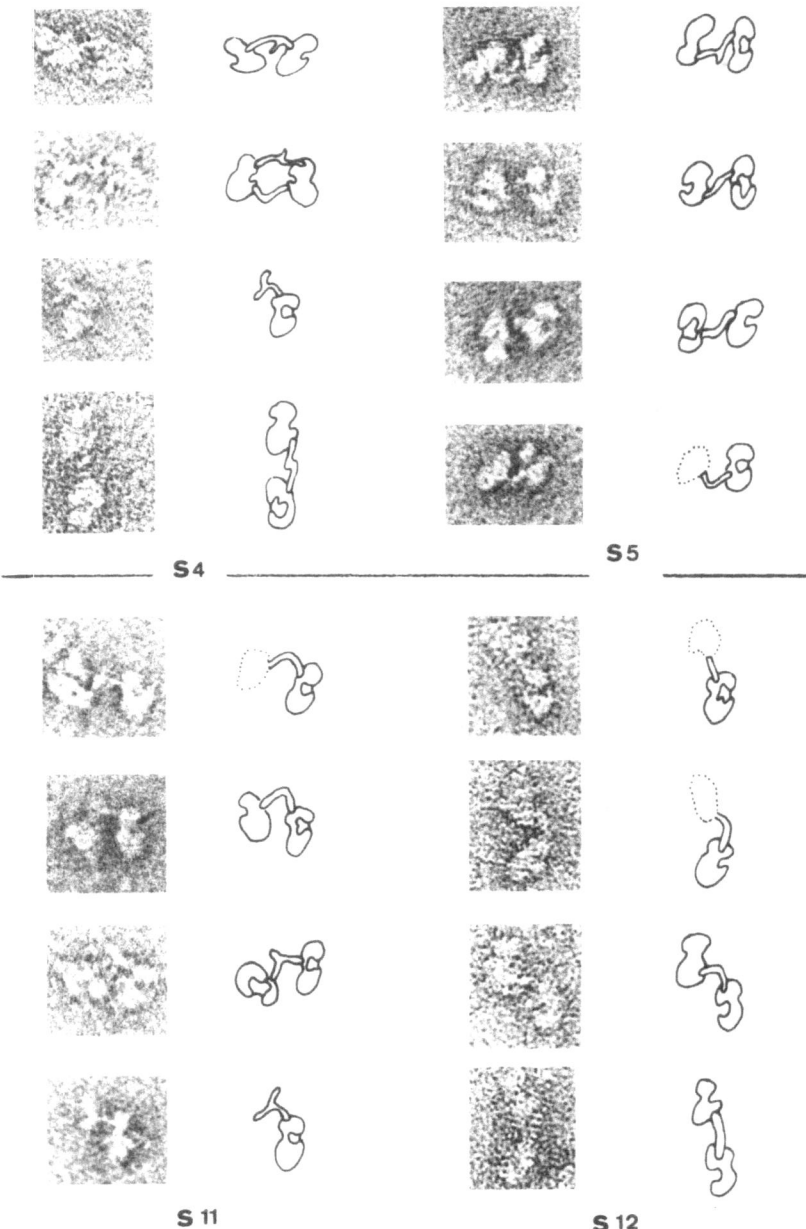

Fig. 4. Selected images and their interpretive drawings of 30S-IgG-30S complexes obtained with anti-S4, -S5, -S11 and -S12. X 300.000.

129

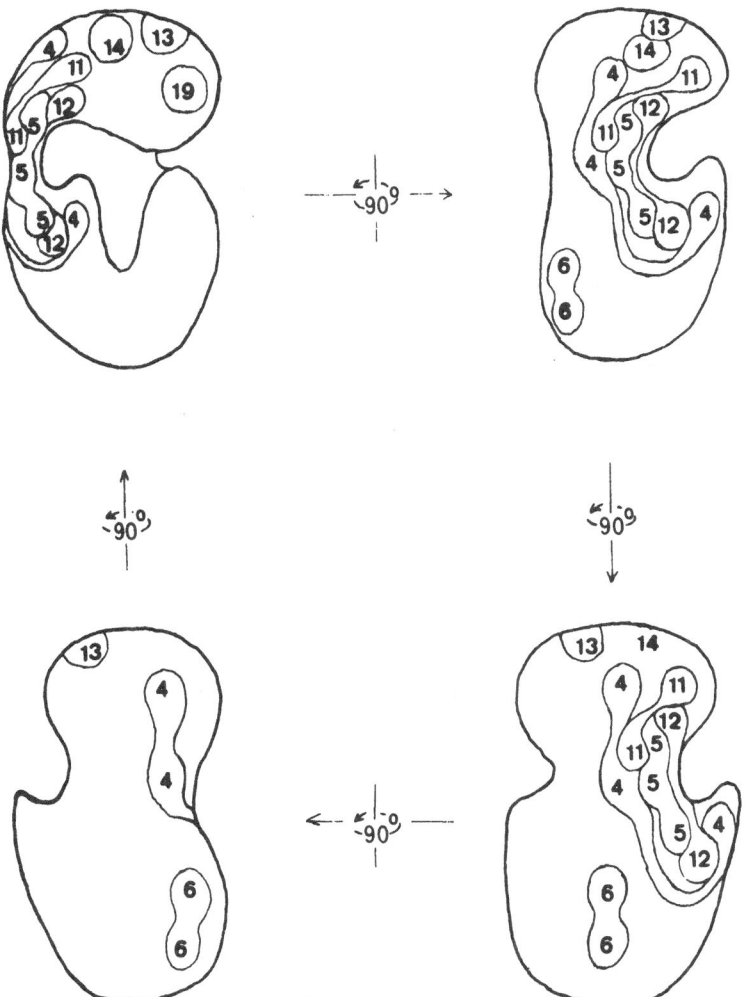

Fig. 5. Three-dimensional model of the 3OS ribosomal subunit with the
locations of eight proteins in four views. The arabic numbers correspond to the actual binding site of the respective antibody. Encircled
numbers refer to proteins located at a single site; numbers not in
rings refer to proteins located at the rear side of the particular
view. Multiple antibody binding sites found for one protein are connected into a hypothetical protein shape. Data from Tischendorf *et al.*,
1974a and Tischendorf, Zeichhardt and Stöffler, unpublished data.

These mutant S4 proteins gave a reduced cross-reaction with an anti-serum against wild type S4 (Hasenbank *et al.*, 1973). Antibodies to cyanogen bromide fragments of S4 have been prepared to localize the various antigenically different regions of S4 on the ribosomal surface.

Protein S5 is like S4, also altered in revertants from strepto-mycin dependence to independence. It is required for the binding of streptomycin to the 30S subunit and is located near S4 in the neck region (see above).

Protein S12 was found to be at two separate sites on the surface of the 30S subunit (Fig. 4). It seems to confine the left edge of the hollow between the two heads (Figs. 4 and 5).

Protein S11 is also located at multiple sites and extends from the small head to the neck region (Fig. 4). A third site for S11 has been seen in a few electron micrographs (Tischendorf, Zeichhardt and Stöffler, unpublished observations).

Protein S3 which is required for the binding of streptomycin to 30S ribosomal subparticles seems to be exposed in the vicinity of one of the sites of protein S4 (Tischendorf, Zeichhardt and Stöffler, unpublished results; see Fig. 5).

Protein S6 occupies two adjacent sites on the larger globular section of the 30S subunit (Figs. 3 and 5). The two antibody binding sites are best discernible when two 30S subunits are linked by two IgG molecules (Fig. 3).

Protein S6 is altered in mutants resistant to the aminoglycosides kanamycin and neomycin; both antibiotics induce miscoding. It was hence anticipated that S6 would be near to the proteins of the fidelity group; this notion was not proven by the results. However, the data do not disprove this assumption. S6 could still continue into the neck region either unexposed or exposed with a region that has no antigenic determinant. So far at least five proteins of the 30S subunit have been found to have extended conformations (Fig. 5). This leads to new considerations for the interpretation of results on the structure and function of the ribosome. For example: A strepto-mycin analogue was bound to protein S4 by affinity labeling (Pongs and Erdmann, 1973). Assuming the protein to be globular the drug binding site should be in a confined area of 30 Å. The finding that S4 is elongated and extends over 150 Å, however, limits the use of affinity labels as topographical probes. The occurrence of elongated proteins in the ribosome also limits the interpretation of protein neighborhoods as obtained by cross-linking or by the use of fluores-cent markers.

The finding that the five proteins of the fidelity group are lo-cated in close vicinity to each other in the neck region of the 30S ribosomal subunit provide at least an explanation for the complexity of proteins which contribute to translational fidelity. So far there is only limited information on the physical localization of the streptomycin binding site. All data on streptomycin binding taken together make it likely that streptomycin binds close to the transi-tion of the upper and smaller section to the neck region. This possi-bility could be tested by cross-linking streptomycin (or any other drug) to the ribosome and then localizing it with antibodies to streptomycin by immune electron microscopy.

50S INHIBITORS

Few mutants resistant to antibiotics which exhibit their action on the 50S subunit are available for study.

Resistance to macrolide antibiotics. Erythromycin resistant mutants have an altered 50S ribosomal protein, namely 50-8 (Tanaka *et al.*, 1971) which is identical with protein L4 (Wittmann et al., 1973). Tryptic peptide analysis revealed that single amino acids are replaced in each mutant; the replacements are located within the same peptide (Otaka *et al.*, 1971). Ribosomes isolated from these mutants do not bind erythromycin *in vitro*; their ability to form N-acetyl-phenylalanyl-puromycin is also strongly impaired (Wittmann *et al.*, 1973). Protein L4 was shown to be altered in mutants resistant to leucomycin, spiramycin and tylosin. These mutants were, however, relatively sensitive to the action of erythromycin (Tanaka *et al.*, 1971). It remains open whether the amino acid substitutions in L4 are different in these cases. Another group of mutants was isolated which were resistant to erythromycin *in vivo* but not *in vitro*. Protein L22 was altered in these strains (Wittmann *et al.*, 1973).

Antibiotic resistant mutants of B. subtilis. Mutants resistant to antibiotics such as erythromycin, chloramphenicol, fusidic acid, thiostrepton and micrococcin, having an altered 50S ribosomal protein, were isolated from *B. subtilis* (Dubnau *et al.*, 1967; Smith *et al.*, 1969; Goldthwaite and Smith, 1972; Osawa *et al.*, 1973; Tanaka *et al.*, 1973; S. Pestka, personal communication). Neither chemical analysis of the altered proteins nor correlation to the corresponding *E. coli* proteins has so far been performed.

THE THREE-DIMENSIONAL ARRANGEMENT OF TWELVE RIBOSOMAL PROTEINS ON THE SURFACE OF THE 50S SUBUNIT

The structure of the 50S subunit as studied by electron microscopy. Electron microscopy of the 50S subunit revealed an armchair-like structure; this was observed in two main forms which reflect different projections of one and the same structure (Tischendorf *et al.*, 1974b; Fig. 6). "Crown-forms" were seen from the front and the rear. The larger protuberance in the middle is envisaged as the seatback which confines together with the lateral crests (the "arms" of the chair) the region of a vaulted seat (Fig. 6). "Crown-forms" revealed a bilateral symmetry: if we consider the long axis of the 50S subunits, the particle is divided into two mirror image parts. "Kidney-forms" are crescent shaped asymmetric particles with a notch. The notch is on the concave side of the particle and is located at the more condensed pole (Fig. 6). "Kidney-forms" were also seen in two projections as judged from the orientation of the notch. The condensed pole of "kidney-forms" corresponds to the central protuberance of "kidney-forms". The different forms are interconvertible by rotation through an angle of 90°. The projectional forms of the 50S subunit provide sufficient distinctive features of orientation to localize IgG-antibodies bound to their specific proteins (Figs. 6 and 8).

The location of proteins L4 and L22 and the Ery[R] site. The two proteins L4 and L22 occur with unique sites on the surface of the 50S subunit (Tischendorf *et al.*, 1974b and unpublished results). They appear to be in close vicinity to each other on the rear of the "armchair". Anti-L4 attaches near the angle formed by the central and the left peripheral protuberance (Fig. 7). Anti-L22 was bound at the same level as the notch but on the opposite, convex side of

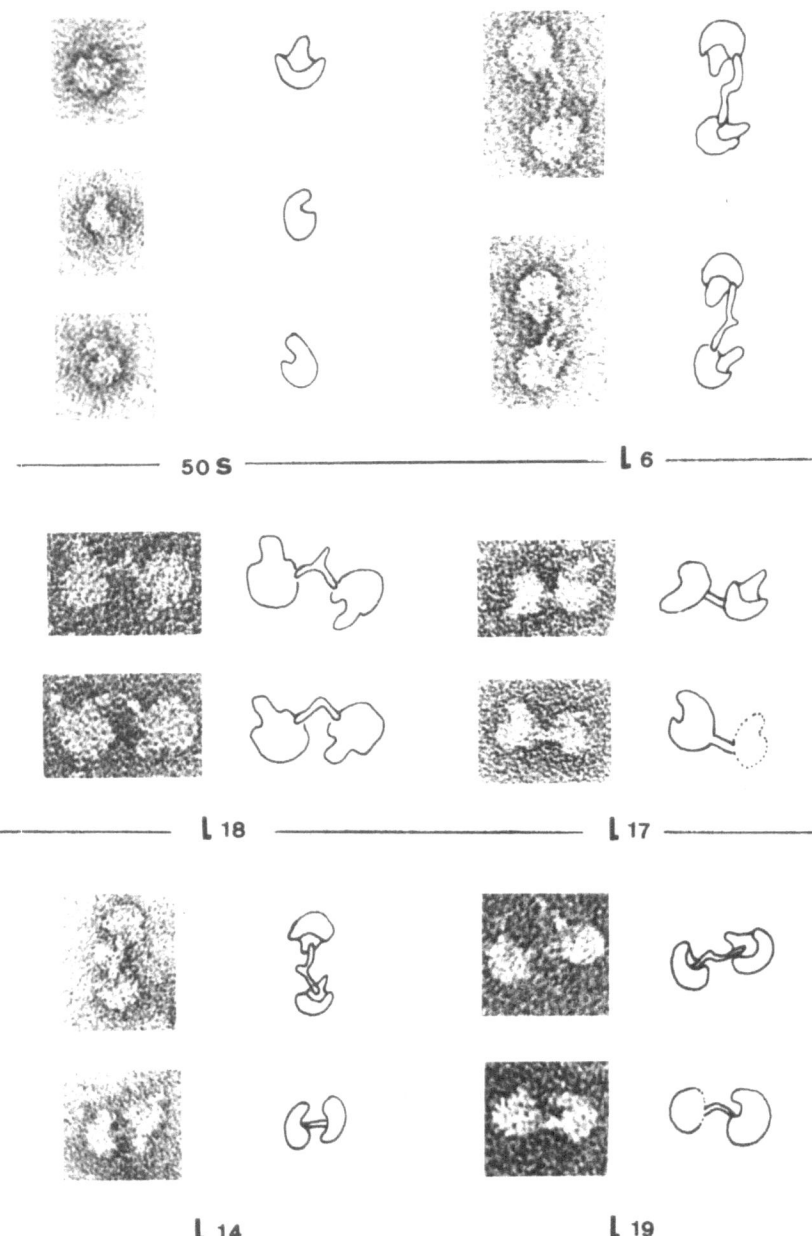

Fig. 6. Selected images and their interpretive drawings of 50S subunits and 50S-IgG-50S complexes obtained with anti-L6, -L18, -L17,
-L14 and -L19. X 260.000 - X 320.000.

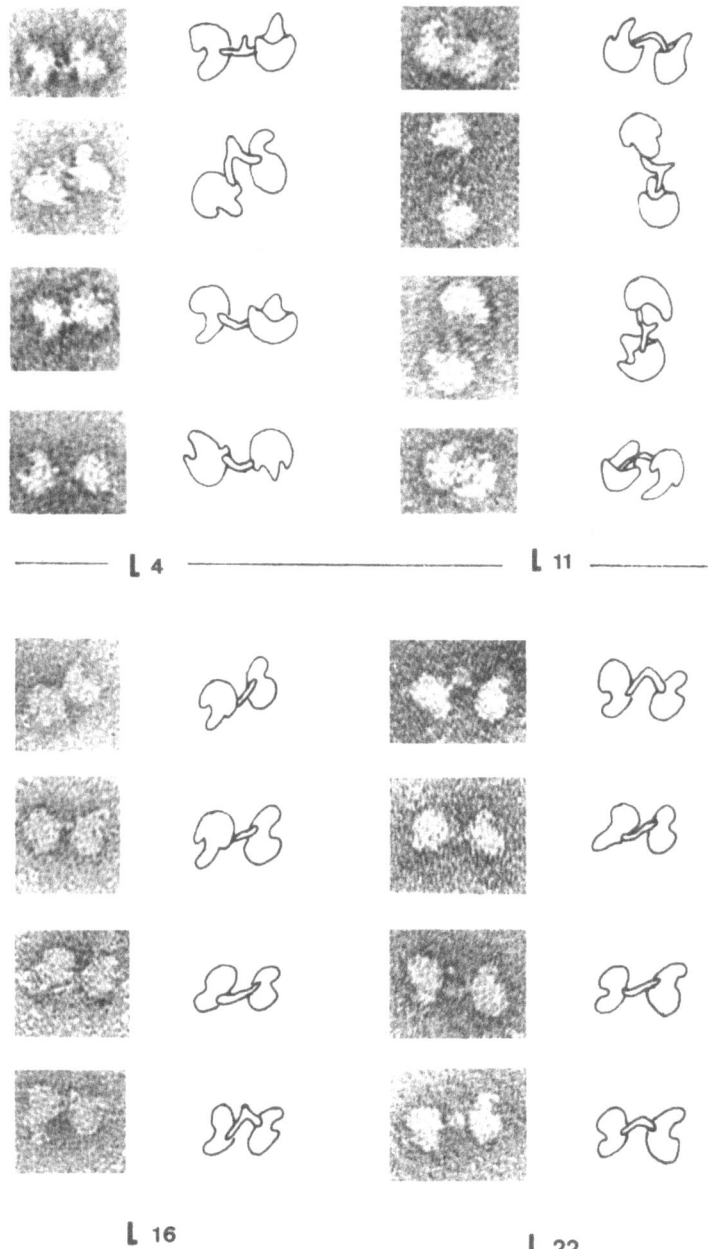

Fig. 7. Selected images and their interpretive drawings for 50S-IgG-50S complexes obtained with anti-L4, -L11, -L16 and -L22. X 280.000 - X 300.000.

the particle (Fig. 7). Like L17, L22 is opposite the side of the 50S subunit which interacts with the 30S subunit to form a 70S ribosome (Figs. 6, 7 and 8; see below). It is possible that the change in protein L22 interferes with the interaction of the 50S ribosome with the cell membrane which then could lead to a reduction of the permeability of erythromycin (Wittmann *et al.*, 1973). It remains to be seen whether this explanation is true. The ribosomal site which is occupied by L22 would allow an interaction with the membrane.

Proteins L14, L19 and L23 are located at the subunit interface. The notation as to which proteins occupy positions at the interface between the two subunits is not only essential for a conception of ribosome structure and function but is also crucial for an understanding of the mode of action of antibiotics. Tetracycline is only one example: although it predominantly affects the 30S subunit, it also influences 50S functions.

Specific antibodies to a number of 50S subunit proteins inhibited the formation of 70S ribosomes, both in structural and functional tests. Among them were proteins L14, L19 and L23 (Morrison *et al.*, 1973; Highland *et al.*, 1974; Stöffler, 1974). These three proteins were found by immune electron microscopy to be located in the vaulted seat region (Tischendorf *et al.*, 1974b; Figs. 6 and 8). Electron micrographs of 70S ribosomes clearly showed that this region corresponds to the interacting surface of the two subunits (unpublished results).

The location of proteins L7/L12. The role of proteins L7 and L12 was investigated during the last several years by two different lines of experiments. Convenient and simple partial reconstitution (Kischa *et al.*, 1971; Hamel *et al.*, 1972) and antibody-blocking tests (Kischa *et al.*, 1971; Highland *et al.*, 1973, 1974) were successfully applied to show that these proteins, which occur in at least three copies per ribosome, are required for the interaction both with elongation factors EF-G and EF-Tu, and with release factors RF-1 and RF-2. They are also required for IF-2 dependent GTP hydrolysis (for literature see reviews: Möller, 1974; Stöffler, 1974).

Proteins L7/L12 which are immunologically not distinguishable are located at several sites on the central protuberance of the 50S subunit (Fig. 8; unpublished results). It is not yet established whether these proteins actually form a garland around the central protuberance or whether the garland is interrupted as indicated in Figure 8.

Location of the "chloramphenicol binding-protein" L16. Protein L16 is located on the base of the central protuberance and is an immediate neighbor of L7/L12 (Figs. 7 and 8). Protein L16 is required for chloramphenicol binding and should, therefore, be a constituent of the ribosomal A-site (Nierhaus and Nierhaus, 1973; Pongs *et al.*, 1973). The same anti-L16 IgG preparation used for these experiments was shown to inhibit the peptidyltransferase step during termination (Tate *et al.*, 1975). Inhibition of chloramphenicol binding with antibodies has not yet been performed.

L11 Peptidyltransferase and "thiostrepton-binding protein". Protein L11 is among the few proteins of the 50S subunit which is exposed at two sites (Fig. 7). One of them is located in the middle of the base of the central protuberance in close proximity to one of the sites for L7/L12. It seems then to continue through the entire seat region and appears at a second site on the anterior surface of the ribosome almost exactly at the edge of the seat. A line connecting the two sides follows almost exactly the longitudinal and symmetry

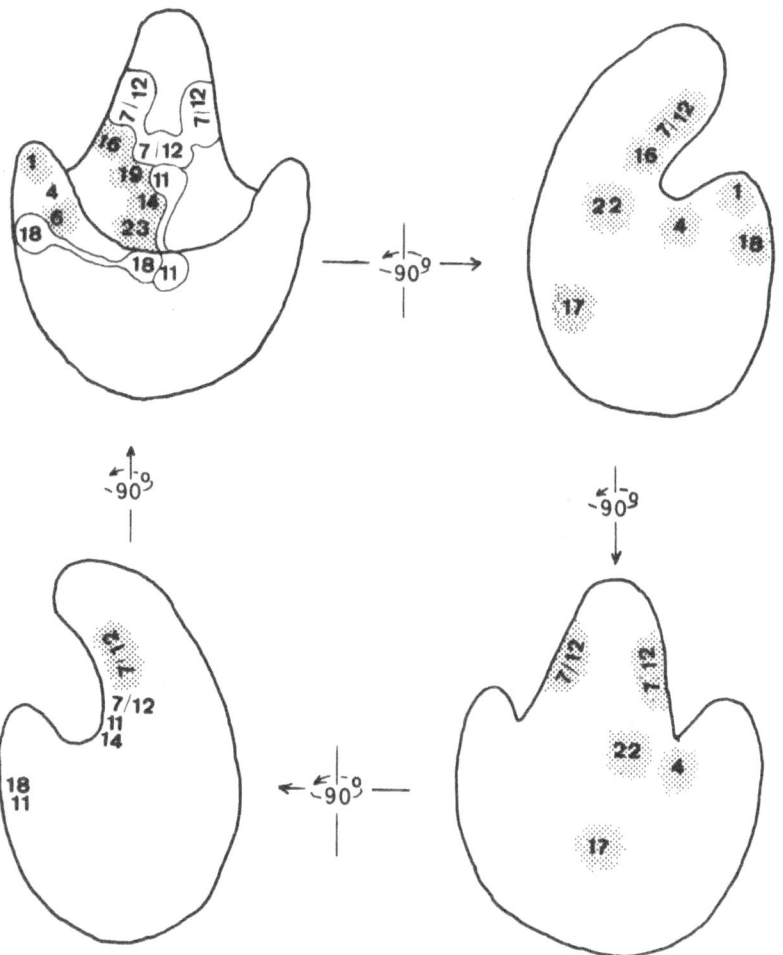

Fig. 8. Three-dimensional model of the 50S ribosomal subunit with the location of twelve proteins in four different views. Dotted areas refer to proteins located at a single site. For further details see legend to Fig. 5. Data from Tischendorf *et al*., 1974b and Tischendorf, Zeichhardt and Stöffler, unpublished data.

axis of the 5OS ribosome (Figs. 7 and 8). Protein L18 is a close neighbor with one of these sites. Experiments with a peptidyl-tRNA photoaffinity analogue strongly indicated that these two proteins are located adjacent to the peptidyltransferase center of the 5OS ribosome (Hsiung *et al.*, 1974). That protein L11 is crucial for the expression of peptidyltransferase activity was shown earlier by partial reconstitution experiments (Montejo and Nierhaus, 1973). Anti-L11 also inhibited peptidyltransferase during termination (Tate *et al.*, 1975). Despite a recent controversy on the role of L11 (Ballesta and Vazquez, 1974; Howard and Gordon, 1974) these results strongly support the idea that L11 is at least part of the peptidyl-transferase center. It was recently shown that the binding of thio-strepton to ribosomes is dependent on the presence of L11 (Highland *et al.*, 1975). It is, however, necessary to remove proteins L7 and L12 from the 5OS ribosome before anti-L11 is inhibitory for thio-strepton binding, whereas peptidyltransferase activity is inhibited in the presence of L7/L12 (Tate *et al.*, 1975). A separation of pepti-dyltransferase activity and antibiotic binding site on protein L11 could be expected since thiostrepton does not inhibit the peptidyl-transferase reaction.

The site of 5S rRNA and the GTPase-center as deduced from the locali-zation of proteins L18 and L6. Three or four proteins of the 5OS sub-unit interact *in vitro* with 5S rRNA: L18, L25, L5 and/or L6 (Gray *et al.*, 1972, 1973; Monier, 1974). In an attempt to identify the nucleotide sequences involved in the interaction between *Escherichia coli* 5S rRNA and the two 5OS subunit proteins L18 and L25, specific fragments of the 5S rRNA molecule were obtained after partial diges-tion of the protein-RNA complex with pancreatic RNase. The sequences of the isolated fragments have been determined. From the results, it can be concluded that sequence 69 to 120 and, possibly the sequence of the stem 1 to 11, are involved in the 5S rRNA-protein interaction (Gray *et al.*, 1973). If we assume that the same proteins which bind to 5S rRNA *in vitro* are also in close contact with each other in the ribosome *in situ*, then the localization of a binding protein should indirectly allow the localization of the 5S rRNA molecule. So far proteins L18 and L6 have been localized on the 5OS ribosomal surface. L18 was located at two sites, separated by approximately 80 Å. Both sites are on the anterior surface of the ribosome (Figs. 6 and 8). An elongated shape of protein L18 cannot be concluded from the occur-rence of two sites, since L18 occurs in two copies per 5OS ribosome (Weber, 1972). The two sites could be, therefore, provided by the two copies of L18. Intraribosomal links of antibodies, characteristic for repeat structures were, however, not observed. Anti-L6 binds at a single site in proximity to L18 on the left peripheral protuberance (Figs. 6 and 8).

A 5S rRNA-protein complex was also isolated from *B. stearothermo-philus* 5OS ribosomes (Horne and Erdmann, 1972). Such 5S rRNA-protein complexes exhibit enzymatic activities and hydrolyze GTP and ATP (Horne and Erdmann, 1973). Fusidic acid and thiostrepton are inhibit-ory to these enzymatic activities (Horne and Erdmann, 1974). These data were interpreted as indicating that the 5S rRNA binding proteins are part of the GTPase center of the ribosome. The proteins in the complex should be located in the vicinity of the A-site of the pepti-dyltransferase center. Proteins L11 and L6 were indeed found in close proximity to L18 and hence 5S rRNA (Fig. 8).

137

CONCLUSION

Several techniques have so far been used for the localization of antibiotic action to a particular site on the ribosome. In some cases the
action of antibiotics could be localized to a specific protein. Until
recently, however, we had little idea as to their exact position in
intact ribosomes. Knowledge of the structure of the ribosome is necessary for elucidation of the molecular mechanism of protein synthesis,
in particular of these structures on the ribosome that contribute to
functionally active sites.

Immune electron microscopy provided a means to vizualize and to
locate proteins within the large macromolecular structure of the
ribosome (Tischendorf *et al.*, 1974a,b; Wabl, 1974). The location of
several ribosomal proteins, previously associated with the action
of various antibiotics, has been recently determined (Tischendorf,
Zeichhardt and Stöffler, unpublished results) and has been described
in this article. The data provide a first conception of the three-
dimensional arrangement of ribosomal proteins on the ribosomal surface and of the physical location of active sites in ribosomes.

Antibodies to several proteins have been shown to bind at more
than one ribosomal site. The distances between these sites strongly
suggest that the respective proteins have extended conformations in
intact ribosomes. This finding is in contrast to the general view
that ribosomal proteins are globular *in situ*. The notion of extended
protein conformations in the ribosome leads to new considerations
for the interpretation of results on the structure and function of
the ribosome. This knowledge also provides essential information for
the construction of ribosomal models.

The availability of specific, non-crossreacting antibodies to each
ribosomal protein, together with the finding that at least one determinant for each protein is at the ribosomal surface assure further
progress of this work (Stöffler and Wittmann, 1971a,b; Stöffler *et
al.*, 1973; Stöffler, 1974).

Our goal is to map the positions of the 55 ribosomal proteins on
the surface of the three-dimensional structure of the ribosome and
to construct a structural model for the ribosome at 30 Å resolution.

Acknowledgment. The authors are pleased to thank Prof. Dr. H.G.
Wittmann for his helpful suggestions and criticism. We thank Drs.
H. Cronenberger and R. Brimacombe for reading the manuscript. The
authors are particularly indebted to Heinz Zeichhardt for his per-
mission to use results of unpublished experiments. This work was
supported in parts by grants of the Deutsche Forschungsgemeinschaft.

REFERENCES

BALLESTA, J.P.G. and D. Vazquez: Activities of ribosomal cores de-
    prived of proteins L7, L10, L11 and L12. FEBS Letters 48, 266
    (1974).
BENJAMINI, E., D. Michaeli and J.D. Young: Antigenic determinants of
    proteins of defined sequences. In Current Topics in Microbiology
    and Immunology 58, 85 (1972).
BIRGE, E.A. and C.G. Kurland: Altered ribosomal protein in strepto-
    mycin-dependent *Escherichia coli*. Science 166, 1282 (1969).
BIRGE, E.A. and C.G. Kurland: Reversion of a streptomycin-dependent
    strain of *Escherichia coli*. Mol. Gen. Genet. 109, 356 (1970).

BISWAS, D.K. and L. Gorini: The attachment site of streptomycin to the 30S ribosomal subunit. Proc. Natl. Acad. Sci. USA 69, 2141 (1972).

BJARE, U. and L. Gorini: Drug dependence reverted by ribosomal ambiguity mutation, *ram*. J. Mol. Biol. 57, 423 (1971).

BODE, U., L.C. Lutter and G. Stöffler: Proteins S14 and S19 are nearneigbors in the *E. coli* ribosome. FEBS Letters 45, 232 (1974).

BOLLEN, A., T. Helser, T. Yamada and J. Davies: Altered ribosomes in antibiotic-resistant mutants of *E. coli*. Cold Spring Harb. Symp. Quant. Biol. 34, 95 (1969).

BRECKENRIDGE, L. and L. Gorini: Genetic analysis of streptomycin resistance in *Escherichia coli*. Genetics 65, 9 (1970).

BUCKEL, P., D. Ruffler, W. Piepersberg and A. Böck: RNA overproducing revertants of an alanyl-tRNA synthetase mutant of *Escherichia coli*. Mol. Gen. Genet. 119, 323 (1972).

BURNS, D.J.W. and E. Cundliffe: Bacterial-protein synthesis. A novel system for studying antibiotic action *in vivo*. Eur. J. Biochem. 37, 570 (1973).

CANTOR, C.R.: Fluorescence spectroscopic approaches to the studies of three-dimensional structure of ribosomes. In Ribosomes, Nomura, Tissières and Lengyel, Edts.; Cold Spring Harbor, New York (1974).

COX, E.C., J.R. White and J.G. Flaks: Streptomycin action and the ribosome. Proc. Natl. Acad. Sci. USA 51, 703 (1964).

DAVIES, J.E.: Studies on the ribosomes of streptomycin-sensitive and resistant strains of *Escherichia coli*. Proc. Natl. Acad. Sci. USA 51, 659 (1964).

DAVIES, J., W. Gilbert and L. Gorini: Streptomycin, suppression, and the code. Proc. Natl. Acad. Sci. USA 51, 883 (1964).

DAVIES, J., L. Gorini and B.D. Davis: Misreading of RNA codewords induced by aminoglycoside antibiotics. Mol. Pharmacol. 1, 93 (1965).

DEKIO, S. and R. Takata: Genetic studies of the ribosomal proteins in *Escherichia coli* II. Altered 30S ribosomal protein component specific to spectinomycin-resistant mutants. Mol. Gen. Genet. 105, 219 (1969).

DEUSSER, E., G. Stöffler, H.G. Wittmann and D. Apirion: Ribosomal Proteins XVI. Altered S4 proteins in *Escherichia coli* revertants from streptomycin dependence to independence. Mol. Gen. Genet. 109, 298 (1970).

DE WILDE, M. and B. Wittmann-Liebold: Localization of the amino acid exchange in protein S5 from *Escherichia coli* mutant resistant to spectinomycin. Mol. Gen. Genet. 127, 273 (1973).

DONNER, D. and C.G. Kurland: Changes in the primary structure of a mutationally altered ribosomal protein. Mol. Gen. Genet. 115, 49 (1972).

DUBNAU, D., C. Goldthwaite, I. Smith and J. Murmur: Genetic mapping in *Bacillus subtilis*. J. Mol. Biol. 27, 163 (1967).

ERDÖS, T. and A. Ullmann: Effect of streptomycin on the incorporation of amino acids labelled with carbon-14 into ribonucleic acid and protein in a cell-free system of a mycobacterium. Nature 183, 618 (1959).

FELLNER, P.: Structure of the 16S and 23S ribosomal RNAs. In Ribosomes, Nomura, Tissières and Lengyel, Edts.; Cold Spring Harbor, New York (1974).

FITZGERALD, R.J., F. Bernheim and D.B. Fitzgerald: The inhibition by streptomycin of adaptive enzyme formation in mycobacteria. J. Biol. Chem. 175, 195 (1948).

FLAKS, J.G., E.C. Cox, M.L. Witting and J.R. White: Polypeptide synthesis with ribosomes from streptomycin-resistant and dependent *E. coli*. Biochem. Biophys. Res. Commun. 7, 390 (1962).

FUNATSU, G., K.H. Nierhaus and H.G. Wittmann: Determination of allele types and amino acid exchange in protein S12 of three streptomycin resistant mutants of *Escherichia coli*. Biochim. Biophys. Acta 287, 282 (1972).

FUNATSU, G., K. Nierhaus and B. Wittmann-Liebold: Ribosomal Proteins XXII. Studies on the altered protein S5 from a spectinomycin-resistant mutant of *Escherichia coli*. J. Mol. Biol. 64, 201 (1972).

FUNATSU, G., W. Puls, E. Schiltz, J. Reinbolt and H.G. Wittmann: Ribosomal Proteins XXXI. Comparative studies on altered proteins S4 of six *Escherichia coli* revertants from streptomycin dependence. Mol. Gen. Genet. 115, 131 (1972).

FUNATSU, G., E. Schiltz and H.G. Wittmann: Ribosomal Proteins XXVII. Localization of the amino acid exchanges in protein S5 from two *E. coli* mutants resistant to spectinomycin. Mol. Gen. Genet. 114, 106 (1971).

FUNATSU, G. and H.G. Wittmann: Ribosomal Proteins XXXIII. Location of amino acid replacements in protein S12 isolated from *Escherichia coli* mutants resistant to streptomycin. J. Mol. Biol. 68, 547 (1972).

GARRETT, R.A. and H.G. Wittmann: Protein-RNA interaction in bacterial ribosomes. In Protein Synthesis in Reproductive Tissue, Diczfalusy, Ed.; Karolinska Symposia on Research Methods in Reproductive Endocrinology, 6th Symp., Stockholm, 1973, P. 75.

GRAY, P.N., G. Bellemare, R. Monier, R.A. Garrett and G. Stöffler: Identification of the nucleotide sequences involved in the interaction between *Escherichia coli* 5S RNA and specific 50S subunit proteins. J. Mol. Biol. 77, 133 (1973).

GRAY, P.N., R.A. Garrett, G. Stöffler and R. Monier: An attempt at the identification of the proteins involved in the incorporation of 5-S RNA during 50-S ribosomal subunit assembly. Eur. J. Biochem. 28, 412 (1972).

GOLDTHWAITE, C. and I. Smith: Genetic mapping of aminoglycoside and fusidic acid resistant mutations in *Bacillus subtilis*. Mol. Gen. Genet. 114,181 (1972).

GORINI, L. and E. Kataja: Phenotypic repair by streptomycin of defective genotypes in *E. coli*. Proc. Natl. Acad. Sci. USA 51, 487 (1964).

GUTHRIE, C., H. Nashimoto and M. Nomura: Studies on the assembly of ribosomes *in vivo*. Cold Spring Harb. Symp. Quant. Biol. 34, 69 (1969).

HAHN, F.E. and J. Ciak: Studies on the mode of action of streptomycin. I. Inhibition of bacterial protein synthesis by streptomycin. Bact. Proc. 131 (1959).

HAHN, F.E. and C.L. Wisseman: Inhibition of adaptive enzyme formation by antimicrobial agents. Proc. Soc. Exptl. Biol. Med. 76, 533 (1951).

HAMEL, E., M. Koka and T. Nakamoto: Requirement of an *E. coli* 50S ribosomal protein component for effective interaction of the ribosome with T and G factors and with guanosine triphosphate. J. Biol. Chem. 247, 805 (1972).

HASELKORN, R. and L.B. Rothman-Denes: Protein Synthesis. Ann. Rev. Biochem. 42, 397 (1973).

HASENBANK, R., C. Guthrie, G. Stöffler, H.G. Wittmann, L. Rosen and D. Apirion: Electrophoretic and immunological studies on ribosomal proteins of 100 *Escherichia coli* revertants from streptomycin dependence. Mol. Gen. Genet. 127, 1 (1973).

HASHIMOTO, K.: Streptomycin resistance in *Escherichia coli* analyzed by transduction. Genetics 45, 49 (1960).

HELSER, T.L., J.E. Davies and J.E. Dahlberg: Change in methylation of 16S ribosomal RNA associated with mutation to kasugamycin resistance in *Escherichia coli*. Nature New Biology 233, 12 (1971).

HELSER, T.L., J.E. Davies and J.E. Dahlberg: Mechanism of kasugamycin resistance in *Escherichia coli*. Nature New Biology 235, 6 (1972).

HIGHLAND, J.H., J.W. Bodley, J. Gordon, R. Hasenbank and G. Stöffler:
    Identity of the ribosomal proteins involved in the interaction with
    elongation factor G. Proc. Natl. Acad. Sci. USA 70, 142 (1973).
HIGHLAND, J.H., G.A. Howard, E. Ochsner, G. Stöffler, R. Hasenbank
    and J. Gordon: Identification of the ribosomal proteins responsible
    for the binding of thiostrepton to *E. coli* ribosomes. J. Biol.
    Chem. (1975) in press.
HIGHLAND, J.H., E. Ochsner, J. Gordon, J.W. Bodley, R. Hasenbank and
    G. Stöffler: Coordinate inhibition of elongation factor G function
    and ribosomal subunit association by antibodies to several ribo-
    somal proteins. Proc. Natl. Acad. Sci. USA 71, 627 (1974).
HORNE, J.R. and V.A. Erdmann: Isolation and characterization of 5S
    RNA-protein complexes from *Bacillus stearothermophilus* and *Escheri-
    chia coli* ribosomes. Mol. Gen. Genet. 119, 337 (1972).
HORNE, J.R. and V.A. Erdmann: ATPase and GTPase activities associated
    with a specific 5S RNA-protein complex. Proc. Natl. Acad. Sci. USA
    70, 2870 (1973).
HORNE, J.R. and V.A. Erdmann: Effects of ethanol, methanol and dif-
    ferent antibiotics on the ATPase and GTPase activities associated
    with *B. stearothermophilus* 5S RNS-protein complex. FEBS Letters
    42, 42 (1974).
HOWARD, G.A. and J. Gordon: Peptidyltransferase activity of ribosomal
    particles lacking protein L11. FEBS Letters 48, 271 (1974).
HSIUNG, N., S.A. Reines and C.R. Cantor: Investigation of the ribo-
    somal peptidyl transferase center using a photoaffinity label.
    J. Mol. Biol. 88, 841 (1974).
HUANG, K.H. and C.R. Cantor: Surface topography of the 30S *Escherichia
    coli* ribosomal subunit: Reactivity towards fluorescein isothio-
    cyanate. J. Mol. Biol. 67, 265 (1972).
ITOH, T. and H.G. Wittmann: Amino acid replacement in protein S5 and
    S12 from streptomycin dependence to independence. Mol. Gen. Genet.
    127, 19 (1973).
KAJI, H. and Y. Tanaka: Binding of dihydrostreptomycin to ribosomal
    subunits. J. Mol. Biol. 32, 221 (1968).
KALTSCHMIDT, E. and H.G. Wittmann: Ribosomal proteins XII. Number of
    proteins in small and large ribosomal subunits of *Escherichia coli*
    as determined by two-dimensional gel electrophoresis. Proc. Natl.
    Acad. Sci. USA 67, 1276 (1970).
KISCHA, K., W. Möller and G. Stöffler: Reconstitution of a GTPase
    activity by a 50S ribosomal protein from *E. coli*. Nature 233,
    62 (1971).
KREIDER, G. and B.L. Brownstein: A mutation suppressing streptomycin
    dependence. II. An altered protein in the 30S ribosomal subunit.
    J. Mol. Biol. 61, 135 (1971).
KREIDER, G. and B.L. Brownstein: Ribosomal proteins involved in the
    suppression of streptomycin dependence in *Escherichia coli*.
    J. Bact. 109, 780 (1972).
KURLAND, C.G.: Functional organization of the 30S ribosomal subunit.
    In Ribosomes, Nomura, Tissières and Lengyel, Edts.; Cold Spring
    Harbor, New York (1974).
LELONG, J.C., H.A. Cousin and F. Gros, R. Miskin, Z. Vogel, Y. Groner
    and M. Revel: Protection of *Escherichia coli* ribosomes against
    streptomycin by purified initiation factors. Eur. J. Biochem. 27,
    174 (1972).
LELONG, J.C., D. Gros, F. Gros, A. Bollen, R. Maschler and G. Stöffler:
    Function of individual 30S subunit proteins of *E. coli*. The effect
    of specific immunoglobulin fragments (Fab) on the activities of
    ribosomal decoding sites. Proc. Natl. Acad. Sci. USA 71, 248 (1974).
LUTTER, L.C., U. Bode, C.G. Kurland and G. Stöffler: Ribosomal protein
    neighborhoods III. Cooperativity of assembly. Mol. Gen. Genet.
    129, 167 (1974).

LUTTER, L.C., H. Zeichhardt, C.G. Kurland and G. Stöffler: Ribosomal
protein neighborhoods I. S18 and S21 as well as S5 and S8 are
neighbors. Mol. Gen. Genet. 119, 357 (1972).
MASUKAWA, H.: Localization of sensitivity to kanamycin and strepto-
mycin in 30S ribosomal proteins of *Escherichia coli*. J. Antibiotics
22, 612 (1969).
MÖLLER, W.: The ribosomal components involved in EF-G-and EF-Tu-
dependent GTP hydrolysis. In Ribosomes, Nomura, Tissières and
Lengyel, Edts., Cold Spring Harbor, New York (1974).
MOMOSE, H. and L. Gorini: Genetic analysis of streptomycin dependence
in *Escherichia coli*. Genetics 67, 19 (1971).
MONIER, R.: 5S RNA. In Ribosomes, Nomura, Tissières and Lengyel, Edts.,
Cold Spring Harbor, New York (1974).
MORGAN, J. and R. Brimacombe: A preliminary three-dimensional arrangement of the proteins in the *Escherichia coli* 30S ribosomal sub-
particle. Eur. J. Biochem. 37, 472 (1973).
MORRISON, C.A., R.A. Garrett, H. Zeichhardt and G. Stöffler: Proteins
occurring at, or near the subunit interface of *E. coli* ribosomes.
Mol. Gen. Genet. 127, 359 (1973).
NASHIMOTO, H., W. Held, E. Kaltschmidt and M. Nomura: Structure and
function of bacterial ribosomes. XII. Accumulation of 21S particles
by some cold-sensitive mutants of *Escherichia coli*. J. Mol. Biol.
62, 121 (1971).
NASHIMOTO, H. and M. Nomura: Structure and function of bacterial ribosomes XI. Dependence of 50S ribosomal assembly on simultaneous
assembly of 30S subunits. Proc. Natl. Acad. Sci. USA 67, 1440
(1970).
NEWCOMBE, H.B. and M.H. Nyholm: The inheritance of streptomycin resistance and dependence in crosses of *Escherichia coli*. Genetics
35, 603 (1950).
NIERHAUS, K.H. and O. Montejo: A protein involved in the peptidyltransferase activity of *Escherichia coli* ribosomes. Proc. Natl.
Acad. Sci. USA 70, 1931 (1973).
NIERHAUS, D. and K.H. Nierhaus: Identification of the chloramphenicol-
binding protein in *Escherichia coli* ribosomes by partial reconsti-
tution. Proc. Natl. Acad. Sci. USA 70, 2224 (1973).
NOMURA, M. and V.A. Erdmann: Reconstitution of 50S ribosomal subunits
from dissociated molecular components. Nature 228, 744 (1970).
NOMURA, M., S. Mizushima, M. Ozaki, P. Traub and C.V. Lowry: Structure
and function of ribosomes and their molecular components. Cold
Spring Harb. Symp. Quant. Biol. 34, 49 (1969).
OSAWA, S., E. Otake, R. Takata, S. Dekio, M. Matsubara, T. Itoh and
A. Muto: Ribosomal protein genes in bacteria. FEBS Symp. 23, 313
(1972).
OSAWA, S., R. Takata, K. Tanaka and M. Tamaki: Chloramphenicol resistant mutants of *Bacillus subtilis*. Mol. Gen. Genet. 127, 163
(1973).
OTAKA, E., T. Itoh and S. Osawa: Ribosomal proteins of bacterial
cells: Strain- and species-specificity. J. Mol. Biol. 33, 93
(1968).
OTAKA, E., T. Itoh, S. Osawa, K. Tanaka and M. Tamaki: Peptide analyses
of a protein component, 50-8, of 50S ribosomal subunits from
erythromycin resistant mutants of *Escherichia coli* and *Escherichia
freundii*. Mol. Gen. Genet. 114, 14 (1971).
OZAKI, M., S. Mizushima and M. Nomura: Identification and functional
characterization of the protein controlled by the streptomycin-
resistant locus in *E. coli*. Nature 222, 333 (1969).
PESTKA, S.: Inhibitors of ribosome functions. Ann. Rev. Microbiol.
25, 487 (1971).
PESTKA, S. and J.W. Bodley: In Antibiotics, Gottlieb and Shaw, Edts.,
Springer, Berlin-Heidelberg-New York (1974).

PONGS, O., R. Bald and V.A. Erdmann: Identification of chloramphenicol-binding protein in *Escherichia coli* ribosomes by affinity labeling. Proc. Natl. Acad. Sci. USA 70, 2229 (1973).

PONGS, O. and V.A. Erdmann: Affinity labeling of *E. coli* ribosomes with a streptomycin-analogue. FEBS Letters 37, 47 (1973).

PONGS, O., K.H. Nierhaus, V.A. Erdmann and H.G. Wittmann: Active sites in *Escherichia coli* ribosomes. FEBS Letters 40, S28 (1974).

REINBOLT, J. and E. Schiltz: The primary structure of ribosomal protein S4 from *Escherichia coli*. FEBS Letters 36, 250 (1973).

ROSSET, R. and L. Gorini: Ribosomal ambiguity mutation. J. Mol. Biol. 39, 95 (1969).

SCHREINER, G. and K.H. Nierhaus: Protein involved in the binding of dihydrostreptomycin to ribosomes of *Escherichia coli*. J. Mol. Biol. 81, 71 (1973).

SMITH, I., C. Goldthwaite and D. Dubnau: The genetic of ribosomes in *Bacillus subtilis*. Cold Spring Harb. Symp. Quant. Biol. 34, 85 (1969).

SPEYER, J.F., P. Lengyel and V. Basilio: Ribosomal localization of streptomycin sensitivity. Proc. Natl. Acad. Sci. USA 48, 684 (1962).

SPOTTS, C.R. and R.Y. Stanier: Mechanism of streptomycin action on bacteria: A unitary hypothesis. Nature 192, 633 (1961).

STAEHELIN, T., D. Maglott and R.E. Monro: On the catalytic center of peptidyl transfer: A part of the 50S ribosome structure. Cold Spring Harb. Symp. Quant. Biol. 34, 39 (1969).

STAEHELIN, T. and M. Meselson: Determination of streptomycin sensitivity by a subunit of the 30S ribosome of *Escherichia coli*. J. Mol. Biol. 19, 207 (1966).

STÖFFLER, G.: Structure and function of the *Escherichia coli* ribosome: Immunological analysis. In Ribosomes, Nomura, Tissières and Lengyel, Edts., Cold Spring Harbor, New York (1974).

STÖFFLER, G., E. Deusser, H.G. Wittmann and D. Apirion: Ribosomal Proteins XIX. Altered S5 ribosomal protein in an *Escherichia coli* revertant from streptomycin dependence to independence. Mol. Gen. Genet. 111, 334 (1971).

STÖFFLER, G., R. Hasenbank, M. Lütgehaus, R. Maschler, C.A. Morrison, H. Zeichhardt and R.A. Garrett: The accessibility of proteins of the *Escherichia coli* ribosomal subunit to antibody binding. Mol. Gen. Genet. 127, 89 (1973).

STÖFFLER, G. and H.G. Wittmann: Sequence differences of *Escherichia coli* 30S ribosomal proteins as determined by immunochemical methods. Proc. Natl. Acad. Sci. USA 68, 2283 (1971a).

STÖFFLER, G. and H.G. Wittmann: Ribosomal Proteins, XXV. Immunological studies on *Escherichia coli* ribosomal proteins. J. Mol. Biol. 62, 407 (1971b).

SZÉKELY, M., R. Brimacombe and J. Morgan: A specific ribonucleoprotein fragment from *Escherichia coli* 30S ribosomes. Location of the RNA component in 16S RNA. Eur. J. Biochem. 35, 574 (1973).

TANAKA, N., H. Masukawa and U. Umezawa: Structural basis of kanamycin for miscoding activity. Biochem. Biophys. Res. 26, 544 (1967).

TANAKA, K., M. Tamaki, A. Kimura, R. Takata and S. Osawa: Erythromycin resistant mutants from *Bacillus subtilis*. Mol. Gen. Genet. 127, 157 (1973).

TANAKA, K., H. Teraoka, M. Tamaki, R. Takata and S. Osawa: Phenotypes represented by a mutational change in a 50S ribosomal protein component, 50-8, in *Escherichia coli*. Mol. Gen. Genet. 114, 9 (1971).

TATE, W.P., C.T. Caskey and G. Stöffler: Inhibition of peptide chain termination by antibodies specific for ribosomal proteins. J. Mol. Biol. (1975) in press.

TISCHENDORF, G.W., H. Zeichhardt and G. Stöffler: Location of proteins S5, S13 and S14 on the surface of the 30S ribosomal subunit from *Escherichia coli* as determined by immune electron microscopy. Mol. Gen. Genet. 134, 209 (1974a).

TISCHENDORF, G.W., H. Zeichhardt and G. Stöffler: Determination of the location of proteins L14, L17, L18, L19, L22 and L23 on the surface of the 50S ribosomal subunit of *Escherichia coli* by immune electron microscopy. Mol. Gen. Genet. 134, 187 (1974).

TRAUB, P., K. Hosokawa and M. Nomura: Streptomycin sensitivity and the structural components of the 30S ribosomes of *Escherichia coli*. J. Mol. Biol. 19, 211 (1966).

TRAUB, P. and Nomura, M.: Structure and function of *E. coli* ribosomes. V. Reconstitution of functionally active 30S ribosomal particles from RNA and protein. Proc. Natl. Acad. Sci. USA 59, 777 (1968).

TRAUT, R.R.: Protein topography by ribosomal subunits from *Escherichia coli*. In Ribosomes, Nomura, Tissières and Lengyel, Edts., Cold Spring Harbor, New York (1974).

VAZQUEZ, D.: Inhibitors of protein synthesis. FEBS Letters 40, S63 (1974).

WABL, M.R.: Electron microscopic localization of two proteins on the surface of the 50S ribosomal subunit of *Escherichia coli* using specific antibody markers. J. Mol. Biol. 84, 241 (1974).

WEBER, H.J.: Stoichiometric measurements of 30S and 50S ribosomal proteins from *Escherichia coli*. Mol. Gen. Genet. 119, 233 (1972).

WEISBLUM, B. and J. Davies: Antibiotic inhibitors of the bacterial ribosome. Bacteriol. Rev. 32, 493 (1968).

WITTMANN, H.G.: Purification and identification of *Escherichia coli* ribosomal proteins. In Ribosomes, Nomura, Tissières and Lengyel, Edts., Cold Spring Harbor, New York (1974).

WITTMANN-LIEBOLD, B. and H.G. Wittmann: Ribosomal Proteins XX. Isolation and analysis of the tryptic peptides of proteins S5 from strain K and B of *Escherichia coli*. Biochim. Biophys. Acta 251, 44 (1971).

WITTMANN, H.G., G. Stöffler, D. Apirion, L. Rosen, K. Tanaka, M. Tamaki, R. Takata, S. Dekio, E. Otake and S. Osawa: Biochemical and genetic studies on two different types of erythromycin resistant mutants of *Escherichia coli* with altered ribosomal proteins. Mol. Gen. Genet. 127, 175 (1973).

WITTMANN, H.G. and B. Wittmann-Liebold: Chemical structure of bacterial ribosomal proteins. In Ribosomes, Nomura, Tissières and Lengyel, Edts., Cold Spring Harbor, New York (1974).

ZIMMERMANN, R.A. and Fellner, P.: RNA-protein interactions in the ribosome. In Ribosomes, Nomura, Tissières and Lengyel, Edts., Cold Spring Harbor, New York (1974).

ZIMMERMANN, R.A., R.T. Garvin and L. Gorini: Alteration of a 30S ribosomal protein accompanying *ram* mutation in *Escherichia coli*. Proc. Natl. Acad. Sci. USA 68, 2263 (1971).

ZIMMERMANN, R.A., Y. Ikeya and P.F. Sparling: Alteration of ribosomal protein S4 by mutation linked to kasugamycin resistance in *Escherichia coli*. Proc. Natl. Acad. Sci. USA 70, 71 (1973).

Altered Methylation of Ribosomal RNA in Erythromycin-Resistant Staphylococcus Aureus

Bernard Weisblum

"This is not an antagonism in the ordinary sense, but a kind of interaction of which, so far as I am aware, no previous example has been
seen."

L.P. Garrod, Brit.Med.J. $\underline{2}$: 57 (1957)

Methylation of 23S ribosomal RNA, a structural component of the
50S ribosome subunit, the receptor for macrolide and lincosamide and
streptogramin-B type ("MLS") antibiotics has been identified as the
chemical change responsible for resistance to these antibiotics in
clinical isolates of *Staphylococcus aureus* and *Streptococcus pyogenes*.
In this work, I would like to review microbiological, biochemical, and
genetic studies of resistance to these antibiotics. This review is
organized under four main headings:

(A) Conclusions regarding rRNA methylation and erythromycin
    resistance.
(B) A summary of works of previous investigators interpreted in
    terms of the methylation reaction.
(C) A summary of work on which the conclusions regarding rRNA
    methylation are based.
(D) Epidemiological and clinical implications of these studies.

A. MY CONCLUSIONS ARE THE FOLLOWING:

(1) Certain strains of *S. aureus* have the capacity to N^6-dimethylate
    specific adenine residue(s) in 23S rRNA.
(2) Ribosomes in which adenine is thus specifically methylated bind
    MLS antibiotics with reduced affinity.
(3) Cells in which the dimethylation reaction occurs are co-resistant
    to all MLS antibiotics.
(4) Methylation can be expressed in an inducible or a generalized con-
    stitutive mode. In either case, induced cells are co-resistant to
    all MLS antibiotics; when erythromycin is removed, adenine methyl-
    ation ceases in inducible cells.
(5) In the natural resistant isolate, eryhtromycin is the most effective
    inducer compared to other commonly available MLS antibiotics.

The features of this model are summarized in the figure below.

Abbreviations used are: MLS, macrolide and lincosamide and streptogramin-B type antibiotics.

MODEL OF ERYTHROMYCIN-INDUCED RESISTANCE IN STAPHYLOCOCCUS AUREUS

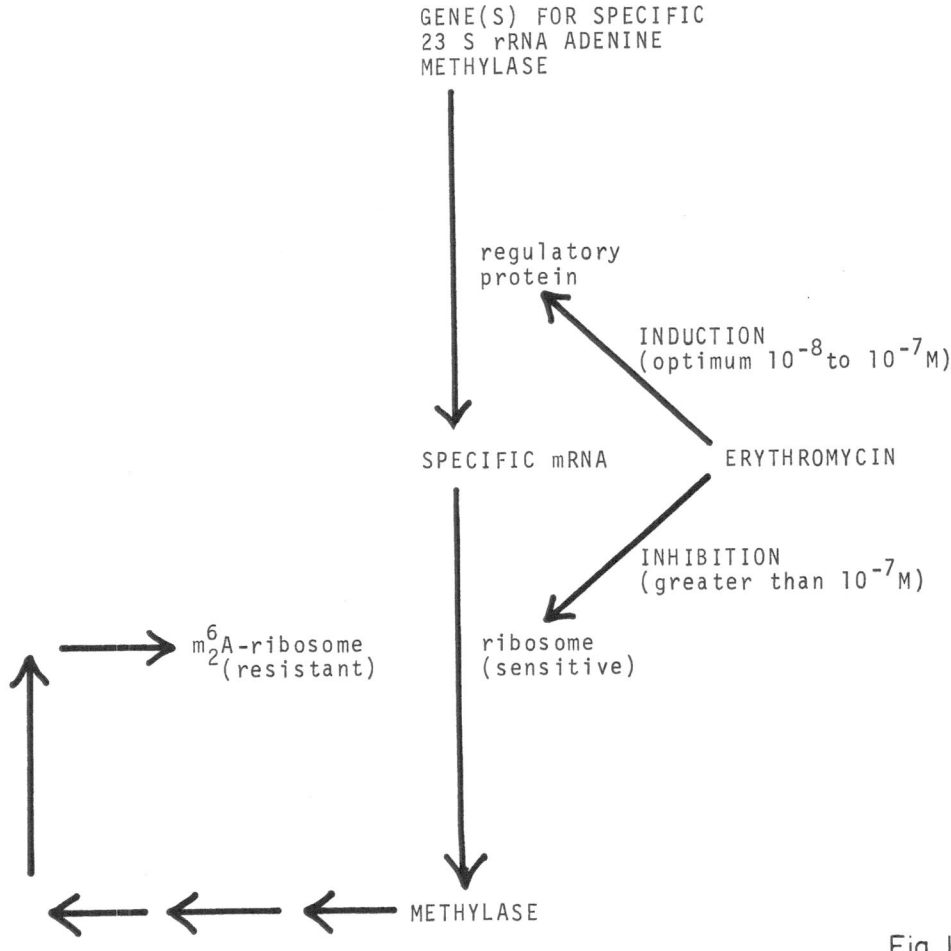

Fig. I.

The following model is proposed in an attempt to describe and explain erythromycin-induced resistance in biochemical terms. It is postulated that erythromycin acts simultaneously at two sites in the cell and elicits two different types of effects. One effect is a specific one which affects the ability of a hypothetical regulatory protein (possibly a repressor or an activator, acting at the transcription level) to control synthesis of mRNA specific for adenine methylation in 23S rRNA, e.g. a specific adenine-N^6-dimethylase; however, synthesis of other proteins associated with methylase function can also be postulated. The receptors for this reaction are saturated at 10^{-8} to 10^{-7} M external concentration; attempts to induce resistance in intact cells by exposure to higher or lower erythromycin concentrations resulted in a smaller fraction of cells induced. Above 10^{-7} M external concentration, erythromycin exerts a second effect, specific with respect to inhibition of ribosome (50S subunit) function but not specific with respect to the type of translation that is affected; under these conditions translation of all mRNAs is inhibited including those associated with erythromycin resistance. Over the range of erythromycin concentrations, 10^{-8} to 10^{-7} M, adenine methylase-specific mRNA synthesis is optimally induced and because this range falls below the minimal inhibitory concentration for erythromycin, the specific mRNA is efficiently translated.

From the studies of Lai (1972), it is likely that a precursor of the 50S subunit (rather than the mature 50S subunit or the 70S ribosome) is the substrate on which the postulated methylase acts. When the fraction of ribosomes containing methylated adenine exceeds a critical level (estimated to be 50 - 75 % because it has been demonstrated experimentally [Weisblum *et al.*, 1971] that growth for 1 - 2 generations under optimal inducing conditions is required for full expression) cells manifest the resistant phenotype. Continued growth under inducing conditions for longer periods eventually results in replacement of all sensitive ribosomes with resistant ones. It is also inferred that induction takes place at high concentrations (greater than 5×10^{-4} M erythromycin) if the culture is first induced with subinhibitory concentrations. This would explain the ability of induced cells to form colonies on solid medium which contains otherwise inhibitory concentrations of erythromycin. In constitutively resistant cells, methylase-specific mRNA is synthesized in the absence of erythromycin, as a consequence of which ribosomes containing m_2^6A in 23S rRNA and therefore resistant to erythromycin are constitutively synthesized.

B. PREVIOUS WORK

In a study of resistance to macrolide antibiotics in *S. aureus*, Chabbert (1956) noted that certain clinical isolates "resistant" to erythromycin were sensitive to spiramycin. He also observed that low concentrations of erythromycin apparently antagonized the action of spiramycin because of the reduced size of the inhibition zone produced by a spiramycin-impregnated filter paper strip in proximity to an erythromycin-impregnated strip on solid medium innoculated with the test organism. Garrod (1957) extended these observations to another macrolide pair, erythromycin-oleandomycin. By means of a slightly different assay, it was shown that erythromycin-resistant staphylococci could grow on oleandomycin-containing solid medium only in a circular zone surrounding the erythromycin disc. Elsewhere on the plate, oleandomycin inhibited growth. The strains resistant to erythromycin but sensitive to either oleandomycin or spiramycin were said by Garrod to have "dissociated" resistance to erythromycin.

Another extension of Chabbert's work was the observation of Weaver and Pattee (1964) that erythromycin induced resistance to _itself_ in "dissociated" strains. They observed that inducible cells grown initially in erythromycin-free medium and then transferred to medium containing 5 x 10⁻⁴ M erythromycin only began to grow (measured turbidimetrically) after a lag of approximately 6 hours, indicating sensitivity to erythromycin. On the other hand, exposure of the innoculum to inducing concentrations of erythromycin reduced the lag in relation to the length of the induction period.

A unified explanation based on the observed behavior of the "dissociated" strains in liquid and solid media can be proposed, as follows: In the "dissociated" strains, erythromycin serves as an inducer _in situ_, i.e. the low levels of erythromycin initially attained as erythromycin diffuses from the test disc into the agar, induce cells such that an otherwise inhibitory concentration (> 1 µg/ml) once attained is no longer effective. Surrounding the erythromycin test disc is a circular zone of cells in which adenine methylation has been induced. These cells, susceptible to erythromycin prior to testing, actually become resistant as a consequence of the testing procedure. Spiramycin is ineffective as an inducer at subinhibitory concentrations so that antibiotic test discs which contain 20 µg produce a zone of inhibition. Genetic information which specifies or regulates the methylation reaction is at least partially encoded by a plasmid in strains such as RN 453 (Rush _et al._, 1969); such information cannot be obtained by the process of random mutation plus selection in the laboratory, but can only be obtained in nature from another bacterium which acts as donor either directly by conjugation or indirectly by transformation or by phage-mediated transduction. The phylogenetic origins of this type of genetic information remain obscure. Erythromycin-resistant mutants of _S. aureus_ can be selected in the laboratory; however, from more definitive studies of _E. coli_ ribosomes (Otaka _et al._, 1970) such mutants are presumed to have altered ribosomal proteins as a consequence of which macrolide antibiotics are bound with reduced affinity. In this way, co-resistance to erythromycin and spiramycin seen in mutant strains can arise by the mutational alteration of a preexisting gene template for a ribosomal protein with a resultant amino acid substitution.

In order to explain the behavior of the inducible strains, it is postulated that a circular zone about 2 cm in diameter surrounding the erythromycin disc consists of cells induced _in situ_ by the erythromycin which diffuses from the sensitivity disc. Erythromycin induction thus provides a protective "umbrella" of methylation. When this zone intersects the zone of potential inhibition by spiramycin, induced cells proximal to the erythromycin disc which are covered by this umbrella grow despite the presence of spiramycin because of a continuous inductive stimulus provided by erythromycin. Other geometric arrangements of testing materials are possible in studies of antibiotic antagonisms. Chabbert (1957), for example, placed two antibiotic impregnated paper strips perpendicular to each other on a lawn of uninduced cells. Discs may be preferable because their use allows simultaneous testing of several different antibiotics per plate.

Barber and Waterworth (1964) further extended the studies of Garrod (1957) to include erythromycin-induced resistance to lincomycin and pristinamycin (presumably "component I"), while Bourse and Monier (1967) reported that _only_ pristinamycin I (the Streptogramin B component) and not pristinamycin II (the Streptogramin A component) was involved. Griffith _et al._ (1965) similarly noted antagonism (i.e., erythromycin-induced resistance) if a lincomycin disc was placed in the proximity of an erythromycin disc.

For antagonism by erythromycin to occur, it is necessary (but not sufficient) that the test antibiotic act on the 50S ribosome subunit. In the works cited above, the involvement of two new classes of 50S subunit inhibitors, distinct from each other as well as from the macrolides, were discovered. The pristinamycins are members of a group of antibiotics known as the streptogramins; a review of the streptogramins has been prepared by Vazquez (1967). The streptogramins have been subdivided into two classes - one class consists of large heterocyclic lactones, while the other class consists of cyclic polypeptides. These have been referred to as the streptogramin A and streptogramin B groups, respectively. Erythromycin antagonizes the action of streptogramin B-group antibiotics but not of streptogramin A-group antibiotics. Both the A- and B-group antibiotics inhibit 50S subunit function. Pristinamycin I belongs to the streptogramin B-group while pristinamycin II belongs to the streptogramin A-group. Another pair of streptogramin antibiotics, the staphylomycins, named M-type and S-type, have been described; they correspond structurally and functionally to the streptogramin A, and B-groups, respectively. A possible source of confusion is the fact that staphylomycin M was so designated because the heterocyclic lactone was found to consist of a ring-structure about 20 atoms in length. Such structures are referred to as "macrolides"; however, in the context of this discussion, it is important to recognize that the staphylomycin M antibiotics are macrolides in name only and that from a functional point of view, it is the staphylomycin S-group along with other streptogramin B-type antibiotics as well as lincosamides and macrolides (*sensu strictu*) to which erythromycin induces resistance. Other streptogramins are designated as A-type or B-type in direct parallel to the name compounds. These include, respectively, mikamycin A and B, PA 114 A and B, osteogrycin A and B, and many more.

The antagonism described by Chabbert (1956) when assayed by the test disc method provides a simple way to determine whether erythromycin induces resistance to a given antibiotic. We first undertook a survey, using the disc method, of many different antibiotics in order to determine the range of antibiotics to which erythromycin induced resistance (Weisblum & Demohn, 1969). The conclusion that emerged from these studies was that erythromycin induced resistance to macrolides, lincosamides, and streptogramin B-type antibiotics but not to streptogramin A-type antibiotics, nor to chloramphenicol, amicetin, or several other classes of 50S subunit inhibitors. These findings pointed to the fact that only antibiotics which act on the 50S subunit were involved and that these belonged to three out of at least eight classes of antibiotics which act on the 50S subunit.

If erythromycin-induced resistance was related to some type of ribosome modification, the modification could involve ribosomal RNA, or ribosomal protein, or both. In preparation for such analytical studies, we undertook to determine the requirements for induction, namely, those optimal conditions of cultivation which one would employ in order to obtain induced cells efficiently (Weisblum *et al.*, 1971). Moreover, it was also important to isolate constitutively resistant mutants from an inducible parent strain. Biochemical studies of such mutants grown in the absence of erythromycin would have to reveal the same chemical modifications as those induced by erythromycin in the inducible parent strain.

From these studies, we concluded that: (a) following growth in the presence of 0.1 μg/ml (10^{-7} M) erythromycin for 1 hour, a culture of *S. aureus* could be induced to the extent that every cell in the population was capable of forming a colony when plated on solid medium containing 50 μg/ml erythromycin; (b) the optimum for induction was in the range 0.01 to 0.1 μg/ml (10^{-8} to 10^{-7} M) erythromycin while higher or lower concentrations of erythromycin used for induction produced a sharp decline in the number of colony forming units on solid medium containing 50 µg/ml erythromycin, without a corresponding effect on cell viability; (c) inhibition of RNA and protein synthesis by the antibiotics streptovaricin and chloramphenicol respectively, inhibited induction (measured by colony-forming ability on 50 µg/ml erythromycin medium) without proportional reduction in cell viability; on the other hand, inhibition of DNA synthesis by novobiocin inhibited induction only insofar as it reduced cell viability. These observations suggested that RNA and protein synthesis but not DNA synthesis were required for induction.

In a search for the biochemical alteration responsible for erythromycin inducible resistance, Mitsuhashi and his coworkers reported that induced and constitutively resistant cells showed a reduced uptake of erythromycin and furthermore, that ribosomes from these strains had reduced affinity for macrolides. Their results have been summarized by Saito *et al.* (1972). Studies of Nakajima *et al.* (1968) were unable to demonstrate erythromycin metabolites if labelled erythromycin was incubated with erythromycin-resistant cells or cell-free extracts derived from them which was consistent with the idea that a structural modification of the ribosome rather than an "erythromycinase" might be responsible for the resistant phenotype. Ribosomal proteins extracted from sensitive and resistant cells failed to show any differences when fractionated on CM cellulose (Saito *et al.*, 1972) or by electrophoresis on acrylamide gels (Lai, 1972). Neither of these techniques completely resolved all the ribosomal proteins (approximately 35), and even if they could, putative mutations involving uncharged amino acids might results in ribosomal protein differences undetectable by electrophoretic methods.

C. STUDIES OF rRNA METHYLATION

In parallel with these studies of ribosomal proteins, we also compared the extent of rRNA methylation, with [*methyl*-^{3}H]methionine as methyl donor, in uninduced inducible, induced inducible, and constitutively resistant cells (Lai & Weisblum, 1971). In preliminary studies, a 10 - 20 % consistently higher degree of aggregate methylation (methyl cpm/OD$_{260}$ unit) of 23S rRNA from induced and constitutively resistant cells (compared to 23S rRNA from uninduced cells) was noted, while 16S rRNA showed only 0 - 5 % increase. Although the observed changes were reproducible, we inferred that a more unequivocal type of change might be seen if methyl-labelled rRNAs were degraded and differences in the extents of methylation of individual bases were compared. For this purpose, a double label experiment was performed in which rRNAs from induced or constitutive cells grown in the presence of [*methyl*-^{3}H]methionine were compared with rRNAs from uninduced cells grown in the presence of [*methyl*-^{14}C]methionine. In these studies, we discovered a dramatic change in the amounts of N^6, N^6-dimethyl adenine (m$_2^6$A) which rose from < 0.1 residue per molecule of 23S RNA to approximately 1-2 residues per molecule of 23S rRNA. No detectable changes in methylation of guanine or of the pyrimidines was seen, nor were any changes detectable in the 16S rRNA, particularly in the levels of m$_2^6$A, which is a "normal" constituent of 16S rRNA in induced, uninduced, and constitutively resistant cells.

In an attempt to identify other possible changes in the pattern of 23S rRNA methylation, [*methyl*-^{14}C]-labelled 23S rRNA from sensitive and resistant cells was prepared and degraded to oligonucleotides with T$_1$ ribonuclease. The digests were fractionated by two-dimensional fingerprinting techniques and methyl-labelled fragments located by autoradiography (Lai *et al.*, 1973a). Seven methyl-labelled fragments were found to be common to rRNA from uninduced, induced, and constitutive cells, while a single additional fragment was found only in the digests from the induced and constitutively resistant cells. Analysis of the 8 fragments revealed that the additional fragment was derived by dimethylation of a single adenine residue in the sequence AAAG, that this fragment was the only one which contained m_2^6A, and that m_2^6A was the only methyl-labelled component present in this fragment. Further structural studies in which the [*methyl*-^{14}C]-labelled RNA was degraded with pancreatic RNAase permitted identification of a heptamer sequence, tentatively identified as GGAAAGC or GAAAGGC, as the site of adenine methylation in 23S rRNA (Tanaka & Weisblum, unpublished data). In order to determine whether altered methylation of adenine was the cause or the result of erythromycin resistance we attempted to reconstitute 50S ribosome subunits using proteins and 5S rRNA from sensitive cells, and 23S rRNA from sensitive or resistant cells. From the work of Nomura and his colleagues, it had recently become technically feasible to reconstitute functionally active 50S subunits from constituent proteins and RNAs in *Bacillus stearothermophilus*. Attempts to reconstitute 50S subunits from *S. aureus* were unsuccessful so that heterologous reconstitution was attempted in which proteins and 5S rRNA were purified from an erythromycin-sensitive strain of *B. stearothermophilus* while 23S rRNA was purified from erythromycin-sensitive or resistant *S. aureus* (Lai *et al.*, 1973b). This type of reconstitution was found to produce a phenotype which corresponded to that of the *S. aureus* preparation from which the 23S rRNA was obtained. These studies pointed to the fact that the 23S rRNA plays an important role in specifying the state of sensitivity or resistance of the ribosome toward erythromycin.

Constitutive methylating strains which also display the MLS-resistant phenotype can be isolated in the laboratory from inducible strains by placing the latter on solid medium containing 10 µg/ml lincomycin, carbomycin, streptogramin B, or any other noninducing MLS antibiotic. Strains isolated in this manner fall into three classes:

(1) Generalized constitutive strains which show co-resistance to all MLS antibiotics tested.

(2) Partial constitutive strains which show co-resistance to several but not all MLS antibiotics tested. In these strains, resistance is inducible by erythromycin to those MLS antibiotics to which the organism remains sensitive.

(3) Mutants with reversed specificity of induction. In one such example, a colony which grew on carbomycin medium (10 µg/ml) was found to be inducible by carbomycin and lincomycin; induction by erythromycin was to a much lesser degree, if at all (Tanaka & Weisblum, 1974). So far, constitutive methylation has only been examined in a strain which showed generalized constitutive resistance. In the strain studied, it was found that m_2^6A as well as the tetranucleotide sequence (A,A, m_2^6A)G were present without a requirement for induction by erythromycin (Lai *et al.*, 1973a). From a biochemical point of view, constitutive mutants are useful because they permit us to study the interaction of erythromycin with a system not previously perturbed by erythromycin.

D. EPIDEMIOLOGICAL AND CLINICAL IMPLICATIONS OF THESE STUDIES

1. *Erythromycin Resistance in Other Bacteria*

The MLS phenotype has been found in *Streptococcus pyogenes* group A (Lai, 1972; Clewell & Franke, 1974) and group D (Courvalin *et al.*, 1972). The studies of Clewell and Franke and of Courvalin *et al.* demonstrated the association of MLS resistance with the presence of a plasmid. Upon elimination of the plasmid, cells displayed MLS sensitivity. In the studies of Lai (1972), m_2^6A was shown to be present in 23S rRNA of an MLS-resistant strain but absent from the 23S rRNA of a (non-isogenic) sensitive strain. By extrapolation from our experience with *S. aureus*, these strains are all presumed to be constitutive methylators. Apparently an erythromycin-inducible strain of *S. pyogenes* group A has been found by Hyder and Streitfeld (1973); unfortunately, they only tested erythromycin and lincomycin but did not test streptogramins.

By means of a simple sensitivity disc assay, a presumptive identification of methylating strains can be made. The ease of identification of this unique property in common organisms pathogenic to man is of obvious epidemiological importance. The exact relationship between the chemical structures of MLS antibiotics and resistance of ribosomes which contain methylated 23S rRNA is not yet clear; however, in view of the ease with which the determination of MLS-resistance can be made, it is unfortunate to note the number of independent reports calling attention to the pattern of co-resistance to erythromycin and lincomycin which omit an additional test of streptogramins.

A study of the organization of genetic elements which specify inducible resistance has not been possible because of: (a) the inherent difficulties involved in genetic studies of *S. aureus* and (b) the failure to isolate an extrachromosomal element involved in this process. The only hard evidence available concerns a form of erythromycin resistance conferred by the plasmid pI 258 in *S. aureus*. The resistance specified by this plasmid appears to be of the constitutive type both with respect to MLS resistance (disc method) and 23S rRNA methylation; by deletion mapping, Novick (1967) has ordered a set of genes which specify resistance to erythromycin, penicillin, and metal ions. This plasmid has a molecular weight of approximately 18×10^6 daltons.

In attempting to ascertain whether erythromycin induces the synthesis of specific messenger RNA, unlabelled RNA from uninduced, induced and constitutively resistant cells has been used in competition hybridization assays involving pI 258 and its ^{3}H-labelled transcript (deHaseth & Weisblum, unpublished data). Preliminary results show RNA from resistant cells to be more effective in the competitive reaction.

2. *Recognition of the MLS Phenotype*

In view of the prevalence of staphylococci, it is of interest to have epidemiological information concerning the type of erythromycin resistance present when resistant organisms are obtained from a patient. Clinical isolates of erythromycin-resistant *S. aureus* appear to fall into at least two classes. These are: (a) inducible methylators, and (b) constitutive methylators. Having defined these phenotypes, it would be of interest to determine whether additional mechanisms of clinical resistance exist. The ease with which disc testing can be done suggests a means by which methylating resistant strains can be identified.

In the early studies of Garrod (1957) and of Barber and Waterworth (1964) on erythromycin resistance in clinical isolates of *S. aureus*, strains were described as having either "dissociated" resistance on the one hand or "double" resistance on the other. The basis for this designation suggested by Garrod (1957) was, respectively, sensitivity or resistance to spiramycin or oleandomycin in addition to erythromycin resistance. Unfortunately the term "double" resistance was applied both to <u>natural</u> isolates co-resistant to both erythromycin and spiramycin as well as to mutant strains selected in the laboratory from initially sensitive (but erythromycin-inducible) parent strains. In view of our present understanding of the role of rRNA methylation, it is likely that the double resistant strains obtained as such from natural isolates were constitutive methylators while the double resistant strains, selected in the laboratory, acquired the resistant phenotype by mutation in a ribosomal protein structural gene with consequent amino acid replacement. In any case, both the dissociated and double resistant natural isolates appear to be methylators, differing only in the regulation of the same biochemical reactions.

Presumptive identification of an inducible methylator can easily be made with sensitivity discs appropriately placed on a test plate, as described above. From making inquiries at a local hospital diagnostic bacteriology laboratory, it was learned that technicians place erythromycin and lincomycin test discs on diametrically opposite sides of a test plate because of distortions occasionally seen in the inhibitory zones which preclude measurement of the inhibitory zone diameter. In point of fact, even the most extreme examples of "antagonism" should not preclude making such a measurement. Much useful epidemiological information pertaining to erythromycin resistance is thus deliberately discarded. The possible clinical significance of knowing whether a particular isolate of *S. aureus* is an inducible methylator will be discussed in the next section.

3. *An Exception to the Kirby-Bauer Method of Antibiotic Sensitivity Determination*

The "Kirby-Bauer method" (Bauer *et al.*, 1966) is a widely used technique for ascertaining clinical sensitivity of a bacterial strain to a particular antibiotic. This technique is based on the assumption that, under defined conditions (medium, inoculum size, disc potency), the diameter of an inhibitory zone produced by a specific antibiotic can be correlated with the minimum inhibitory concentration of that antibiotic determined in liquid culture. It is assumed that this latter figure, considered in the light of attainable serum levels of antibiotic, affords some idea whether a specific organism can be treated with a specific antibiotic. The case of inducible methylators provides an instructive <u>exception</u> to the Kirby-Bauer method.

For most (if not all) inducible methylators, the diameter of the inhibitory zone surrounding a lincomycin disc is large enough for the strain to be reported by the clinical bacteriology laboratory to be lincomycin-sensitive. If a determination of minimum inhibitory concentration in broth is attempted, there is a high probability that a mutant constitutive methylator is present which would then be selected by the presence of lincomycin. Such mutants are capable of growing at lincomycin concentrations of at least 50 ug/ml and overgrow the culture, but if present in the inoculum used for sensitivity disc testing only appear as single colonies arising within the inhibitory zone, and do not interfere with measurement of the inhibitory zone diameter. In the treatment of infections caused by erythromycin-resistant lincomycin-sensitive staphylococci, it would be useful to know whether the causative agent is a methylator and to anticipate the possible replacement of the original population by constitutive methylators if lincomycin is used.

4. *Macrolides in the Environment*

Although not as widely used in agriculture as the tetracyclines, the macrolide antibiotic tylosin has found wide application in the control of mycoplasma infections of livestock. Resistance to macrolides has not yet assumed the proportions of resistance to tetracyclines found in gram-negative fecal flora of livestock, however, the widespread use of this antibiotic would be expected to introduce some selective pressure for the emergence of methylating strains.

CRITIQUE

The role of erythromycin as inducer of rRNA methylation has been conceived in terms of a model similar to the extensively studied system of induced beta galactosidase synthesis. To date, there is no direct evidence for the existence of a putative repressor nor for a methylase. Only preliminary evidence is available for the existence of RNA whose synthesis is induced by erythromycin.

Acknowledgment. This work was supported by a Research Grant from the National Science Foundation (GB-17108) and from funds provided by the Upjohn Co. and from Eli Lilly and Co.

REFERENCES

BARBER, M. and WATERWORTH, P.M.: Antibacterial activity of lincomycin and pristinamycin: A comparison with erythromycin. Brit. Med. J. 2, 603-606 (1964).

BAUER, A.W., KIRBY, W.M.M., SHERRIS, J.C. and TURCK, M.: Antibiotic susceptibility testing by a standardized single disc method. Amer. J. Clin. Pathol. 45, 493-496 (1966).

BOURSE, R. and MONIER, J.: Effect de l'erythromycine sur la croissance de *S. aureus* "resistant dissocié" en bacteriostase par un autre macrolide ou un antibiotique apparanté. Ann. Inst. Pasteur 110, 67-79 (1967).

CHABBERT, Y.: Antagonisme *in vitro* entre l'erythromycine et la spiramycine. Ann. Inst. Pasteur 90, 787-790 (1956).

CLEWELL, D.B. and FRANKE, A.E.: Characterization of a plasmid determining resistance to erythromycin, lincomycin, and vernamycin Bα in a strain of *Streptococcus pyogenes*. Antimicrobial Ag. Chemother. 5, 534-537 (1974).

COURVALIN, P.M., CARLIER, C. and CHABBERT, Y.A.: Plasmid-linked tetracycline and erythromycin resistance in group D *"Streptococcus"*. Ann. Inst. Pasteur 123, 755-759 (1972).

GARROD, L.P.: The erythromycin group of antibiotics. Brit. Med. J. 2, 57-63 (1957).

GRIFFITH, L.J., OSTRANDER, W.E., MULLINS, C.G. and BESWICK, D.E.: Drug antagonism between lincomycin and erythromycin. Science 147, 746-747 (1965).

HYDER, S.L. and STREITFELD, M.M.: Inducible and constitutive resistance to macrolide antibiotics and lincomycin in clinically isolated strains of *Streptococcus pyogenes*. Antimicrobial Ag. Chemother. 4, 327-331 (1973).

LAI, C.J.: Ph.D. Thesis. University of Wisconsin, Madison (1972).

LAI, C.J., DAHLBERG, J. and WEISBLUM, B.: Structure of an inducibly methylatable nucleotide sequence in 23S ribosomal ribonucleic acid from erythromycin-resistant *Staphylococcus aureus*. Biochemistry 12, 457-460 (1973a).

LAI, C.J. and WEISBLUM, B.: Altered methylation of ribosomal RNA in an erythromycin-resistant strain of *Staphylococcus aureus*. Proc. Nat. Acad. Sci. U.S.A. 68, 856-886 (1971).

LAI, C.J., WEISBLUM, B., FAHNESTOCK, S. and NOMURA, M.: Alteration of 23S ribosomal RNA and erythromycin-induced resistance to lincomycin and spiramycin in *Staphylococcus aureus*. J. Mol. Biol. 74, 67-72 (1973b).

NAKAJIMA, Y., INOUE, M., OKA, Y. and YAMGISHI, S.: A mode of resistance to macrolide antibiotics in *Staphylococcus aureus*. Japan J. Microbiol. 12, 248-250 (1968).

NOVICK, R.P.: Penicillinase plasmids of *Staphylococcus aureus*. Fed. Proc. 26, 29-38 (1967).

OTAKA, E., TERAOKA, H., TAMAKI, M., TANAKA, K. and OSAWA, S.: Ribosomes from erythromycin-resistant mutant of *Escherichia coli*. J. Mol. Biol. 48, 499-510 (1970).

RUSH, M.G., GORDON, C.N., NOVICK, R.P. and WARNER, R.C.: Penicillinase plasmid DNA from *Staphylococcus aureus*. Proc. Nat. Acad. Sci. U.S.A. 63, 1304-1310 (1969).

SAITO, T., SHIMIZU, M. and MITSUHASHI, S.: Macrolide resistance in Staphylococci. Ann. N.Y. Acad. Sci. 182, 267-278 (1972).

TANAKA, T. and WEISBLUM, B.: Mutant of *Staphylococcus aureus* with lincomycin- and carbomycin-inducible resistance to erythromycin. Antimicrobial Ag. Chemother. 5, 538-540 (1974).

VAZQUEZ, D.: The Streptogramin family of antibiotics. In: Antibiotics I, Mechanisms of Action (D. Gottlieb and P.D. Shaw, ed.) Springer-Verlag, Berlin-Heidelberg-New York (1967).

WEAVER, J.R. and PATTEE, P.A.: Inducible resistance to erythromycin in *Staphylococcus aureus*. J. Bacteriol. 88, 574-580 (1964).

WEISBLUM, B. and DEMOHN, V.: Erythromycin-inducible resistance in *Staphylococcus aureus*: Survey of antibiotic classes involved. J. Bacteriol. 98, 447-452 (1969).

WEISBLUM, B., SIDDHIKOL, C., LAI, C.J. and DEMOHN, V.: Erythromycin-inducible resistance in *Staphylococcus aureus*: Requirements for induction. J. Bacteriol. 106, 835-847 (1971).

Binding of Tetracyclines and Other Antibiotics to Ribosomes

H. Kersten

I. INTRODUCTION

Tetracyclines inhibit ribosomal functions. From the observed interference of the antibiotics with initiation and elongation steps in
cell-free systems of peptide synthesis, it was concluded that tetracyclines block the A-site of the 30S ribosomal subunit (see Pestka,
1971, for summarizing references).

Another function of the ribosome in which the A-site is involved
is the *rel* gene dependent regulatory control of RNA synthesis in
bacteria (Haseltine & Block, 1973). In *rel*[+] strains on deprival of
an essential amino acid the rate of protein synthesis and concomi-
tantly the rate of transcription of stable RNA decreases, whereas in
rel[−] strains transcription proceeds normally while protein synthesis
is decreased. The *rel* gene product causes the formation of guanosine
tetraphosphate (ppGpp). This unusual nucleotide is formed at the
ribosome from GTP or GDP + ATP. The signal for making this compound
is the presence of an uncharged tRNA in the ribosomal A-site. The
formation of ppGpp in bacteria and in cell-free systems can be inhibited by tetracyclines as well as by other inhibitors of ribosome
A-site function (Lund & Kjeldgaard, 1972).

The inhibitory potency of tetracyclines on ribosomal functions and
the differences in the permeability of microbial and mammalian membranes for this class of inhibitors has made them useful as drugs
against infectious diseases. Unfortunately, however, tetracyclines
belong to the group of antibiotics for which extrachromosomal transferable drug resistance, localized on R-factors has been shown. The
design of chemically modified tetracyclines, which cannot be inacti-
vated by extrachromosomal gene products but which still retain the
ability to inhibit ribosomal functions, might be one of several
approaches to overcome R-factor mediated tetracycline resistance. For
the design of new tetracyclines it is certainly of help to know in
more detail: (a) The particular activities of the drug in biological
systems and the molecular mode of interaction of tetracyclines and
known derivatives with the ribosome. A rapid test should be available
which would allow the study of the interaction of several derivatives
with ribosomes. In this paper we shall discuss:

1. a biological aspect, namely the general effect of several ribosome
   inhibitors on the biosynthesis of RNA,

2. a fluorometric investigation, which permits studies of the interaction of tetracyclines and derivatives with ribosomes to be made.

II. RESULTS AND DISCUSSION

1. *Particular activities of ribosome inhibitors on the biosynthesis of RNA.*

In bacteria and mammalian cells the biosynthesis of ribosomal and transfer RNAs involves several processes, namely transcription, post-transcriptional processing and modification. Among several modifications, the transfer of methyl groups from methionine via S-adenosyl-methionine to tRNA plays an important role. Some modifications occur before, others after processing.

Direct evidence was obtained that antibiotics inhibiting ribosomal functions uncouple the transcription of tRNA genes and subsequent methylation of tRNA. Parallel cultures of *B. subtilis* were incubated with [^{3}H]uridine or [^{3}H]methionine in the presence or absence of an appropriate amount of pactamycin or tetracycline. The specific activities of the different types of RNA were determined and the ratio of methyl-/uridine labelling calculated (Table 1).

Table 1

VARIATION OF METHYL-/URIDINE LABELLING OF TRANSFER RNAS AND RIBOSOMAL RNAS UPON TREATMENT WITH PACTAMYCIN.

	ratio of CH$_3$-/uridine incorporation		
	tRNA	16S	23S RNA
control	1.00	0.33	0.26
pactamycin	0.53	0.13	0.08

Pactamycin treatment: log phase cultures of *B. subtilis* with 0.1 µg/ml pactamycin (PA) 20 min. Concentrations of PA or tetracyclines must be chosen, which stimulate the rate of transcription and lead to an accumulation of tRNA. (Usually between 0.1 - 0.25 µg/ml for PA and 0.1 - 0.4 µg/ml for oxytetracycline). The values are referred to the ratio of CH$_3$-/uridine labelling of tRNA set at 1 (Schmidt, Kersten unpublished).

In the presence of the antibiotics the ratio of methyl-/uridine labelling decreases for tRNA by about 50 %, for 16S rRNA by 60 % and for 23S rNA by 70 %.

As expected, total tRNA populations from pactamycin or tetracycline treated cells can be methylated in an *in vitro* system with S-adenosyl-methionine and homologous tRNA methyltransferases. This *in vitro* methylation occurs at a relatively low, but highly reproducible, frequency.

A rough calculation of the amount of incorporated methyl groups into submethylated tRNA revealed, on average, one methyl group per 15 tRNA molecules. Thus in the population of tRNAs, either one or only very few tRNA species accepted methyl groups, or about 10 % of the total tRNA is submethylated.

To distinguish between these possibilities tRNAs from antibiotic treated cells were methylated *in vitro* on a preparative scale and analyzed by RPC 5 column chromatography (Fig. 1).

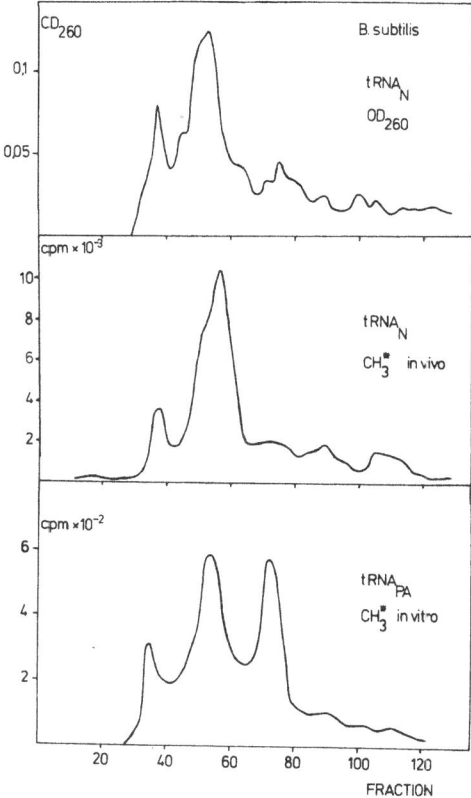

Fig. 1. RPC 5 column chromatography of tRNAs from *B. subtilis*.
(a) Elution profile of mature (normal) tRNA = tRNAs plotted as OD_{260}nm,
(b) plotted as incorporated [$^{14}CH_3$]activity after labelling *in vivo*,
(c) plotted as incorporated [$^{14}CH_3$]activity after *in vitro* methylation
of submethylated tRNAs from pactamycin treated cells (tRNA PA).

The upper curve in Fig. 1 represents the distribution of tRNAs from
untreated controls upon reverse phase column chromatography, as measured by the optical density in each fraction (a). When tRNAs were
labelled in untreated cultures with [$^{14}CH_3$]methionine and the radioactivity measured in each fraction a similar elution profile was obtained (b). However when tRNAs from pactamycin, chloramphenicol or
tetracycline treated cells were methylated *in vitro* the elution profiles always showed an additional peak between fraction 70-80 (c).
tRNAs from these fractions exhibited rather high methyl group accep-
tance properties relative to the other tRNAs. These tRNAs were then
tested for amino acid specificity.

To see what base specific tRNA methylations are disturbed, when
transcription proceeds normally under conditions of reduced translation, the normal base specific methylation pattern of *B. subtilis*
tRNAs was compared with the pattern obtained by *in vitro* methylation
of tRNA from antibiotic treated cells.

On in vitro methylation of submethylated tRNA from pactamycin
treated *B. subtilis*, mainly guanine residues are methylated. Neither
1-methyladenine nor 2-methyladenine which occur in *B. subtilis* tRNAs

with a relatively high frequency were found to be labelled. The methylated adenines were either already present in the tRNAs from treated cells or 1-methyladenine and 2-methyladenine tRNA methyltransferases cannot recognize the partially unmodified substrate.

Table 2

RELATIVE FREQUENCY OF METHYLATED BASES OBTAINED BY *IN VITRO* METHYLATION OF SUBMETHYLATED TRNAS FROM *B. SUBTILIS* WITH *B. SUBTILIS* ENZYMES.

| | percentage of total radioactivity recovered | |
compound	*in vitro*	*in vivo*
7-methylguanine	71.0	43.8
1-methylguanine		
2-methylguanine	3.6	4.9
1-methyladenine	1.0	22.8
P-unidentified	17.5	3.0
X-unidentified	3.4	3.7
2-methyladenine	−	13.0
6-methyladenine	−	3.0
6-dimethyladenine	−	

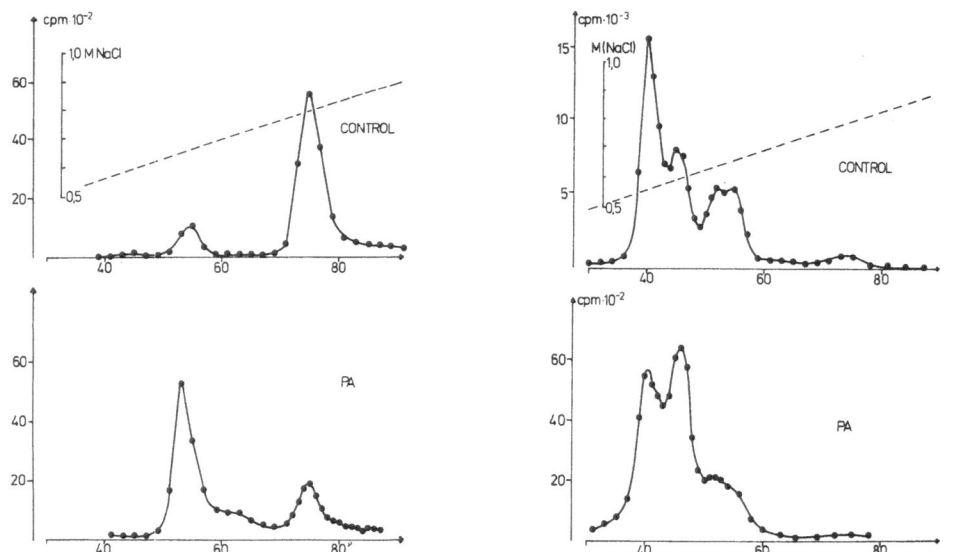

Fig. 2. Patterns of tRNA [Tyr] (a), tRNA[Leu] (b), after RPC 5 column chromatography of tRNA isolated from *B. subtilis* normal (control and pactamycin treated (PA) *B. subtilis* (Raettig & Kersten 1974, unpublished).

Ribosome inhibitors cause the accumulation of submodified tRNAs. Moreover several alterations in the patterns of isoaccepting species of phenylalanine, tyrosine and leucine specific tRNAs occur (Fig. 2). In tRNA populations from pactamycin treated *B. subtilis* the relative distributions of isoacceptors for tRNA^{Phe} (Kersten, 1971), tRNA^{Tyr} and tRNA^{Leu} (Fig. 2) are changed. Isoaccepting tRNA species are either premature (submodified) tRNAs or isoacceptors, coded for by different genes. Mann and Huang (1973) and Waters *et al.* (1973) have found isoacceptors of tRNA^{Phe} in chloramphenicol treated *E. coli*, the isoacceptors are premature tRNAs. Schellberger and Kersten (1974) showed that one isoaccepting tRNA^{Phe} cochromatographs with a tRNA^{Phe} accumulating in *E. coli arg⁻ rel⁺* upon deprival of arginine.

SUMMARY

The particular activity of ribosome-inhibitors on the ribosome dependent regulatory control of RNA synthesis causes significant disturbances in the posttranscriptional maturation process of ribonucleic acids. Low drug concentrations which only cause 10 % inhibition of *in vivo* protein synthesis are adequate to produce this effect. In general, it might be worthwhile in future to draw attention especially to drug action on regulatory mechanisms of cell metabolism.

2. *Fluorometric analysis of tetracycline binding to E. coli ribosomes.*

Earlier binding studies with labelled tetracyclines revealed that the drugs exhibit two types of binding: one type of strong interaction by which about one molecule or less is bound per ribosome and another type of weaker, reversible association by which up to 300 molecules can bind per ribosome. These results were obtained by Maxwell, Connamacher and Mandel and Day. White and Cantor (1971) also performed fluorescence analysis of tetracycline binding to ribosomes and concluded from their studies that the strong binding of tetracyclines to 70 S ribosomes involves chelation to the ribosomal RNA phosphate groups via magnesium ions.

We have studied the interaction of three tetracycline derivatives to ribosomes and ribosomal subunits, using a fluorometric technique. Inhibitor concentrations as low as 10^{-7} M were used with a tetracycline to ribosome ratio of 0.1. The tetracycline derivatives used were oxytetracycline, tetracycline methiodide and tetracycline nitrile (kindly supplied by Dr. Schmidt Thomé and Dr. Summ, Hoechst). The antibiotics exhibit correlated effects on growing bacteria and on an *in vitro* system of phenylalanine incorporation into polyphenylalanine. They differ in their biological effects by two orders of magnitude, as can be seen from their inhibitor constants (Fig. 3).

The three tetracycline derivatives were found to exhibit nearly identical absolute fluorescence emission intensities. Oxytetracycline exhibits an excitation maximum at 375 nm in standard buffer and a fluorescence emission of maximum intensity at 520 nm. Excitation at 366 nm used in these experiments is only slightly less effective. Upon excitation at this wavelength tetracycline methiodide and tetracycline nitrile showed emission maxima at 525 nm.

The tetracyclines are nearly free in solution at 0.1 mM Mg^{2+} and chelated to Mg^{2+} at 10 mM Mg^{2+}. The dependence of the emission intensities on the Mg^{2+} concentration of the three derivatives was studied first, since the interaction with undissociated 70S ribosomes was measured at 10 mM Mg^{2+} and the interaction with the subunits at

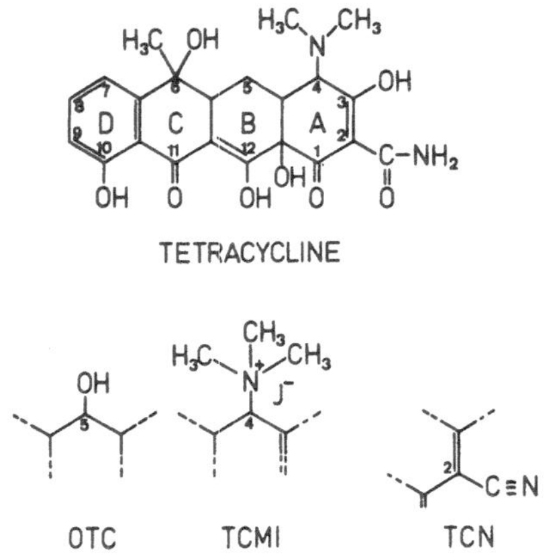

Fig. 3. Chemical formulas of tetracycline, oxytetracycline (OTC), tetracycline methiodide (TCMI), and tetracycline nitrile (TCN).

10 mM Mg^{2+} and at 0.5 mM Mg^{2+}. The relative fluorescence intensity of oxytetracycline was found to be about five times higher at 10 mM than at 0.1 mM Mg^{2+}. Maximum intensity is reached at Mg^{2+} concentrations of 10 mM.

All three compounds were found to exhibit nearly identical absolute emission intensities for a given inhibitor concentration at both high and low Mg^{2+} concentrations. The curves for all compounds have identical slopes. Thus the quantum yields of the three compounds when free or chelated to Mg^{2+} are nearly equal.

Association of ribosomal particles with oxytetracycline at 10 mM Mg^{2+} results in a considerable enhancement of the emission intensity of the drug. If the relative fluorescence enhancement $\Delta I/I_0$, (for definition see legend of Fig. 4), is plotted versus the molar concentration ratio (D/R) of total drug to ribosome characteristic curves are obtained for 70S ribosomes, 50S and 30S subunits. The relative fluorescence enhancements increase continuously with D/R up to 10 for 70S and 30S particles and reach maximum values of 30 % for 70S and 18 % for 30S particles. With the 50S subunit a maximum of the relative enhancement of 30 % is obtained with a D/R value of 1. Thus the maximum relative fluorescence enhancement for the 70S complex is closer to the value of the 50S complex than to the value of 30S complex and is considerably lower than the sum of both. This was reproducible for different ribosome and subunit preparations.

Since we have plotted $\Delta I/I_0$ versus D/R, the plateau does not indicate that oxytetracycline binding to ribosomes has reached saturation, but that on further binding of drug molecules to ribosomes the interaction must occur in the same well-defined binding mode. For 70S ribosomes the slope remains constant for D/R ratios up to 200. When the complexes of oxytetracycline with ribosomes were sedimented for 6 hours through 1.1 M sucrose the fluorescence analysis revealed that after this process only very few molecules remain bound. We therefore take the region of the steep increase in this plot as reflecting the strong irreversible binding type, whereas the plateau region represents the second, weak, reversible, mode of interaction.

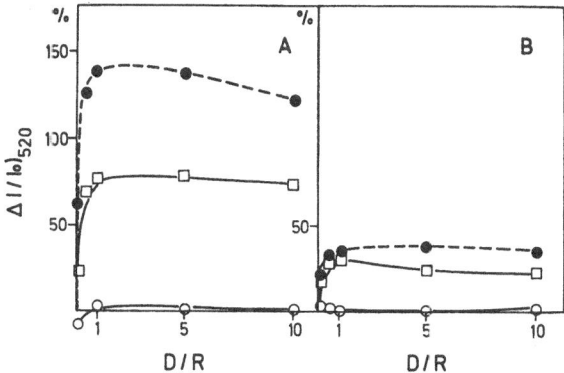

Fig. 4. Fluorescence enhancements of tetracycline derivatives by addition of 50S ribosomal subunits at (A) 5×10^{-4} M Mg^{2+} and (B) 10^{-2} M Mg^{2-}. Standard conditions for fluorescence measurement: constant concentration of ribosomal particles 1×10^{-6} M in 0.01 M Tris·HCl-0.06 M KCl-0.01 M Mg^{2+} (unless otherwise stated), pH 7.2 at 20°C. D/R = molar concentration ratio drug to ribosomes. (A) 70S ribosomes; (B) 50S subunits (O-O) and 30S subunits (O-O). $\Delta I = I_c - I_o$; $I_o = I_d + I_r - I_b$; I_c = fluorescence intensity of the complex as % of the emission intensity of the fluorescein standard set at 100%. I_d = fluorescence intensity of free drug at the given concentration of Mg^{2+}; I_r = fluorescence intensity of free ribosomes; I_b = fluorescence intensity of the solute (buffer). (Fey *et al.*, 1973).

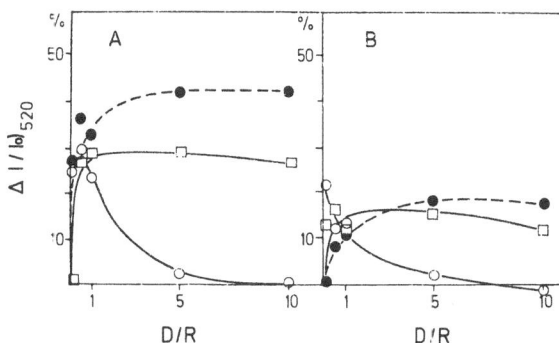

Fig. 5. Fluorescence enhancements of tetracycline derivatives by 30S subunits at (A) 5×10^{-4} M Mg^{2+} and (B) 10^{-2}M Mg^{2+}. For further details see legend of Fig. 4. (Fey *et al.*, 1973).

The fluorescence changes with D/R for the three derivatives upon addition of the 50S or 30S subunits were measured at 10 and 0.5 mM Mg^{2+} (Fig. 4 and Fig. 5). In Fig. 4 the fluorescence changes of all three tetracycline derivatives upon addition of 50S subunits are shown.

The plateau values of the relative fluorescence enhancements at 0.5 mM Mg^{2+} upon complex formation with the 50S subunit at a D/R ratio of 1:1 are highest for oxytetracycline (145 %), medium for tetracycline methiodide (75 %) and zero for tetracycline nitrile. Analogous experiments with the 30S subunit (Fig. 5) reveal that at D/R ratios greater than 5, oxytetracycline causes a relative increase of 40 %, tetracycline methiodide of 30 % whereas tetracycline nitrile has no effect. However, in the D/R regions between 0.1 and 1 tetracycline nitrile shows considerable fluorescence enhancement at high and also at low levels of Mg^{2+}, indicating interactions with the 30S ribosomal subunit.

With native and reassociated 70S ribosomes the influence on the fluorescence of the three tetracycline derivatives was measured only at 10 mM Mg^{2+} to avoid dissociation of the ribosomes into subunits. At a D/R value of 10 the fluorescence enhancement of oxytetracycline is 30 %, while that of tetracycline methiodide is about 22 %. Tetracycline nitrile interacts with the 70S ribosome at low D/R values as with the 30S subunits. Surprisingly, corresponding experiments with 70S ribosomes, reassociated from isolated 30S and 50S subunits show, that the particles behave like 50S particles. Fluorescence enhancement reflects well the inhibitory potencies of the drugs.

What can be concluded from these studies? White and Cantor (1971) concluded from a fluorescence analysis that Mg^{2+} ions are involved in the strong interaction of tetracyclines with ribosomes. The threefold increase of the original fluorescence intensity is comparable in magnitude with the value we have found upon interaction of oxytetracycline with the 50S subunit at low Mg^{2+}. Since the transition of partially chelated to totally chelated drug also results in a threefold increase of the relative fluorescence intensity of the molecule a Mg^{2+} chelation bridge might be involved in the strong binding of oxytetracycline and tetracycline methiodide to the 50S subunit. Binding studies with 50S subunits at 10 mM Mg^{2+} gave evidence that oxytetracycline could gain an additional 30 % fluorescence increase. We therefore suggest that interactions other than chelation by Mg^{2+} are involved in binding of tetracyclines with the 50S particle.

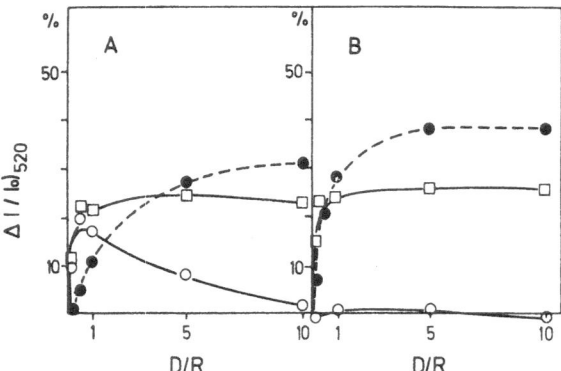

Fig. 6. Fluorescence enhancements of tetracycline derivatives by addition of 70S native ribosomes (A) and 70S reassociated ribosomes (B). For further details see legend of Fig. 4 (Fey *et al.*, 1973).

The fluorescence enhancement for oxytetracycline upon association with the 30S subunit at 0.5 mM Mg^{2+} is about 30 % and at 10 mM Mg^{2+} about 10 % higher than the original fluorescence. Since at 10 mM Mg^{2+} nearly all tetracycline molecules are in the chelated state they are already immobilized and cannot gain as much fluorescence increase as the free molecules upon binding to the subunit.

Since tetracycline nitrile does not inhibit cell-free systems and bacterial growth in the low concentration range the strong binding site for tetracycline at the 30S subunit is probably not important for the inhibitory potencies of tetracyclines. The strong binding site at the 50S subunit is possibly not available at the native 70S subunit (Fig. 6) and is probably not important for the inhibitory potencies of these drugs. As yet there is no way to determine which type of tetracycline-ribosome interaction is responsible for the inhibition of bacterial growth. Different interactions are probably involved depending on the ratio of drug/ribosome or subunits within the intact cell.

REFERENCES

FEY, G., M. REISS, and H. KERSTEN: Interaction of tetracyclines with ribosomal subunits from *Escherichia coli*. A fluorometric investigation. Biochemistry 12, 1160-1164 (1973).

HASELTINE, W.A., and R. BLOCK: Synthesis of guanosine tetra- and pentaphosphate requires the presence of a codon-specific, uncharged transfer ribonucleic acid in the acceptor site of ribosomes. Proc. Nat. Acad. Sci. USA 70, 1564-1568 (1973).

KERSTEN, H.: Changes in the properties of ribosomes and transfer RNA induced by inhibitors of protein synthesis. In: Progress in Molecular and Subcellular Biology, Vol. 2, (Hahn, F.E., ed.) pp. 58-68, Berlin-Heidelberg-New York: Springer 1971.

LUND, E., and N.O. KJELDGAARD: Metabolism of guanosine tetraphosphate in *Escherichia coli*. Eur. J. Biochem. 28, 316-326 (1972).

MANN, M.B., and P.C. HUANG: Behavior of chloramphenicol-induced phenylalanine transfer ribonucleic acid during recovery from chloramphenicol treatment in *Escherichia coli*. Biochemistry 12, 5289-5294 (1973).

PESTKA, S.: Inhibitions of ribosome functions. Ann. Rev.Microbiol. 25, 487-562 (1971).

SCHELLBERGER, H., and H. KERSTEN: Arginine dependent occurrence of a new isoaccepting tRNA [Phe] in *E. coli*. Abstr. FEBS Meeting, Budapest 1974.

WATERS, L.C., L. SHUGART, W.-K. YANG, and A.N. BEST: Some physical and biological properties of 4-thiouridine- and dihydro-uridine-deficient tRNA from chloramphenicol-treated *Escherichia coli*. Arch. Biochem. Biophys. 156, 780-793 (1973).

WHITE, J.P., and C.R. CANTOR: Role of magnesium in the binding of tetracycline to *Escherichia coli* ribosomes. J. Mol. Biol. 58, 397-400 (1971).

Acknowledgement

We are indebted to the "Deutsche Forschungsgemeinschaft" and the "Fonds der Chemischen Industrie" for the support of this work.

Ribosomal Effects of Thiostrepton and Related Antibiotics

Eric Cundliffe, Janet E. Beven, and Peter D. Dixon

I. INTRODUCTION

Thiostrepton (alias bryamycin) is a polypeptide antibiotic of sixteen residues with several modifications to the amino acids, for example cyclization of cysteine residues. A portion of the molecule is cyclic and there is an ester linkage to a terminal quinaldic acid derivative (Anderson *et al.*, 1970). Thiostrepton inhibits protein synthesis on procaryotic ribosomes by binding firmly to the 50s ribosomal subunit (Weisblum & Demohn, 1970a) with 1:1 stoichiometry (Sopori & Lengyel, 1972; Gordon & Highland, 1974) and recently (Highland *et al.*, 1974), ribosomal protein L11 of *E. coli* was implicated in the thiostrepton-binding reaction. To date however, no detailed analysis of thiostrepton-resistant ribosomes has been reported although a mutant of *E. coli*, resistant to the related antibiotic, thiopeptin, possesses altered 50s ribosomal subunits (Liou *et al.*, 1973). Other antibiotics, chemically related to thiostrepton and thiopeptin, include siomycin and sporangiomycin, and although the complete structure is only available for thiostrepton it is already apparent that this group of compounds have identical (or closely similar) biochemical modes of action. (For a review, see Cundliffe 1972a; also Pirali *et al.*, 1972).

Initially (Pestka, 1970), thiostrepton was found to inhibit ribosomal GTPase reactions dependent upon elongation factor G (EF-G) without affecting certain other ribosomal activities. Subsequently (Weisblum & Demohn, 1970b; Bodley *et al.*, 1970), thiostrepton was shown to prevent the formation of [ribosome·EF-G·GDP] complexes which are normally stabilized by another antibiotic, fusidic acid (Bodley *et al.*, 1969). Taken together these observations suggested that thiostrepton binds to 50s subunits at or near the site utilized by EF-G and/or guanine nucleotides as did the further observation (Highland *et al.*, 1971) that ribosomes carrying EF-G and GDP in the presence of fusidic acid were protected from inactivation by thiostrepton. Consequently, since the hydrolysis of GTP by EF-G is known to occur on the ribosome as part of the so-called "translocation reaction", thiostrepton became known as an inhibitor of translocation although this was not commonly demonstrated directly. A somewhat similar mode of action was also widely postulated for fusidic acid, particularly since certain fusidic acid-resistant mutants of *E. coli* were found to possess an altered G-factor (Kinoshita *et al.*, 1968). According to this scheme, fusidic acid inhibited translocation by sequestering EF-G and GDP on ribosomes.

The notion that thiostrepton inhibits translocation required modification when the drug was shown to inhibit the binding of aminoacyl-

tRNA into the ribosomal A-site in intact bacterial protoplasts
(Cundliffe, 1971) without affecting translocation. Concurrently,
thiostrepton and siomycin (Modolell *et al.*, 1971) and thiopeptin
(Kinoshita *et al.*, 1971) were shown to inhibit *in vitro* both the binding of aminoacyl-tRNA to ribosomes and hydrolysis of GTP dependent
upon EF-Tu, and the hydrolysis of GTP by ribosomes and EF-G when these
activities were each assayed independently of other ribosomal events.
However, when the action of thiostrepton was followed in a complete
protein-synthesizing system *in vitro* (Cannon & Burns, 1971), results
similar to those seen *in vivo* were obtained. To explain these various
results, the "single ribosomal GTPase" hypothesis was put forward,
according to which, ribosomes possess a single GTPase site with which
both EF-G and EF-Tu (the latter in complex with aminoacyl-tRNA and
GTP) interact (Cundliffe, 1971; Modolell *et al.*, 1971; Kinoshita *et
al.*, 1971). According to our particular version of this model, the
GTPase site, in the 50s moiety of the ribosomal A-site, is only available for the binding of drugs such as thiostrepton when the A-site is
empty, i.e. after translocation and prior to the binding of aminoacyl-
tRNA. This at once rationalizes the lack of effect of thiostrepton
upon translocation described above.

The single GTPase model was both strengthened and refined when one of
its predictions was tested namely, that by sequestering EF-G and GDP
on the ribosome, fusidic acid might inhibit protein synthesis by preventing [aminoacyl-tRNA·EF-Tu·GTP] complexes from binding into the
A-site. That fusidic acid <u>could</u> cause such effects was demonstrated
in vitro (Richman & Bodley, 1972; Miller, 1972; Richter, 1972; Cabrer
et al., 1972); that the drug <u>does</u> cause such effects in a complete
protein-synthesizing system was demonstrated *in vivo* (Cundliffe, 1972b).
These findings are widely assumed to have established the concept
that EF-G and EF-Tu cannot interact simultaneously with the single
GTPase site. Among many experimental observations which support this
scheme is one intriguing result which may refine the model further.
In the presence of 20% (v/v) methanol, ribosomes and EF-Tu catalyse
an "uncoupled" hydrolysis of GTP (in the absence of aminoacyl-tRNA)
which is resistant to thiostrepton (Ballesta & Vazquez, 1972) although
the GTPase activity of ribosomes associated with EF-G remains sensitive
to the drug under similar conditions. The requirement for methanol in
these experiments makes a detailed interpretation hazardous but various tempting conclusions concerning the possible ability of methanol
to influence the conformation of EF-Tu, or of the complex ribosomal
A-site come obviously to mind.

Since studies with thiostrepton and related antibiotics have been so
fruitful in helping to elucidate various aspects of ribosomal function
we have continued to follow the modes of action of such drugs *in vivo*.
Also, we have begun to examine the effects of some of these compounds
on the organisms which produce them and to study the ribosomes of
thiostrepton-resistant bacterial mutants. Some recent results are
discussed below.

II. MODES OF ACTION OF ANTIBIOTICS RELATED TO THIOSTREPTON

As reviewed elsewhere (Cundliffe, 1972a), there are a number of antibiotics which resemble thiostrepton chemically - at least to the extent of being sulphur-containing polypeptides containing modified
amino acids and non-amino acid residues. Most prominent among these
compounds have been siomycin and its derivatives, studied in detail
by Drs. Modolell, Vazquez and collaborators (references cited above;
see also Celma *et al.*, 1972) and by Dr. K. Tanaka and associates
(Tanaka *et al.*, 1970). Other compounds of interest include thiopeptin,

studied mainly in the laboratory of Dr. N. Tanaka (Kinoshita *et al.*, 1971; Liou *et al.*, 1973) and sporangiomycin (Pirali *et al.*, 1972). These antibiotics resemble thiostrepton in their ability to inhibit protein synthesis on procaryotic ribosomes by binding to the 50s ribosomal subunit and thereby interfering with both the EF-G-dependent ribosomal GTPase reaction and also the binding of [aminoacyl-tRNA·EF-Tu·GTP] complexes into the ribosomal A-site together with the associated GTPase event.

When added to complete protein-synthesizing systems *in vitro* siomycin specifically inhibits the binding of aminoacyl-tRNA into the ribosomal A-site and is without effect upon translocation (Celma *et al.*, 1972) and, as shown in Table 1, sporangiomycin acts similarly *in vivo*. In these latter experiments, carried out in intact protoplasts of *Bacillus megaterium*, sporangiomycin inhibited protein synthesis so as to preserve polyribosomes intact with very little loss of nascent peptides from the ribosomes. Even when sporangiomycin was used at concentrations well in excess of those required to stop protein synthesis, subsequent addition of puromycin was followed by rapid release of 80% of the nascent peptides from the ribosomes. We have previously argued (Cundliffe, 1971) that this pattern of behaviour implies inhibition of the binding of aminoacyl-tRNA into the ribosomal A-site and, indeed, sporangiomycin closely resembles thiostrepton in this system (Table 1). Two other compounds were also tested, thermothiocin - which clearly inhibits the puromycin reaction *in vivo* and micrococcin (Heatley & Doert, 1951) which acts similarly to both thiostrepton and sporangiomycin *in vivo*.

TABLE 1

EFFECTS OF ANTIBIOTICS ON THE PUROMYCIN REACTION *IN VIVO*

ADDITIONS	NASCENT PEPTIDES ON RIBOSOMES (% of those present when puromycin added)
THERMOTHIOCIN	60
SPORANGIOMYCIN	21
MICROCOCCIN	26
THIOSTREPTON	10

The methods used here have been described fully elsewhere (Cundliffe & McQuillen, 1967; Cundliffe, 1971). Protoplasts were prepared from cells of *B. megaterium KM* previously grown in [^{32}P]phosphate for several generations to steady-state label their ribosomes. Nascent peptides were labelled by incubating protoplasts at 37°C with [^{3}H]leucine (50 c/mM) for 30 sec. before the addition of an antibiotic to stop protein synthesis. Puromycin was added 2 min. later and incubation was continued at 37°C for a further 60 sec. At appropriate intervals samples were taken for lysis, mild treatment with RNAse and analysis on sucrose density gradients. Nascent peptides present on ribosomes were estimated from the specific radioactivity (^{3}H in 70s monosomes/ ^{32}P in total ribosomes).

Puromycin was used at a final concentration of 25 µg/ml, other antibiotics at 100 µg/ml (stock solutions of the latter being 10 mg/ml in dimethyl sulphoxide).

The effects of these compounds upon the formation of [ribosome·EF-G· GDP] complexes and their stabilization by fusidic acid *in vitro* are shown in Table 2. In agreement with the work of others (references cited above), thiostrepton and sporangiomycin inhibited complex formation, as did micrococcin and micrococcin P, albeit not as potently. In contrast, thermothiocin had no effect on complex formation even at very high concentrations. These results with micrococcin and micrococcin P appear to conflict with others reported elsewhere. These antibiotics (which appear to be identical - J. Walker, personal communication 1974) were found to inhibit neither the EF-G-dependent GTPase, nor the formation of complexes as above (Pestka & Brot, 1971). However, in agreement with the results presented here, these latter workers found thermothiocin to be without effect on complex formation. From the results presented so far, we conclude that the "thiostrepton group" of antibiotics properly includes siomycin, sporangiomycin, micrococcin and micrococcin P but not thermothiocin. This latter antibiotic, being capable of inhibiting the puromycin reaction *in vivo* may well turn out to resemble althiomycin, another compound of this general type, which has been shown to inhibit the peptidyl transferase reaction (Burns & Cundliffe, 1973).

TABLE 2

EFFECTS OF ANTIBIOTICS ON THE FORMATION OF RIBOSOME·EF-G·GDP COMPLEXES
IN THE PRESENCE OF FUSIDIC ACID

DRUG		COMPLEX FORMATION (% of control)
SPORANGIOMYCIN	150 pmol	9
THIOSTREPTON	150 pmol	10
THERMOTHIOCIN	5.4 nmol	93
MICROCOCCIN	200 pmol	61
MICROCOCCIN	21 nmol	44
MICROCOCCIN P	200 pmol	65

Ribosomes were from *B. megaterium KM*, EF-G was from *E. coli*, complex formation in controls was 30 % of that observed with homologous *E. coli* ribosomes. A heterologous system was used here since *bacillus* ribosomes are more sensitive to each of the above antibiotics than are those from *E. coli*.

Incubation 1. Ribosomes (44 pmol) in complex buffer with or without antibiotic as indicated in the Table. 5 min. 0°C. Volume 15 µl. Incubation 2. The following components were added, each dissolved in complex buffer: EF-G (50 pmol), ring-[^{3}H]GTP (49 pmol, 13.3 c/mM), fusidic acid (2.5 mM final concentration). 5 min. 0°C. Total volume 65 µl. Incubation 2 was terminated by the addition of 3 ml ice-cold complex buffer containing 1.5 x 10^{-4}M fusidic acid. Ribosomes were collected by filtration on cellulose nitrate "Millipore" filters (0.45 µ pore size) which were washed several times with cold complex buffer containing fusidic acid. Radioactivity retained on filters was estimated by liquid-scintillation counting and was assumed to represent [ribosome·EF-G·GDP] complexes. In all cases "blank" estimations (lacking ribosomes) were performed and these were substracted from experimental values. "Complex buffer" was Tris HCl (pH 7.5) 10 mM, magnesium acetate 20 mM, ammonium chloride 10 mM, dithiothreitol 1 mM.

III. COMPETITION BETWEEN ANTIBIOTICS FOR RIBOSOMAL BINDING SITES

In an attempt to determine whether thermothiocin, while distinguishable in its action from other members of the "thiostrepton group" might still compete for ribosomal binding sites, we examined the ability of thiostrepton and sporangiomycin to prevent the formation of [ribosome· EF-G·GDP] complexes on thermothiocin-treated ribosomes. As shown in Table 3, there was no evidence that thermothiocin was able to inter- fere with the action of those drugs. In more recent, and very prelim- inary, experiments (data not given) we have ascertained that exposure of ribosomes to members of the "thiostrepton group" of antibiotics (namely microccin and sporangiomycin) prevents the subsequent bind- ing of [^{35}S]thiostrepton to those ribosomes, as expected.

TABLE 3

LACK OF EFFECT OF THERMOTHIOCIN ON THE BINDING OF THIOSTREPTON AND
SPORANGIOMYCIN TO RIBOSOMES

ADDITIONS	FORMATION OF RIBOSOME·EF-G·GDP COMPLEXES (normalised to % of control values)
THERMOTHIOCIN 5.4 nmol	90
SPORANGIOMYCIN 150 pmol	5
THIOSTREPTON 150 pmol	8
THERMOTHIOCIN 5.4 nmol then SPORANGIOMYCIN 150 pmol	16
THERMOTHIOCIN 5.4 nmol then THIOSTREPTON 150 pmol	2

Experiments carried out as in Table 2 again utilising ribosomes from *B. megaterium*. Here two or three incubations, each for 5 min. at 0°C, were carried out as indicated in the Table. Additions for the final incubation were as in Table 2, Incubation 2.

IV. PROBLEMS OF SELF-DEFENCE

Various authors have considered at some length the possible natural functions of antibiotics. Resisting the (naive?) temptation to assume that antibiotics automatically confer upon the producing organisms a survival advantage in the wild, an hypothesis has been developed, which we find plausible and attractive, according to which antibiotics are to be considered as "secondary metabolites" along with many other compounds devoid of biological activity. Of course, under certain circumstances (and always pre-supposing that the producing-organism is insensitive to its product), production of an antibiotic might be advantageous in removing competitors from some ecological niche, but it has also been argued persuasively that the advantages gained from secondary metabolism may be more obscure. Thus (Bu'Lock, 1961), sec- ondary metabolism may allow a cell to maintain essential enzymes and entire uptake or synthetic systems in working order following the cessation of primary metabolism (i.e. integrated cell growth). Thus, a more rapid resumption of growth might be possible if conditions became more favourable. Alternatively, Woodruff (1966) has considered the advantages to a cell (but not necessarily at the expense of its neighbours) of excreting secondary metabolites of no direct value to itself. These would arise from the action of enzymes upon normal meta-bolic intermediates following their accumulation in abnormal amounts after inhibition of growth. According to this hypothesis, biological activity of excreted secondary metabolites might be accidental, but not necessarily surprising since many of them will resemble normal metabolic intermediates and may be potent antimetabolites. Both of these hypotheses (others are not excluded) leave open the question of whether antibiotic producers should be expected to be sensitive or resistant to their products.

The organisms which produce thiostrepton (*Streptomyces azureus* ATCC 14,921), micrococcin (*Su's micrococcus* NCTC 7218; see Su, 1948) and micrococcin P (*Bacillus pumilis*; see Brookes *et al.*, 1957) are clearly faced with a problem of self defence since, being procaryotes, they all contain 70s ribosomes. Having first ascertained that each of these organisms does indeed produce an antibiotic, we then tested their sensitivities on agar to a range of antibiotics applied on paper discs (Table 4). Also included in Table 4 are the antibiotic sensitivities of two spontaneously-arising mutants of *B. megaterium* selected for resistance to thiostrepton. These mutants were resistant to the entire thiostrepton group but not to any other one of a wide range of 70s ribosome-inhibitors which included thermothiocin and althiomycin. Interestingly, *B. pumilis* and *Su's micrococcus* were resistant only to the antibiotic they produce (as mentioned above, micrococcin and micrococcin P are thought to be identical) whereas *S. azureus* was re-sistant to a small number of compounds including the thiostrepton group and amicetin but sensitive to many others. As a control, to establish the fact that streptomycetes in general are not resistant to the thiostrepton group, we tested the streptomycin-producer *Strepto-myces griseus* CUB 94. This organism was sensitive to the thiostrepton group of antibiotics and also to streptomycin, giving a large clear zone of inhibition around the streptomycin-disc after 48 hrs incuba-tion. However, on prolonged incubation at 25°C, the organism grew through this zone (i.e. after 5 days the "zone" was detectable only from the thickness of mycelium covering it) probably due to the pres-ence of an enzyme in this organism capable of inactivating strepto-mycin (for a discussion and details see Benveniste & Davies, 1973).

The sensitivity or otherwise of the ribosomes of these organisms to-wards the thiostrepton group of antibiotics is detailed in Tables 5 and 6 and in Fig. 1. Here we assayed the formation of [ribosome·EF-G ·GDP] complexes in the presence of fusidic acid utilising, in each case, purified EF-G derived from *E. coli*. The efficiencies with which various ribosomes responded to *E. coli* G factor are given in Tables 5 and 6. As shown in Table 5, ribosomes of *S. azureus* appear to be totally resistant to all members of the thiostrepton group of anti-biotics explaining, at a stroke, the resistance of this organism to its own toxic product. (This does not exclude the possibility that the cell membranes of *S. azureus* may also be impermeable to thio-strepton or that the cell may be able to inactivate the drug enzy-mically).Conversely, ribosomes of the thiostrepton-resistant mutant of *B. megaterium*, designated PDI, were tolerant of thiostrepton rather than totally resistant (Fig. 1). In other, preliminary, experiments utilising [^{35}S]thiostrepton, we examined, and disproved, the simple hypothesis that ribosomes of *S. azureus* (and to a lesser extent those of mutant PDI) might be resistant to thiostrepton by virtue of being unable to bind the drug. Rather, under conditions where ribosomes were present in a large molar excess with respect to the radioactive

TABLE 4

SENSITIVITIES OF VARIOUS MICRO-ORGANISMS TO SELECTED ANTIBIOTICS

ANTIBIOTIC	ORGANISM		
	Streptomyces azureus	*Streptomyces griseus*	*Su's micrococcus*
CHLORAMPHENICOL	S	S	S
THIOSTREPTON	R	S	S
SIOMYCIN	R	S	S
SPORANGIOMYCIN	R	S	S
MICROCOCCIN	R	S	R
MICROCOCCIN P	R	–	R
THERMOTHIOCIN	S	S	S
ALTHIOMYCIN	S	–	S
FUSIDIC ACID	S	–	S
STREPTOMYCIN	S	S/R*	–

	Bacillus pumilis	*Bacillus megaterium* mutants PD1 & PD14	*Bacillus megaterium* wild type
CHLORAMPHENICOL	S	S	S
THIOSTREPTON	S	R	S
SIOMYCIN	S	R	S
SPORANGIOMYCIN	S	R	S
MICROCOCCIN	R	R	S
MICROCOCCIN P	R	–	–
THERMOTHIOCIN	S	S	S
ALTHIOMYCIN	–	S	S
FUSIDIC ACID	S	–	S
STREPTOMYCIN	–	–	S

Filter paper discs (5 mm diameter) containing antibiotics (10 µg - 25 µg per disc) were placed on freshly-spread lawns of each micro-organism on rich agar plates. These were then incubated at 37 °C (bacteria) or 25 °C (streptomycetes). Clear zones around discs indicated sensitivity to particular antibiotics. The results were unequivocal and not dependent upon the duration of incubation except for *S. griseus* growing around a disc containing streptomycin (25 µg) indicated S/R* in the Table. As discussed in the text, a clear zone appeared at early times but subsequently the organism grew through this area.

TABLE 5

EFFECTS OF ANTIBIOTICS ON FORMATION OF RIBOSOME·EF-G·GDP COMPLEXES
WITH RIBOSOMES FROM *STREPTOMYCES AZUREUS*

| DRUG ADDED | pmol GTP* complexed/pmol Ribosomes | |
	(i)	(ii)
NONE	0.11	0.10
THIOSTREPTON	0.09	0.11
SIOMYCIN	0.10	0.08
MICROCOCCIN	0.10	0.10
SPORANGIOMYCIN	0.11	0.08

Experiments carried out as in Table 2 except for origin of ribosomes.
i.e. EF-G from *E. coli* was used. Control experiments indicated that
streptomyces ribosomes supported 17 % of the complex formation observed with *E. coli* ribosomes. 50 pmol of ribosomes were used per
assay. *As in Table 2, ring-[^{3}H]GTP was used but it was assumed that
radioactivity retained on filters was present as GDP. Drugs were present in 70-fold molar excess over ribosomes.

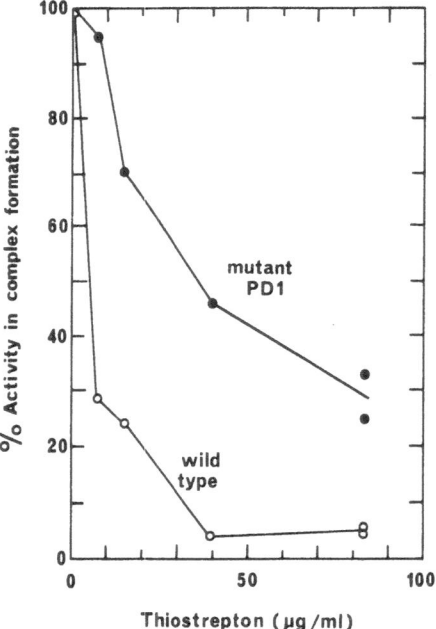

Fig. 1. Effects of thiostrepton on formation of ribosome·EF-G·GDP
complexes with ribosomes from *B. megaterium* and mutant PD1.
Experiments were carried out as in Table 2 utilising ribosomes from
either *Bacillus megaterium KM* wild type or from a spontaneously-
arising mutant of this organism selected for thiostrepton-resistance
and designated PD1.

drug, we were unable to distinguish ribosomes of *S. azureus* or PDI
from those of *E. coli* or *B. megaterium* wild type in their ability to
bind the drug (data not given). When experiments are carried out with
limiting quantities of ribosomes, it will be interesting to compare
the binding constants for the interaction between the drug and ribosomes from various sources.

In contrast, *Su's micrococcus* possesses ribosomes which are sensitive
to the thiostrepton group of antibiotics and, moreover are more sensitive to micrococcin than are ribosomes from *E. coli* or *B. megaterium*
wild types (Table 6). Obviously, the resistance of this micrococcus
to its own antibiotic must be derived either from the permeability
properties of its cell membrane or upon the presence of an enzyme
capable of inactivating the drug. This latter point remains to be investigated.

TABLE 6

EFFECT OF MICROCOCCIN ON FORMATION OF RIBOSOME·EF-G·GDP COMPLEXES WITH
RIBOSOMES FROM VARIOUS SOURCES

DRUG ADDED	COMPLEX FORMATION (normalised)		
	Ribosomes from *E. coli*	Ribosomes from *Su's micrococcus*	Ribosomes from *B.megaterium* w.t.
NONE	100	100	100
MICROCOCCIN 200 pmol	80	48	61
MICROCOCCIN 4 nmol	43	38	50
MICROCOCCIN 21 nmol	33	14	44
THIOSTREPTON 150pmol	51	5	8

Experiments carried out utilising EF-G from *E. coli* as on Table 2. In
controls, micrococcus ribosomes were 83 % as efficient and bacillus
ribosomes 30 % as efficient as *E. coli* ribosomes in supporting complex
formation. In each assay 44 pmol of ribosomes and 50 pmol of EF-G were
used.

V. CONCLUDING REMARKS

Our demonstration that *S. azureus* possesses thiostrepton-resistant
ribosomes is, to our knowledge, the first demonstration that a strepto-
mycete producing an inhibitor of 70s ribosomes possesses ribosomes
specifically resistant to its own product. It is curious, to us, that
this point has not been examined before, particularly in view of the
current interest in aminoglycoside-inactivating enzymes found in amino-
glycoside-producing streptomycetes (Benveniste & Davies, 1973). Obviously, in view of our results above, there is no absolute rule
whereby all producers of ribosome inhibitors possess refractory drug
targets although it remains possible that a general rule may exist
among streptomycetes. It will be particularly interesting to examine
the ribosomes from aminoglycoside-producers although our observations
(above) concerning *Streptomyces griseus* suggest that this organism
possesses streptomycin-sensitive ribosomes. Another explanation of

some of those effects might be that the antibiotic-sensitivity of
streptomyces ribosomes might change in the direction of resistance
as the organisms leave the phase of logarithmic growth and commence
antibiotic production. This point needs to be investigated in some
detail, although we utilised ribosomes from *S. azureus* harvested during log. phase, at which time the organism would not have been expected to be engaged in antibiotic production. Any examples of changes
in the sensitivities of ribosomes towards antibiotics related to the
cycle of cell growth would be fascinating if observed, since they
would presumably involve local modifications of the components of pre-
existing ribosomes and might prove particularly useful in the elucidation of ribosomal target sites.

Acknowledgements. This work was supported by grants to Eric Cundliffe
from the Medical Research Council and The Wellcome Trust. An MRC
Research Studentship is held by P.D.D. We are deeply indebted to
Dr. Norman Heatley and Dr. James Walker for gifts of micrococcin,
micrococcin P and bacterial strains. Thiostrepton was obtained from
Miss Barbara Stearns and *S. azureus* from Dr. Edward Meyer, both of
the Squibb Institute for Medical Research, Princeton, N.J. Purified
EF-G from *E. coli* was a generous gift from Jim Bodley.

REFERENCES

ANDERSON, B., HODGKIN, D.C. and M.A. WISWAMITRA: The structure of
    thiostrepton. Nature 225, 233-235 (1970).
BALLESTA, J.P.G. and D. VAZQUEZ: Elongation factor T-dependent hydro-
    lysis of guanine triphosphate resistant to thiostrepton. Proc.
    Nat. Acad. Sci. USA 69, 3058-3062 (1972).
BENVENISTE, R. and J. DAVIES: Aminoglycoside antibiotic-inactivating
    enzymes in actinomycetes similar to those present in clinical
    isolates of antibiotic-resistant bacteria. Proc. Nat. Acad. Sci.
    USA 70, 2276-2280 (1973).
BODLEY, J.W., LIN, L. and J.H. HIGHLAND: Thiostrepton prevents the
    formation of a ribosome·G factor·guanine nucleotide complex.
    Biochem. Biophys. Research Commun. 41, 1406-1411 (1970).
BODLEY, J.W., ZIEVE, F.J., LIN, L. and S.T. ZIEVE: Formation of the
    ribosome·G factor·GDP complex in the presence of fusidic acid.
    Biochem. Biophys. Research Commun. 37, 437-443 (1969).
BROOKES, P., FULLER, A.T. and J. WALKER: Chemistry of micrococcin P.
    Part 1. J. Chem. Soc. p. 689 (1957).
BU'LOCK, J.D.: Intermediary metabolism and antibiotic synthesis.
    Adv. in App. Microbiol. 3, 293-342 (1961).
BURNS, D.J.W. and E. CUNDLIFFE: Bacterial protein synthesis. A novel
    system for studying antibiotic action *in vivo*. Eur. J. Biochem. 37,
    570-574 (1973).
CABRER, B., VAZQUEZ, D. and J. MODOLELL: Inhibition by elongation
    factor G of aminoacyl-tRNA binding to ribosomes. Proc. Nat. Acad.
    Sci. USA 69, 733-736 (1972).
CANNON, M. and K. BURNS: Modes of action of erythromycin and thio-
    strepton as inhibitors of protein synthesis. FEBS Lett. 18, 1-5
    (1971).
CELMA, M.L., VAZQUEZ, D. and J. MODOLELL: Failure of fusidic acid and
    siomycin to block ribosomes in the pretranslocated state. Biochem.
    Biophys. Research Commun. 48, 1240-1246 (1972).
CUNDLIFFE, E: The mode of action of thiostrepton *in vivo*. Biochem.
    Biophys. Research Commun. 44, 912-917 (1971).

CUNDLIFFE, E.: Antibiotic inhibitors of ribosome function, in Molecular basis of antibiotic action. Authors E.F. Gale, E. Cundliffe, P.E. Reynolds, M.H. Richmond and M.J. Waring. Pages 278-379. Wiley and Sons, London (1972a).

CUNDLIFFE, E.: The mode of action of fusidic acid. Biochem. Biophys. Research Commun. 46, 1974-1801 (1972b).

CUNDLIFFE, E. and K.McQUILLEN: Bacterial protein synthesis: The effects of antibiotics. J. Mol. Biol. 30, 137-146 (1967).

GORDON, J. and J.H. HIGHLAND: Binding of thiostrepton to the ribosomes of E. coli: Characterization and stoichiometry of binding. J. Biol. Chem. in press (1974).

HEATLEY, N.G. and H.M. DOERY: The preparation and some properties of purified microccocin. Biochem. J. 50, 247-253 (1951).

HIGHLAND, J.H., HOWARD, G.A., OCHSNER, E., STÖFFLER, G., HASENBANK, R. and J. GORDON: Identification of the ribosomal protein responsible for the binding of thiostrepton to E. coli ribosomes. J. Biol. Chem. in press (1974).

HIGHLAND, J.H., LIN, L. and J.W. BODLEY: Protection of ribosomes from thiostrepton inactivation by the binding of G factor and GDP. Biochemistry 10, 4404-4409 (1971).

KINOSHITA, T., LIOU, Y.-F. and N. TANAKA: Inhibition by thiopeptin of ribosomal functions associated with T and G factors. Biochem. Biophys. Research Commun. 44, 859-863 (1971).

KINOSHITA, T., KUWANA, G. and N. TANAKA: Association of fusidic acid sensitivity with G factor in a protein synthesizing system. Biochem. Biophys. Research Commun. 33, 769-773 (1968).

LIOU, Y.-F., KINOSHITA, T., TANAKA, N. and M. YOSHIKAWA: Studies on the ribosomes of a thiopeptin-resistant mutant of E. coli. J. Antibiotics 26, 711-716 (1973).

MILLER, D.L.: Elongation factors EF-Tu and EF-G interact at related sites on ribosomes. Proc. Nat. Acad. Sci. USA 69, 752-755 (1972).

MODOLELL, J., CABRER, B., PARMEGGIANI, A. and D. VAZQUEZ: Inhibition by siomycin and thiostrepton of both aminoacyl-tRNA and factor G binding to ribosomes. Proc. Nat. Acad. Sci. USA 68, 1796-1800 (1971).

PESTKA, S.: Thiostrepton: A ribosomal inhibitor of translocation. Biochem. Biophys. Research Commun. 40, 667-674 (1970).

PESTKA, S. and N. BROT: Effect of antibiotics on steps of bacterial protein synthesis: Some new ribosomal inhibitors of translocation. J. Biol. Chem. 246, 7715-7722 (1971).

PIRALI, G., LANCINI, G.C., PARISI, B. and F. SALA: Interaction of sporangiomycin with the bacterial ribosome. J. Antibiotics 25, 561-568 (1972).

RICHMAN, N. and J.W. BODLEY: The sites on the 50s ribosomal subunit with which elongation factors Tu and G interact are at least partially identical. Proc. Nat. Acad. Sci. USA 69, 686-689 (1972).

RICHTER, D.: Inability of E. coli ribosomes to interact simultaneously with the bacterial elongation factors EF-Tu and EF-G. Biochem. Biophys. Research Commun. 46, 1850-1856 (1972).

SOPORI, M.L. and P. LENGYEL: Components of the 50s ribosomal subunit involved in GTP cleavage. Biochem. Biophys. Research Commun. 46, 238-244 (1972).

SU, T.L.: Microccocin, an anti-bacterial substance formed by a strain of micrococcus. Brit. J. Exp. Path. 29, 473-481 (1948).

TANAKA, K., WATANABE, S., TERAOKA, H. and M. TAMAKI: Effect of siomycin on protein synthetic activity. Biochem. Biophys. Research Commun. 39, 1189-1193 (1970).

WEISBLUM, B. and V. DEMOHN: Thiostrepton, an inhibitor of 50s ribosome subunit function. Biochem. Biophys. Research Commun. 101, 1073-1075 (1970a).

WEISBLUM, B. and V. DEMOHN: Inhibition by thiostrepton of the formation of a ribosome-bound guanine nucleotide complex. FEBS Lett. 11, 149-152 (1970b).

WOODRUFF, H.B.: The physiology of antibiotic production: The role of the producing organism. Symp. Soc. Gen. Microbiol. 16, 22-46 (1966).

Studies on Active Sites of Ribosomes with Haloacetylated Antibiotic Analogs*

O. Pongs, R. Bald, V. A. Erdmann, and E. Reinwald

1. INTRODUCTION

The technique of affinity labeling allows the direct identification of the sites of interaction between two molecules, for example,
between substrate and enzyme or, just as well, between a drug and
its target. In general, a chemically reactive group is introduced
into a molecule, which then can react preferentially and irreversibly with a properly oriented amino acid functional group in the binding region of the protein(s). We applied this technique to the antibiotics chloramphenicol, puromycin and streptomycin in order to find
out, which ribosomal protein is associated with the binding sites of
these antibiotics. All three antibiotics were modified with bromo-
or iodoacetic acid such that they did not lose their known antibiotic
properties. However, the introduction of a haloacetyl group into the
antibiotics leads to a chemical linkage between the antibiotic and
its ribosomal binding site. The respective labeled ribosomal proteins
were isolated and, thus, the ribosomal protein(s) involved in the
binding of the antibiotic, could be identified.

2. AFFINITY LABELING WITH MONOIODOAMPHENICOL

In our earlier work we employed the chloramphenicol analog, monoiodoamphenicol, in order to elucidate the ribosomal chloramphenicol
binding site by affinity labeling (Bald *et al.*, 1972). Substitution
of this antibiotic's dichloroacetyl group by a monoiodoacetyl group
did not change the antibiotic's specificity, but made its binding
irreversible, as shown by the following *in vivo* and *in vitro* studies.

Chloramphenicol has been known for many years as a strong, but reversible, inhibitor of protein biosynthesis (Wolfe & Hahn, 1965;
Vazquez, 1964; for a review see Pestka, 1971). Similarly, addition
of monoiodoamphenicol to a culture of *E. coli* cells at a concentration of 30 µg/ml immediately stops all growth by inhibiting protein
synthesis (data are not shown). DNA-synthesis, on the other hand,
appears to be unaffected. However, contrary to the action of chloramphenicol, monoiodoamphenicol acts as a bacteriocide and not as a
bacteriostat, since it irreversibly inhibits cell growth. This killing
effect of *E. coli* cells by monoiodoamphenicol is not seen with chlor-

---

* Paper No. 10 on "Affinity Labeling of Ribosomes". Preceding paper:
  Pongs, O., & Lanka, E. (1974) Proc. Nat. Acad. Sci. USA, submitted
  for publication.

amphenicol, which can be washed out, after which the cells resume growth again. These *in vivo* studies indicate that monoiodoamphenicol binds irreversibly to some component, which is essential for protein synthesis.

Monoiodoamphenicol behaves similarly to chloramphenicol *in vitro* (Pongs *et al.*, 1973a). As summarized in Table 1, monoiodoamphenicol strongly inhibits f2-mRNA dependent protein synthesis and, to a lesser degree, poly(U)-dependent polyphenylalanine synthesis. However, again in contrast to chloramphenicol, the inhibitory action is not reversible. The binding of monoiodoamphenicol to *E. coli* ribosomes has been further investigated. These studies showed that chloramphenicol and lincomycin compete with monoiodoamphenicol for the same binding site (Pongs *et al.*, 1973a). It was observed that the affinity of monoiodoamphenicol for 70S ribosomes is one order of magnitude greater than that to 50S subunits. This indicates that upon dissociation of ribosomes into subunits either the conformation of the chloramphenicol binding site is changed or that the 30S subunit contributes to the chloramphenicol binding site.

Table 1

f2mRNA- AND POLY(U)-DIRECTED POLYPEPTIDE SYNTHESIS WITH *E. COLI* 70S RIBOSOMES AFTER REACTION WITH MONOIODOAMPHENICOL

Antibiotic	f2mRNA-directed activity of *E.coli* ribosomes in % [a]	poly(U)-directed activity of *E.coli* ribosomes in % [b]
None	100	100
Monoiodoamphenicol	5	50
Chloramphenicol	8	48

After incubation of *E. coli* 70S ribosomes with a 10-fold molar excess of monoiodoamphenicol for 2 hr at 37°C in 10 mM $MgCl_2$, 30 mM NH_4Cl, 10 mM Tris-HCl (pH 7.8) buffer, the ribosomes were exhaustively dialyzed against the incubation buffer overnight at 4°C. Aliquots containing 1.4 A_{260} units of ribosomes were examined for biological activity. (a) f2mRNA-directed [^{14}C]valine incorporation into protein was measured according to Erdmann *et al.* (1971). (b) Poly(U)-directed polyphenylalanine synthesis was determined as previously described (Pongs *et al.*, 1973a). The concentration of chloramphenicol in the assays was 1 mM.

Since it could be established that monoiodoamphenicol reacted irreversibly and specifically in the chloramphenicol binding site, it was possible to identify the ribosomal protein(s) associated with this binding site. *E. coli* 70S ribosomes were labeled on a large scale with radiomonoiodoamphenicol. Ribosomal subunits were isolated by sucrose gradient centrifugation. The 30S and 50S ribosomal proteins were then extracted with acetic acid and separated by two-dimensional polyacrylamide gel electrophoresis according to Kaltschmidt and Wittmann (1971). It is important to note that no radioactivity could be detected in the RNA material isolated from the labeled subunits. The staining pattern of the gels obtained from the 30S and 50S ribosomal proteins was identical to that of ribosomal proteins of untreated ribosomes, except for that of protein L16. As a result of the labeling reaction, protein L16 was found in a new position, which was between that of unmodified L16 and S9. As can be seen from Fig. 1, almost all the radioactivity was detected in protein L16 of the 50S subunit. In addition, 10 % of the amount of radioactivity contained in protein L16 was detected in proteins L6 and L24. The 30S proteins contained negligible radioactivity except protein S3, which had about 25 % of the radioactivity found in protein L16. These data strongly indicate that monoiodoamphenicol preferentially reacted with protein L16. Therefore, it is concluded that protein L16 is associated with the chloramphenicol binding site. This observation found strong support in reconstitution experiments, which have been reported by Nierhaus & Nierhaus (1973). These experiments showed that *E. coli* 50S subunits bind chloramphenicol only if protein L16 is present in the subunit.

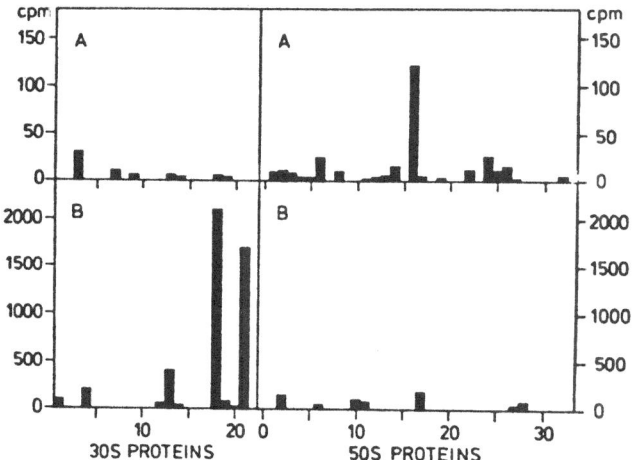

Fig. 1. Radioactivity detected in ribosomal proteins after incubation of 70S ribosomes with monoiodo[14C]amphenicol or with iodo[14C]acetamide. (A) After incubation of *E. coli* 70S ribosomes with a 10-fold excess of monoiodo[14C]amphenicol (4.3 Ci/mol) for 2 hr at 37°C, the ribosomal subunits and proteins were isolated as described (Pongs *et al.*, 1973a). Proteins were separated by two-dimensional gel electrophoresis according to Kaltschmidt & Wittmann (1970). Radioactivity contained in each spot was determined as described (Pongs *et al.*, 1973a). (B) After incubation of *E. coli* 70S ribosomes with a 10-fold molar excess of iodo[14C]acetamide (50 Ci/mol) for 2 hr at 37°C in 10 mM MgCl$_2$, 30 mM NH$_4$Cl, 10 mM Tris-HCl (pH 7.8) buffer, separation of ribosomal proteins and counting of radioactivity was done as in (A).

An investigation was carried out to compare the *in vitro* data with results obtained from *in vivo* studies. *E. coli* cells were incubated with radioactive monoiodoamphenicol. The ribosomes were isolated in the usual manner by high speed centrifugation. The subunits were separated on sucrose gradients. This is shown in Fig. 2. Firstly, it can be seen that radioactive label migrated not only with 50S subunits, but also with 30S particles. Furthermore, a lot of radioactivity is found on top of the gradient. Secondly, the ribosomal "30S" peak is very broad and contains more UV-absorbing material than usual.

This indicates that monoiodoamphenicol treatment causes defective ribosomal particles similar to those described in earlier observations made with chloramphenicol (Nomura and Watson, 1959). The ribosomal proteins were extracted from the 50S and "30S" particles and analyzed by two-dimensional polyacrylamide gel electrophoresis. Besides protein L16, proteins S13 and L24 contained a significant amount of radio-activity. These data indicate that it is difficult to pinpoint the bacteriostatic locus of chloramphenicol action just to one single event, and that it is also difficult to extrapolate from *in vitro* studies to the *in vivo* situation.

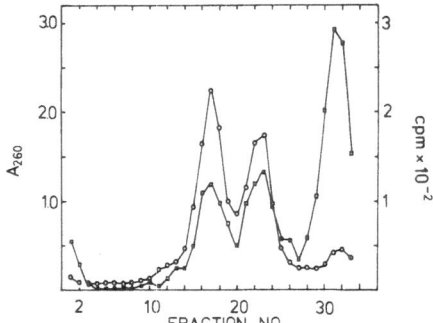

Fig. 2. Sucrose gradient of 70S ribosomes labeled with monoiodo[^{14}C] amphenicol. *E. coli* cell culture was incubated with 30 μg/ml mono-iodoamphenicol at a density of 2×10^8 cells/ml for 10 min at 37°C. After harvest of the cells, ribosomes were isolated and purified as described (Erdmann *et al.*, 1971). On top of the gradient 250 A_{260} units of 70S ribosomes were layered and centrifuged at 24 000 rpm for 14 hr at 4°C in a Spinco SW 27 rotor. 1.3 ml fractions were collected. 50 μl aliquots of each fraction were diluted with 0.5 ml H_2O and ab-sorbance was read at 260 nm. Radioactivity was measured by mixing the diluted aliquots of each fraction with 10 ml of Bray's counting solu-tion. (o———o) A_{260}; (□———□) cpm.

3. AFFINITY LABELING OF *E. COLI* RIBOSOMES WITH A PUROMYCIN ANALOG

Puromycin inhibits protein synthesis by competing with aminoacyl-tRNA as acceptor for the peptidyl moiety. The peptidyl moiety is transferred to puromycin by the ribosomal peptidyltransferase, which then yields N-peptidylpuromycin as a premature termination product of protein synthesis. Since puromycin becomes linked to the released peptides by means of a peptide bond, the reaction has been used ex-tensively as a model of peptide bond formation in protein synthesis (for a review see Pestka, 1971). N-iodoacetylpuromycin was synthe-sized (Pongs *et al.*, 1973b) as an analog of N-peptidylpuromycin, which was expected to have affinity for the peptidyltransferase center. Thereby, it would disclose a ribosomal protein, associated with the puromycin binding site. Puromycin has a close resemblance to the 3'-end of aminoacyl-tRNA (Yarmolinski & de la Haba, 1959). Accordingly, N-iodoacetylpuromycin might have a close resemblance to the 3'- end of N-acetylaminoacyl-tRNA, which binds in the donor site of the peptidyltransferase center.

Experiments were first carried out to test whether the puromycin affinity label bound in the acceptor site like puromycin, or whether the affinity label bound to the donor site like peptidyl-tRNA. Fig. 3 shows the kinetics of the N-iodoacetylpuromycin uptake in the absence and presence of puromycin. It can be seen that puromycin strongly inhibited the labeling reaction at 4°C and 37°C. This indicates that the affinity label reacted in the puromycin binding site, i.e. the acceptor site of the peptidyltransferase center. This observation is further supported by the data in Table 2, which show that the puromycin affinity label inhibits f2-mRNA dependent protein synthesis, but does not inhibit initiation factor dependent fMet-tRNA$_f^{Met}$ binding. This again indicates that binding of N-iodoacetylpuromycin takes place in the acceptor site, since fMet-tRNA$_f^{Met}$ binding in the donor site is not inhibited. Moreover, the reaction of N-iodoacetylpuromycin with 70S ribosomes decreases the binding of puromycin to these ribosomes and also decreases the peptidyltransferase activity as checked by the fragment assay (data are not shown). All these data together show that this affinity label indeed binds in the acceptor site of the peptidyltransferase center and thereby, irreversibly reacts with this site of the ribosome.

Table 2

AUG-DEPENDENT INITIATION AND f2mRNA-DIRECTED PROTEIN SYNTHESIS WITH
E. COLI 70S RIBOSOMES AFTER THE REACTION WITH N-IODOACETYLPUROMYCIN

Antibiotic	AUG-IF-fMet-tRNA$_f^{Met}$ 70S complex formation in % a)	f2mRNA-directed activity of E.coli ribosomes in % b)
None	95	100
N-Iodoacetylpuromycin	100	27
Puromycin	5	12

100 A$_{260}$ units of 70S E. coli ribosomes were incubated with tenfold molar excess of antibiotic (about 30 nmoles dissolved in 10 µl methanol) in 500 µl 10 mM MgCl$_2$, 30 mM NH$_4$Cl and 10 mM Tris-HCl (pH 7.8) buffer for 2 hr at 37°C. After incubation the samples were exhaustively dialyzed against the incubation buffer overnight at 4°C. Aliquots containing 1.5 A$_{260}$ units of ribosomes were then examined for biological activity. (a) Initiation complex formation was measured at 30°C as described by Hershey et al. (1971). (b) f2mRNA-directed [^{14}C]valine incorporation into protein was measured according to Erdmann et al. (1971). The control samples bound 0.6 moles fMet-tRNA$_f^{Met}$ per mole of 70S ribosomes and polymerized 60 - 70 moles phenylalanine per mole of 70S ribosome. Puromycin concentration in the assays was 1 mM.

Ribosomes were incubated with the iodoacetylated puromycin on a preparative scale. Ribosomal subunits were separated by sucrose gradient centrifugation. As can be seen from Fig. 4, label migrated with the 50S and the 30S subunit. Further analysis of the sucrose gradient data showed that approximately 1 mol of label had been attached to the 50S subunit and 0.5 mol to the 30S subunit. It is important to note that reconstitution of 70S ribosomes with either labeled subunit did not restore ribosomal synthesizing activity. In other words, 70S ribosomes, which contained either a labeled 50S or a labeled 30S subunit, exhibited strongly reduced activity. These observations tentatively show that the puromycin label reacts in the peptidyltransferase center at the ribosomal interface with either a 30S or a 50S ribosomal protein.

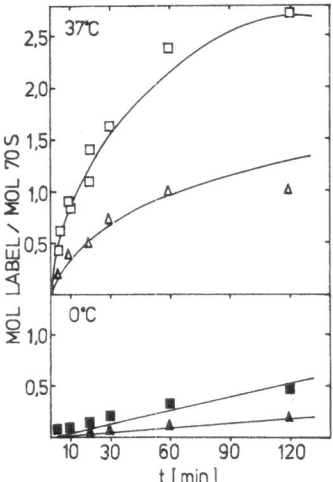

Fig. 3. (A) Time dependence of the reaction of *E. coli* 70S ribosomes with N-iodo-[2-¹⁴C]acetylpuromycin in 10 mM $MgCl_2$, 30 mM NH_4Cl, 10 mM Tris-HCl (pH 7.8) buffer at 37°C ($\square$————$\square$). Concentration of ribosomes were 2×10^{-5} M and of the puromycin analog 10×10^{-5} M. Time dependence of the reaction in the presence of 10^{-2} M puromycin ($\triangle$————$\triangle$). After the times indicated, 10 µl samples were precipitated with 5 % trichloroacetic acid. The precipitate was collected and counted. (B) Time dependence of the reaction of *E. coli* 70S ribosomes with the puromycin analog at 4°C in the absence ($\blacksquare$————$\blacksquare$) and presence ($\blacktriangle$————$\blacktriangle$) of puromycin. Conditions of incubation were the same as in Fig. 1A.

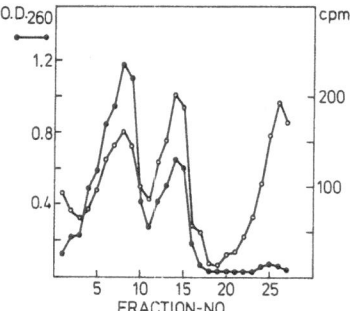

Fig. 4. 10 - 30 % sucrose gradient of 70S ribosomes labeled with N-iodo-[2-¹⁴C]acetylpuromycin for 14 hr at 4°C as described in Fig. 3. Centrifugation, measurement of absorbance and radioactivity was carried out as described in Fig. 2. ($\bullet$————$\bullet$) A_{260}; ($\circ$————$\circ$) cpm.

30S and 50S ribosomal proteins were extracted and then separated by two-dimensional polyacrylamide gel electrophoresis. No radioactivity could be detected in the ribosomal RNA isolated from the labeled subunits. The radioactivity contained in each ribosomal protein was determined and the results are presented in Fig. 5. Protein L6 and to some extent protein L2 were the 50S proteins, which had reacted with the puromycin analog. Therefore, it was concluded that these proteins are associated with the puromycin binding site. Of the 30S proteins, proteins S18 and S14 were found to have most of the radioactivity. Protein S18 contains a very reactive SH-group, which rapidly reacts with iodoacetamide (Moore, 1971). The labeling of S18, therefore, may represent an unspecific reaction rather than a specific one. Proteins S14, L6 and L2, on the other hand, do not readily react with iodoacetamide. S14 is located at the ribosomal interface (Morrison *et al.*, 1974) and stimulates aminoacyl-tRNA binding (Randall-Hazelbauer & Kurland, 1972). This would suggest that the radioactivity detected in protein S14 represents a preferential reaction with the puromycin analog following its binding in the acceptor site.

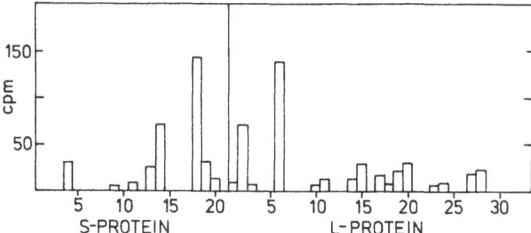

Fig. 5. Radioactivity detected in ribosomal proteins after incubation of 70S ribosomes with N-iodo-[2-^{14}C]acetylpuromycin. *E. coli* 70S ribosomes were incubated with a 10-fold molar excess of affinity label for 12 hr at 4°C in 10 mM MgCl$_2$, 30 mM NH$_4$Cl, 10 mM Tris-HCl (pH 7.8) buffer. Isolation of subunits, separation of proteins and counting of radioactivity was carried out as described (Pongs *et al.*, 1973a).

4. AFFINITY LABELING OF EUKARYOTIC RIBOSOMES WITH N-BROMOACETYL PUROMYCIN

Since puromycin also inhibits protein synthesis in eukaryotes, it was investigated if the puromycin analog did react with proteins of rat liver ribosomes. Fig. 6 shows that this is indeed the case. Furthermore, the amount of labeling depended on the pretreatment of the rat liver ribosomes (Fig. 6). Puromycin treatment of polysomes and breakdown of polysomes to monosomes considerably increased the affinity labeling reaction (Stahl *et al.*, 1974). As observed with *E. coli* ribosomes, the presence of puromycin in the incubation mixture considerably inhibited the labeling reaction. The initial rate of the reaction is lowered by one order of magnitude, if puromycin is added at a 200-fold higher concentration than label. All these data indicate that similar to the reaction with *E. coli* ribosomes, N-bromoacetylpuromycin reacts with rat liver ribosomes in the puromycin binding site of the peptidyltransferase center.

Rat liver ribosomes were treated with the puromycin analog, dissociated into their subunits and the proteins of the subunits were isolated. Again, no significant radioactivity could be detected in the RNA material. The proteins were separated by two dimensional

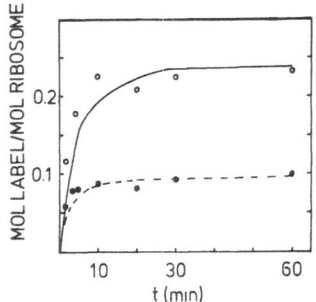

Fig. 6. Time dependence of the labeling of rat liver ribosomes by the puromycin analog. Rat liver polysomes were isolated from a post-mito-chondrial supernatant by the addition of Triton X-100 up to a final concentration of 2 % and were then centrifuged for 90 min at 105 000 xg. The ribosomal pellet was resuspended in 1.5 mM $MgCl_2$, 50 mM KCl, 5 mM Tris-HCl (pH 7.7) buffer. (A) Polysomes (300 A_{260} units/ml) were incubated with the puromycin analog in the resuspension buffer at 37°C. (•————•). At the times indicated, 100 µl aliquots were sampled and the trichloroacetic acid precipitable material was counted.
(B) Polysomes were pretreated with puromycin at 1 mM concentration. Then, they were again incubated with puromycin label under the same conditions as above (o————o).

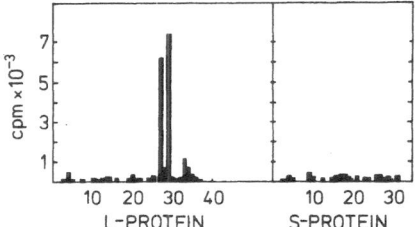

Fig. 7. Radioactivity detected in proteins of rat liver ribosomes after incubation with the puromycin-affinity label. Rat liver ribo-somes were incubated with a fivefold excess of label (54 Ci/mol) for 1 hr at 37°C under the conditions described in Fig. 6. Subunit dis-sociation and isolation and separation of ribosomal proteins were carried out according to Welfle *et al.*, 1971. Each spot, containing a ribosomal protein on the two-dimensional polyacrylamide gels, was cut out and treated with 1 ml 0.5 M hyamine hydroxide in toluene at 50°C overnight. 9 ml toluene-based scintillation fluid, which con-tained 3 % acetic acid and 10 % Triton X-100, were added for counting radioactivity. Similar data have been reported by Stahl *et al.* (1974).

polyacrylamide gel electrophoresis according to Welfle *et al.* (1971). As can be seen from Fig. 7, the puromycin label had almost exclusively reacted with two proteins, namely L27 and L29 of the large subunit. Since the electrophoretic conditions for the separation of rat liver ribosomal proteins and of *E. coli* ribosomal proteins are not identi-cal, it remains to be seen, how much different the *E. coli* and the rat liver puromycin-binding proteins are. It would be interesting to find out if the proteins in the puromycin sensitive site of the pep-tidyltransferase center have been conserved during evolution and if they could possibly be derived from a common ancestor.

5. AFFINITY LABELING WITH A STREPTOMYCIN ANALOG

Streptomycin binds to the small subunit of *E. coli* ribosomes, in contrast to chloramphenicol and puromycin (for a review see Pestka, 1971). Because of its interference with important ribosomal functions, experiments were designed to identify, by affinity labeling, the ribosomal protein(s) which are associated with the streptomycin binding site.

The formyl-residue in position 3 of the streptose moiety of streptomycin was derivatized with p-nitrophenylhydrazine, which yielded the corresponding hydrazone. The hydrazone was reduced to the p-amino compound which then could be bromoacetylated (Reinwald & Pongs, 1974). The antibiotic properties of this bromoacetylated streptomycin were checked in the following manner. Firstly, competition with streptomycin for binding of the streptomycin analog to *E. coli* 70S ribosomes was studied. As can be seen from Fig. 8, the presence of streptomycin inhibits the labeling reaction considerably. Secondly, we investigated the effect of the streptomycin analog on ribosomal activities as compared to that of streptomycin. Thirdly, streptomycin-resistant ribosomes were employed in order to test whether they were also resistant to the streptomycin analog.

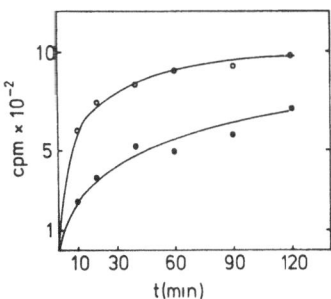

Fig. 8. Time dependence of the reaction of *E. coli* 70S ribosomes with the [2-^{14}C]-bromoacetylated p-aminophenylhydrazone of streptomycin (54 Ci/Mol) in 6 mM MgCl$_2$, 80 mM NH$_4$Cl, 50 mM Tris-HCl (pH 7.4) buffer at 37°C (o———o). Time dependence of the reaction in the presence of 10^{-3} M streptomycin (•———•). Concentrations of ribosomes were 10^{-5} M and of the streptomycin analog 5 x 10^5 M. After the times indicated, aliquots, which contained 1 A$_{260}$ unit of 70S ribosomes, were withdrawn, diluted with 1.5 ml of cold incubation buffer and filtrated over Millipore.

As has already been reported (Pongs & Erdmann, 1973), reaction of the streptomycin analog irreversibly affects the fidelity of protein synthesis. The induction of misreading could be shown to be irreversible. The data of Table 3 show that the bromoacetylated streptomycin also induces release of fMet-tRNA$_f^{Met}$ from the initiation complexes in a manner which is comparable to streptomycin itself (Modolell & Davies, 1970; Lelong *et al.*, 1971). However, this release is not observed in the case of streptomycin resistant ribosomes of the *E. coli* strain L44-1 (kindly provided by Dr. Gorini). The results of experiments which demonstrate that the streptomycin affinity label inhibits f2-mRNA dependent synthesis just as well as streptomycin are summa-

rized in Table 4. Again, no inhibition is seen with streptomycin resistant ribosomes. Furthermore, the inhibition of f2-mRNA dependent
protein synthesis is irreversible. On the other hand, *in vitro* poly(U)
dependent polyphenylalanine synthesis is not inhibited, but misreading
was induced by the affinity label (Pongs & Erdmann, 1973). These data
show that the derivatization of the formyl-moiety of streptomycin
does not alter its *in vitro* antibiotic properties.

Table 3

RELEASE OF fMet-tRNA$_f^{Met}$ FROM THE INITIATION COMPLEX BY STREPTOMYCIN
AND BROMOACETYLATED STREPTOMYCIN ANALOG

Antibiotic	Release of fMet-tRNA$_f^{Met}$ in %	
	Ribosomal source from	
	E.coli A19	*E.coli* L44-1
Streptomycin	76	100
Bromoacetylated p-aminophenyl-hydrazone of streptomycin	68	95
None	100	100

Initiation complex formation was carried out according to Hershey *et
al.* (1971). After initiation 20 µg/ml antibiotic were added and incubations were continued for 15 min at 30°C and then assayed by millipore filtration. Streptomycin-sensitive *E. coli* A19 and streptomycin-
resistant L44-1 ribosomes bound comparable amounts of fMet-tRNA$_f^{Met}$
(0.6 - 0.7 mole tRNA/mole 70S), of which 80 % were puromycin-sensitive.

Table 4

f2mRNA-DIRECTED SYNTHESIS WITH STREPTOMYCIN-RESISTANT AND STREPTO-
MYCIN-SENSITIVE RIBOSOMES AFTER INCUBATION WITH STREPTOMYCIN ANALOG

Antibiotic	f2mRNA-directed ribosomal activity in %	
	E. coli A19	*E. coli* L44-1
Streptomycin	10	86
Streptomycin analog	11	81
None	100	100

After incubation of 70S ribosomes with a 5-fold excess of streptomycin
analog for 2 hr at 37°C in 6 mM MgCl$_2$, 80 mM NH$_4$Cl, 50 mM Tris-HCl
(pH 7.4) buffer, the ribosomes were exhaustively dialyzed against the
incubation buffer overnight at 4°C. Then aliquots containing 1.5 A$_{260}$
units of ribosomes were examined for f2mRNA-directed ribosomal activity as described (Erdmann *et al.*, 1971). Streptomycin concentration
in the assays was 20 µg/ml.

Ribosomes were then incubated on a preparative scale with the streptomycin affinity label in order to identify the ribosomal protein(s), which were close to the streptomycin binding site. The first analyses tentatively show that protein S4 is the major target with which our streptomycin analog preferentially reacts (unpublished results). These data fit quite well with genetic data which showed that protein S4 is the *ram* gene product (Zimmermann *et al.*, 1971). This indicates that protein S4 is located in the neighborhood of the streptomycin binding site and, thereby, can influence the conformation of this site.

6. CONCLUDING REMARKS

Since chloramphenicol, puromycin and streptomycin inhibit protein synthesis by interfering with particular steps of the translational process, the identification of the binding sites of these antibiotics is also a tool to shed light on the detailed structure of the active sites of ribosomes (Pongs *et al.*, 1974). Thus, the data presented in this paper also indicate that proteins L6 and L16 are situated in the acceptor site of *E. coli* ribosomes and that protein S4 is near or at the ribosomal decoding site.

REFERENCES

Bald, R., V.A. Erdmann and O. Pongs: Irreversible binding of chloramphenicol analogues to *E.coli* ribosomes. FEBS Lett. 28, 149-152 (1972).

Erdmann, V.A., S. Fahnestock, K. Higo and M. Nomura: Role of 5S RNA in the functions of 50S ribosomal subunits. Proc. Nat. Acad. Sci. USA 68, 2932-2936 (1971).

Hershey, J.W.B., E. Remold-O'Donnell, D. Kolakofsky, K.F. Dewey and R.E. Thach: Isolation and Purification of Initiation factors. Methods in Enzymology 20, 235-247 (1971).

Kaltschmidt, E. and H.G. Wittmann: Ribosomal proteins. XII.: Number of proteins in small and large ribosomal subunits of *Escherichia coli* as determined by two-dimensional gel electrophoresis. Proc. Nat. Acad. Sci. USA 67, 1276-1282 (1970).

Lelong, J.C., M.A. Cousin, D. Gros, M. Grunberg-Manago and F. Gros: Streptomycin induced release of fmet-tRNA from the ribosomal initiation complex. Biochem. Biophys. Res. Commun. 42, 530-537 (1971).

Modolell, J. and B.D. Davies: Breakdown by Streptomycin of Initiation Complexes Formed on Ribosomes of *Escherichia coli*. Proc. Nat. Acad. Sci. USA 67, 1148-1155 (1970).

Moore, P.B.: Reaction of N-ethyl maleimide with the Ribosomes of *Escherichia coli*. J. Mol. Biol. 60, 169-184 (1971).

Morrison, C.A., R.A. Garrett, H. Zeichhardt and G. Stöffler: Proteins occurring at, or near, the subunit interface of *E.coli* ribosomes. Molec. Gen. Genet., in press (1974).

Nierhaus, D. and K. Nierhaus: Identification of the chloramphenicol-binding protein in *Escherichia coli* ribosomes by partial reconstitution. Proc. Nat. Acad. Sci. USA 70, 2224-2228 (1973).

Nomura, M. and J.D. Watson: Ribonucleoprotein particles within chloromycetin inhibited *E.coli*. J. Mol. Biol. 1, 204-217 (1959).

Pestka, S.: Inhibitors of Ribosome Functions. Ann. Rev. Microbiol. 25, 487-562 (1971).

Pongs, O., R. Bald and V.A. Erdmann: Identification of Chloramphenicol - Binding Protein in *Escherichia coli* Ribosomes by Affinity Labeling. Proc. Nat. Acad. Sci. USA 70, 2229-2233 (1973a).

Pongs, O., R. Bald, T. Wagner and V.A. Erdmann: Irreversible Binding of N-iodoacetylpuromycin to *E.coli* Ribosomes. FEBS Lett. 35, 137-140 (1973b).

Pongs, O. and V.A. Erdmann: Affinity Labeling of *E.coli* ribosomes with a Streptomycin Analog. FEBS Lett. 35, 137-140 (1973).

Pongs, O., K.H. Nierhaus, V.A. Erdmann and H.G. Wittmann: Active Sites in *Escherichia coli* Ribosomes. FEBS Lett. 40, 528-537 (1974).

Randall-Hazelbauer, L.L. and C.G. Kurland: Identification of three 30S proteins contributing to the ribosomal A-site. Molec. Gen. Genet. 115, 234-242 (1972).

Reinwald, E. and O. Pongs: Identification of ribosomal proteins associated with the streptomycin binding site by affinity labeling. Manuscript in preparation (1974).

Stahl, J., K. Dressler and H. Bielka: Studies on proteins of animal ribosomes. XVIII. Affinity labeling of rat liver ribosomes by N-bromoacetylpuromycin. FEBS Lett., in press (1974).

Vazquez, D.: The binding of chloramphenicol by ribosomes from *Bacillus megaterium*. Biochem. Biophys. Res. Commun. 15, 464-468 (1964).

Welfle, H., J. Stahl and H. Bielka: Studies on Proteins of Animal Ribosomes. Biochim. Biophys. Acta 243, 416-428 (1971).

Wolfe, D. and F.E. Hahn: Effects of chloramphenicol upon a ribosomal amino acid polymerization system and its binding to bacterial ribosomes. Biochim. Biophys. Acta 95, 146-155 (1965).

Yarmolinski, M.B. and G. de la Haba: Inhibition by Puromycin of Amino Acid Incorporation into Protein. Proc. Nat. Acad. Sci. USA 45, 1721-1729 (1959).

IV. The Mode of Action of Chloramphenicol

Antibiotic Action on the Ribosomal Peptidyl Transferase Centre

D. Vazquez, M. Barbacid, and R. Fernandez-Muñoz

The peptidyl transferase centre

Peptide bond formation in protein synthesis takes place by linkage of the carboxyl group at the C-terminal end of the peptidyl residue held in the ribosomal P-site with the α-NH_2 group of the amino acid held in the ribosomal A-site.

Since it was originally thought that the peptide bond forming reaction involved GTP, the hypothetical enzyme was termed *peptide synthetase*, by analogy with certain other nucleoside triphosphate-requiring enzymes. However, the demonstration that GTP is not directly involved shows that the enzyme does not belong to the class of enzymes termed synthetases. Since the reaction takes place by simple transfer of a peptidyl group from tRNA to aminoacyl-tRNA it may be classified along with other group transfer reactions, not involving nucleoside triphosphates, which are catalysed by the group of enzymes known generically as *transferases*. For this reason the operational name *peptidyl transferase* has been proposed (Monro *et al.*, 1967) and is widely accepted. The peptidyl transferase is also implicated in the peptidyl-tRNA hydrolytic activity associated with termination and thus any conditions blocking peptidyl transferase activity have been found to block also peptidyl-tRNA hydrolysis (Caskey *et al.*, 1969; Capecchi & Klein, 1969; Beaudet & Caskey, 1972). A detailed model of the active centre of peptidyl transferase has recently been proposed (Harris & Symons, 1973a).

The puromycin reaction

Some well defined experimental systems have been used to study peptide bond formation isolated from other reactions leading to protein synthesis. Most of these systems take advantage of the antibiotic puromycin, an analogue of the 3'-terminal aminoacyl-adenosine moiety of aminoacyl-tRNA and, therefore, a suitable acceptor substrate for peptide bond formation in a reaction in which the α-NH_2 group of puromycin becomes linked to the C-terminal end of the peptidyl group (*puromycin reaction*). Puromycin lacks that part of the molecule of aminoacyl-tRNA responsible for interaction with mRNA, with the small ribosomal subunit and, probably, with some sites on the large subunit. Consequently, the product of the reaction (peptidyl-puromycin) is released from the ribosome and polypeptide chain elongation is interrupted.

The puromycin reaction was initially characterised by incubating washed, polyphenylalanyl-tRNA-charged ribosomes with puromycin (Traut & Monro, 1964; Maden & Monro, 1968; Maden *et al.*, 1968). It was shown that the reaction is unaffected by the washing of the ribosomes or by the presence of aminoacyl-tRNA, deacylated tRNA or poly U, but that it is completely dependent on divalent and monovalent cations. The reaction occurs on the large ribosomal subunit and does not require GTP or supernatant factors. Moreover, the reaction is not impaired by inhibitors of the supernatant factors or by the GTP analogue $Gpp(CH_2)p$.

The validity of these results has been verified with other systems. Binding of either fMet-tRNA$_F$ (directed by AUG) or polylysyl-tRNA (directed by poly A) or Ac-Phe-tRNA (directed by poly U), under suitable ionic conditions, takes place to the ribosomal P-site. When ribosomes charged with fMet-tRNA$_F$ or polylysyl-tRNA are treated with puromycin, fMet-puromycin or polylysyl-puromycin is formed (Rychlik, 1966; Bretscher & Marcker, 1966; Zamir *et al.*, 1966; Haenni & Lucas-Lenard, 1968). The requirements for these reactions are the same as those for the reaction with polyphenylalanyl-tRNA. Moreover no supernatant factors are required, thus confirming the location of the peptidyl transferase on the ribosome. Similar results have been obtained with a system in which oligolysyl-tRNA and lysyl-tRNA are non-enzymically bound to ribosomes at the P- and A-sites, respectively (Gottesman, 1971). The binding is followed by formation of a peptide bond by transfer of the polylysyl-residue to the α-NH$_2$ group of lysyl-tRNA. Although the above experiments have been performed with bacterial systems, similar conclusions have been reached for eukaryotic systems since nascent peptides attached to washed rat liver ribosomes are reactive with puromycin in the absence of supernatant factors (Skogerson & Moldave, 1968a, 1968b). Nascent peptides of polysomes isolated from bacterial and mammalian cells also react with puromycin (Pestka, 1972; Pestka *et al.*, 1972a).

The fragment reaction

Location of the peptidyl transferase centre on the large ribosomal subunit of either prokaryotic (Monro *et al.*, 1969) or eukaryotic (Vazquez *et al.*, 1969) ribosomes was demonstrated by forming peptide bonds with a very simplified system described as the *fragment reaction*. The terminal fragments CACCA-, AACCA-, ACCA- and CCA-Metf from fMet-tRNA$_F$ undergo a ribosome-catalysed reaction with puromycin to yield fMet-puromycin. The reaction requires only the large ribosomal subunit (Monro, 1967; Vazquez *et al.*, 1969), monovalent and divalent cations, and either methanol or ethanol (Monro, 1967; Maden & Monro, 1968; Monro *et al.*, 1969; Vazquez *et al.*, 1969). The small subunit or mRNA are not required, but they can stimulate the peptidyl-transferase activity of the large subunit in certain experimental systems (Berman & Monier, 1971).

The fragment reaction is limited to a region of the large ribosomal subunit in the immediate vicinity of the catalytic centre, since the substrates used (fMet-oligonucleotide and puromycin) are of small size. Hence, it can be expected that interactions which normally take place between tRNA and other regions of the ribosome are absent in the fragment reaction. However, the reaction also works with either fMet-tRNA$_F$, or acetyl-aminoacyl-tRNA, or acetyl-aminoacyl-oligonucleotides as donor substrates (Skogerson & Moldave, 1968a; Monro *et al.*, 1968; Vogel *et al.*, 1969).

A number of protein synthesis inhibitors have been shown to specifically block the peptidyl transferase activity of bacterial ribosomes

(chloramphenicol, lincomycin, spiramycin III, carbomycin, streptogramin A, sparsomycin, amicetin and gougerotin) (Monro, 1967; Monro
& Vazquez, 1967; Contreras *et al.*, 1974) and eukaryotic ribosomes
(anisomycin, trichodermin, tenuazonic acid, sparsomycin, amicetin and
gougerotin (Vazquez *et al.*, 1969; Battaner & Vazquez, 1971; Carrasco
et al., 1973). It is likely that many of these antibiotics interact
specifically with the peptidyl transferase centre.

Binding of substrates to donor site

Considerable efforts have been dedicated to studying the binding
of substrates to the donor and the acceptor sites of the peptidyl
transferase centre. Only 3'-aminoacyl esters are recognised by both
sites (Hussain & Ofengand, 1973). Interaction of substrates with the
donor site is favoured by acylation of the α-amino group of the aminoacyl residue attached to the adenosine and is influenced by the nature
of the amino acid (Monro *et al.*, 1968). Thus, CACCA-Leu-Ac binds to
the donor site of the peptidyl transferase centre (Celma *et al.*, 1970).
This reaction is inhibited by lincomycin, streptrogramin A, spiramycin III and carbomycin in bacterial 50S subunits (Celma *et al.*,
1970) and by anisomycin in eukaryotic ribosomes (Battaner & Vazquez,
1971). Sparsomycin enhances CACCA-Leu-Ac binding, presumably to the
donor site of the peptidyl transferase centre (Monro *et al.*, 1969;
Battaner & Vazquez, 1971). One molecule of the substrate is bound per
50S subunit at saturation, clearly suggesting that there is a single
peptidyl transferase centre per ribosome (Monro *et al.*, 1969). Interaction of substrates at the donor site of the peptidyl transferase
centre is dependent on the length of the oligonucleotide chain. A
minimal requirement for the CCA 3'-terminal oligonucleotide has been
initially suggested (Monro *et al.*, 1968; Mercer & Symons, 1972) since
either CA-Metf or CA-Leu-Ac were found to be inactive as donor substrates. However, it has been more recently reported that pA-Metf can
act as a donor substrate, although it has a much lower affinity than
substrates with longer oligonucleotides (Černá *et al.*, 1973a).

Binding of substrates to acceptor site

CACCA-Phe (Pestka, 1969; Hishizawa & Pestka, 1971) and CACCA-Leu
(Battaner & Vazquez, 1971; Celma *et al.*, 1971) have been found to
interact with the acceptor site of the large subunit from bacterial
and eukaryotic ribosomes. This interaction is inhibited in bacterial
subunits, by chloramphenicol, sparsomycin, amicetin, spiramycin III,
streptogramin A and lincomycin (Hishizawa & Pestka, 1971; Celma *et
al.*, 1971) and in eukaryotic ribosomes by anisomycin, trichodermin
and tenuazonic acid (Battaner & Vazquez, 1971; Carrasco *et al.*, 1973;
Carrasco & Vazquez, 1973). Activity of the acceptor substrate is dependent on the length of the oligonucleotide moiety (Hussain &
Ofengand, 1972) but only the 3'-terminal adenosine seems to be an
absolute requirement. Thus, not only puromycin but also L-Phe- and
L-Tyr-3'-adenosine are active substrates in bacterial and mammalian
systems (Waller *et al.*, 1966; Harbon & Chapeville, 1970; Gottikh *et
al.*, 1970). Further studies (Nathans & Neidle, 1963; Harris *et al.*,
1971; Hengesh & Morris, 1973; Rychlik *et al.*, 1969; Rychlik *et al.*,
1970; Černá *et al.*, 1970) with different nucleotides and puromycin
derivatives have shown that (a) 3'-o-aminoacyl nucleosides are the
simplest acceptor substrates; (b) their activity depends on the nucleoside moiety and it decreases in the sequence A-Phe>I-Phe>C-Phe,
and G-Phe and U-Phe are totally inactive; (c) a free 2-OH group in
the ribose moiety is required; and (d) the acceptor activity depends

on the aminoacyl moiety, the L-configuration being required and substrates with aromatic amino acids being the most active. Moreover, using different CCA-aminoacyl substrates it has been found that the order of activity is:CCA-Phe>CCA-Leu>CCA-Lys>CCA-Ser>CCA-Ala>CCA-Glu (Lessard & Pestka, 1972). Other workers have also confirmed the preferential activity of donor substrates with hydrophobic amino acids (Mao, 1973).

The binding of puromycin to the large ribosomal subunit is inhibited by some puromycin analogues active as acceptor substrates, and by chloramphenicol and lincomycin, antibiotics that affect the acceptor site of the peptidyl transferase centre (Fernandez-Muñoz & Vazquez, 1973a). Conversely, binding of these antibiotics to the ribosome is inhibited by puromycin (Fernandez-Muñoz et $al.$, 1971). It has been shown that a high affinity, single site interaction of chloramphenicol with the 50S subunit is responsible for blocking the activity of the peptidyl transferase centre (Fernandez-Muñoz & Vazquez, 1973b).

Ribosomal components implicated in peptidyl transferase

Ribosomal proteins. A series of protein deficient particles (α,β,γ-cores) can be prepared from 50S subunits by isopycnic centrifugation in CsCl solutions of decreasing Mg^{2+} concentrations (Monro et $al.$, 1969). The cores contain 23S and 5S RNA but lack increasing numbers of 50S proteins. The β-cores, which lack proteins L1, L7, L12, L25 and L23 and have reduced amounts of L6, L16 and L31 (Nierhaus & Montejo, 1973), possess good activity for catalysis of the fragment reaction, for chloramphenicol and lincomycin binding, and for binding of CACCA-Leu-Ac (Monro et $al.$, 1969). In contrast, the γ-cores, which lack proteins L1, L6, L7, L10, L12, L15, L16, L25, L31 and L33 and have reduced amounts of L5, L8, L9, L11, L18, L20, L27, L28 and L30 are devoid of these activities (Monro et $al.$, 1969; Nierhaus & Montejo, 1973). Restoration of activity can be achieved by readdition to the γ-cores of the proteins separated in the conversion β- → γ-core (Monro et $al.$, 1969; Ballesta et $al.$, 1971). Similarly, protein depleted cores, prepared by treatment of 50S subunits with 0.4 or 0.8 M LiCl (Homan & Nierhaus, 1971) lack peptidyl transferase activity (Nierhaus & Montejo, 1973). The activity is reconstituted by addition of the split proteins. Reconstitution with partially purified split protein fractions, has shown that protein L11 is required for peptidyl transferase activity of 0.4 M LiCl cores (Nierhaus & Montejo, 1973) and protein L16 is required for chloramphenicol binding (Nierhaus & Nierhaus, 1973). However a comparison of the 50S proteins resistant to 2-methoxy-5-nitrotropone treatment with those present on CsCl-derived cores points to protein L15 as possibly involved in the peptidyl transferase centre of the ribosome (Ballesta et $al.$, 1974). Proteins other than L11, L15 and L16 may be implicated in the acceptor and the donor sites of the peptidyl transferase centre, since γ-cores, depleted of both proteins, still bind [^{3}H]puromycin (Table 1) and CACCA-Leu-Ac (Nierhaus & Montejo, 1973).

N-bromoacetyl and N-iodoacetyl derivatives of chloramphenicol have been used for affinity labelling of $E.$ $coli$ ribosomes in other attempts to identify the proteins involved in the peptidyl transferase centre. However, there are discrepancies in the results obtained, since ribosomal proteins L2 and L27 were labelled in one work (Sonenberg et $al.$, 1973) and proteins L16 and L24 were labelled in another study (Pongs et $al.$, 1973). It has been found that 2-diazomalonyl-puromycin and chloramphenicol azide mostly label one protein band of the 50S subunit not yet identified but minor labelling of other ribosomal proteins was observed (Leick *et al.*, 1973). Binding of p-nitrophenyl-carbamyl-Phe-tRNA results in the labelling of proteins L27, L16, L15, L14 and/or L13 (Czernilofsky & Kuechler, 1972; Czernilofsky *et al.*, 1973), where-as N-bromoacetyl-Phe-tRNA reacts with proteins L2 and L27 (Pellegrini *et al.*, 1973).

Ribosomal RNA. Digestion of 50S subunits with ribonuclease T_1 results in the loss of peptidyl transferase activity. The inactivation seems to affect only the donor site of the active centre since the treatment prevents binding of CACCA-Leu-Ac to the peptidyl transferase centre without affecting the binding of CACCA-Phe (Černá *et al.*, 1973b). 5S ribosomal RNA is required for peptidyl transferase activity of 50S subunits since reconstituted particles deprived of 5S RNA are not active in peptide bond formation (Erdmann *et al.*, 1971a). However the 3'-end of 5S RNA can be modified without affecting the peptidyl transferase activity of the 50S subunit (Fahnestock & Nomura, 1972; Erdmann *et al.*, 1971b). Affinity labelling experiments using Br-puromycin binds to the RNA of the larger ribosome subunit (Harris *et al.*, 1973). This finding explains the results presented in Table 1 in which [^{3}H]puromycin was observed to bind to γ-cores which are deprived of proteins L11, L15 and L16, reported as implicated.

Table 1

[^3H]*Puromycin binding to 50S ribosomal subunits and derived cores*

Conditions	[^3H]Puromycin bound (pMoles/tube)
Expt. 1	
50S	1.80
γ-cores	2.10
$SP_{50-\gamma}$	0.87
γ-cores + $SP_{50-\gamma}$	2.44
Expt. 2	
50S	2.24
γ-cores	2.04
$SP_{50-\gamma}$	0.11

[^{3}H]Puromycin binding to 50S subunits, 50S-derived γ-cores and the split protein fraction released in the obtention of γ-cores from 50S subunits ($SP_{50-\gamma}$) was studied by equilibrium dialysis (Fernandez-Muñoz & Vazquez, 1973a). Concentration of [^{3}H]puromycin was 10^{-6}M. 50S subunits were added when indicated at 12.5 mg/ml. γ-cores (15 mg/ml) and the corresponding amount of the $SP_{50-\gamma}$ fraction were added when required. Equilibrium dialysis was carried out for 10 hours at 4°C. In Experiment 1 the indicated particles or protein fractions were preincubated, prior to the equilibrium dialysis, in 20 mM Tris-HCl buffer pH 8.0 containing 20 mM Mg, 0.1 M NH₄ and 3 mM 2-mercapto-ethanol for 90 min at 50°C. No such preincubation was performed in Experiment 2. Experiments 1 and 2 were carried out simultaneously with the same batch of ribosomes.

Antibiotics acting on the peptidyl transferase centre

Evidence for antibiotic interaction with the peptidyl transferase centre has been obtained from (a) their inhibitory effect on peptide bond formation and/or substrate binding, (b) direct binding of peptide bond formation inhibitors to ribosomes or ribosomal subunits, (c) inhibition of binding to ribosomes of peptide bond formation inhibitors and (d) identification of some common ribosomal components for the peptidyl transferase centre and the binding site(s) of the inhibitors. Many antibiotics have been reported to inhibit peptide bond formation in certain systems (Table 2) (Vazquez, 1974; Gale *et al.*, 1972; reviews) but very few of them have been confirmed to act on the peptidyl transferase centre according to the four criteria (and) indicated above. The ribosome suffers important conformational changes during translation and it is possible that some inhibitors block peptidyl transferase under certain conditions without specifically acting on the active centre. Therefore only complying with the four criteria indicated above would definitively demonstrate that the site of action of an antibiotic is located on the peptidyl transferase centre.

Antibiotic binding sites of the ribosomal peptidyl transferase

In order to study the ribosomal peptidyl transferase centre and to determine the site of action of the antibiotics presented in Table 2 we have carried out studies on antibiotic binding to the ribosome for the last ten years. Hence we have studied quantitative binding to bacterial ribosomes of [^{14}C]chloramphenicol (Vazquez, 1964; Vazquez, 1966; Fernandez-Muñoz *et al.*, 1971), [^{14}C]thiamphenicol (Contreras *et al.*, 1974), [^{14}C]lincomycin (Fernandez-Muñoz *et al.*, 1971), [^{14}C] clindamycin (Monro *et al.*, 1971), [^{14}C]spiramycin (Vazquez, 1967), [^{14}C]eryhtromycin (Fernandez-Muñoz *et al.*, 1971; Fernandez-Muñoz & Vazquez, 1973c), [^{3}H]streptogramin A (Contreras & Vazquez, unpublished results), [^{3}H]puromycin (Fernandez-Muñoz *et al.*, 1973a) and [^{3}H] gougerotin (Barbacid & Vazquez, 1974a). We have also studied quantitative binding to eukaryotic ribosomes of [^{3}H]gougerotin (Barbacid & Vazquez, 1974a), [^{3}H]anisomycin (Barbacid & Vazquez, 1974b) and [^{14}C]trichodermin (Barbacid & Vazquez, 1974c).

Puromycin is an active acceptor substrate in the fragment reaction assay. Erythromycin does not inhibit the fragment reaction (Monro & Vazquez, 1967), and is not considered an inhibitor of peptidyl transferase (Vazquez, 1974; Gale *et al.*, 1972; reviews), but blocks the inhibitory effect of chloramphenicol (Monro *et al.*, 1970) and lincomycin (Monro *et al.*, 1971) in the fragment reaction assay. All the other antibiotics indicated above are active inhibitors of the fragment reaction. Therefore we have studied binding of the above antibiotics to ribosomes under the ionic and solvent conditions of the fragment reaction. The parameters K_d (dissociation constant) and $\bar{v}$ (number of binding sites) have been determined. In most cases we have also studied the binding of the radioactive antibiotics in the absence of ethanol and under ionic conditions more physiological than those of the fragment reaction assay (see References indicated above). All these studies showed that there is a single site interaction of higher affinity for the antibiotics on the ribosome and hence a single peptidyl transferase centre.

Thus, in order to know the relationship between chloramphenicol binding to the ribosome and its inhibition of the fragment reaction we have studied both reactions under identical conditions (Fig. 1). As shown in Fig. 1A 10^{-4} M chloramphenicol totally blocks the initial rate of the fragment reaction. It is presented in Fig. 1B the Scatchard plot of data obtained in [^{14}C]chloramphenicol binding studies to ribosomes, showing that there is a preferential interaction of one molecule of the antibiotic per ribosome with a $\underline{K}_d$ = 2.2 x 10^{-6} M. At the highest concentrations of the antibiotic used there is a significant deviation from linearity since there are other binding site(s) for the antibiotic with much lower affinity. It is difficult to precisely evaluate the $\underline{K}_d$ of this lower affinity interaction which would be at least of one order of magnitude higher than the other binding.

Table 2

Antibiotics reported to inhibit peptide bond formation in cell-free systems

---

Acting on prokaryotic ribosomes	*Acting on prokaryotic and eukaryotic systems*
Althiomycin	***Actinobolin
Chloramphenicol group:	***Amicetin
Chloramphenicol	Blasticidin S
D-AMP-3	Gougerotin
D-Win-5094	Puromycin
Thiamphenicol	Sparsomycin
Lincomycin group:	
Celesticetin	*Acting on eukaryotic systems*
Clindamycin	Anisomycin
Lincomycin	*Cycloheximide
Macrolides group:	Tenuazonic acid
Carbomycins	Trichodermin group:
*Erythromycin	Fusarenon X
*Forocidins	Trichodermin
Leucomycins	Trichodermol
*Neospiramycins	Trichothecin
Niddamycin	Verrucarin A
*Oleandomycin	
Spiramycins	
Tylosin	
**Streptogramin A group:	
Griseoviridin	
Ostreogrycin G	
Streptogramin A	

---

*Inhibition of peptide bond formation by these antibiotics has been observed only in very specific systems using either certain substrates or special ionic conditions.

**Inhibitors of peptide bond formation in eukaryotic ribosomes using concentrations 100-500 higher than in bacterial ribosomes.

***Rather poor inhibitors in eukaryotic systems.

Data taken from Vazquez (1974).

However, considering that for the higher affinity binding of chloramphenicol, K_d = 2.2 x 10^{-6} M, at a concentration of 10^{-4} M of the antibiotic, which totally inhibits the fragment reaction (Fig. 1A), there is a saturation of $\bar{\nu} \approx$ 0.9 - 1.0 (Fig. 1B). Therefore it is obvious that any possible chloramphenicol binding sites with lower affinities are not relevant for the inhibitory effect of the antibiotic in the fragment reaction (Fernandez-Muñoz *et al.*, 1971; Fernandez-Muñoz & Vazquez, 1973b).

There is a clear evidence of the relationship between the peptidyl transferase centre and the sites of interaction of our peptidyl transferase inhibitors. This evidence comes from our studies on the requirements, characteristics and activities of this ribosomal area. Thus, kinetics of the fragment reaction by yeast ribosomes were studied following the initial rate of the reaction in the presence of different concentrations of anisomycin. The data were plotted as a percentage of the control reaction in the absence of anisomycin (Fig. 2A) showing total identity of this experimental curve with the theoretical one obtained assuming that formation of the anisomycin-ribosome complex in the conditions of the fragment reaction $K_d^{ethanol}$ = 3.6 x 10^{-6} M) by 42 % of the ribosomes (Fig. 2B) is responsible for

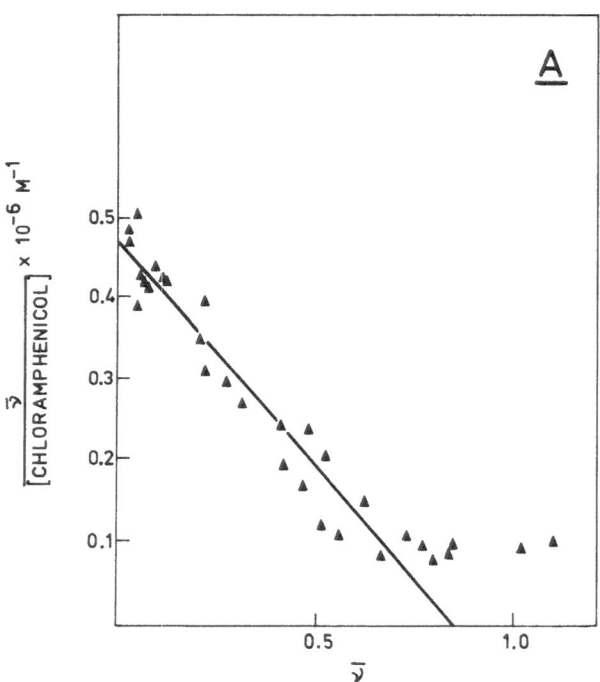

Fig. 1A. Scatchard plot of data for [^{14}C]chloramphenicol binding to *E. coli* ribosomes from an ethanol-precipitation assay (Fernandez-Muñoz *et al*, 1971). The ribosome concentrations were 6.80 and 11.8 mg/ml and the concentrations of added [^{14}C]chloramphenicol were 0.075 to 13 µM. Incubation time was 30 min at 0°C. Extrapolation of the linear portion gives values of $\bar{\nu}$ = 0.81 and $\underline{K}$ = 2.2 x 10^{-6} M.

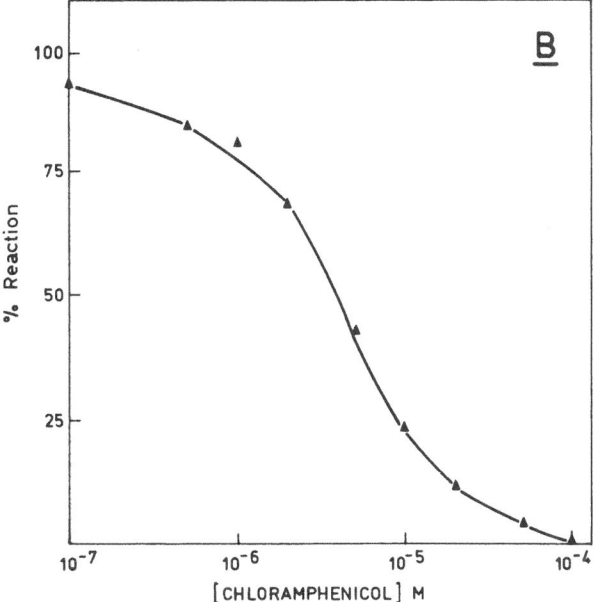

Fig. 1B. Inhibition by chloramphenicol of Ac-[^{14}C]Leu-puromycin formation. Concentrations of CACCA-[^{14}C]Leu-Ac and puromycin were 6 x 10^{-7} M and 5 x 10^{-4} M respectively. Reactions were started by addition of 33% (v/v) ethanol and samples were taken at 3 min of incubation at 0°C.

Ribosome batch and ethanol and ionic conditions were the same in both experiments *A* and *B* (Fernandez-Muñoz and Vazquez, 1973b).

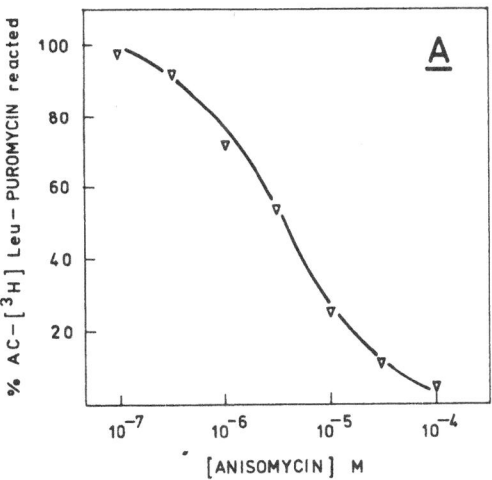

Fig. 2A. The effect of anisomycin on the fragment reaction by yeast ribosomes. 0.24 pmol CACCA-[^{3}H]Leu-Ac was incubated for 20 min at 0°C in the presence of 1 mM puromycin and 25 pmol ribosomes in a total volume of 100 μl; ethanol at a final concentration 33% (v/v) was added to start the reaction.

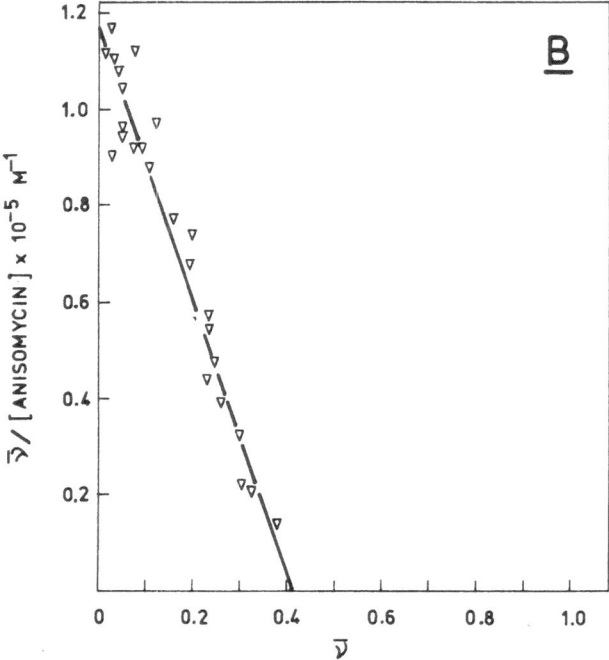

Fig. 2B. Scatchard plot of [³H]anisomycin binding to yeast ribosomes
from an ethanol-precipitation assay. Ribosome concentrations were
2 x 10⁻⁶ M for [³H]anisomycin concentrations ranging from 10⁻⁷ to
10⁻⁶ M for [³H]anisomycin concentrations from 10⁻⁶ to 10⁻⁵ M, and
6 x 10⁻⁶ M for [³H]anisomycin concentrations above 10⁻⁵ M. Extrapolation of the linear plot gives values of $\bar{\nu}$ = 0.42 and K_D = 3.6 x 10⁻⁶
M. Ribosome batch and ethanol and ionic conditions were the same in
both experiments *A* and *B* (Barbacid and Vazquez, 1974b).

the inhibition of peptide bond formation. Since there is a total inhibition of peptide bond formation in the presence of 10⁻⁴ M anisomycin it is obvious that only those ribosomes which are active in the
presence of ethanol for [³H]anisomycin binding can be active for
peptide bond formation (Barbacid & Vazquez, 1974b).

Selectivity in antibiotic interaction with the peptidyl transferase
centre correlates with specificity observed with the antibiotics in
their inhibitory effect on peptide bond formation. Thus tenuazonic
acid and anisomycin inhibit peptide bond formation by human tonsil
ribosomes and bind to this type of ribosomes at mutually exclusive
sites (Fig. 3A). Whereas tenuazonic acid is a good inhibitor of [³H]
anisomycin binding to human tonsil ribosomes, it has a smaller effect
on binding of this radioactive antibiotic to yeast ribosomes (Fig. 3B)
showing that tenuazonic acid has a higher affinity for human tonsil
than for yeast ribosomes (Barbacid & Vazquez, 1974b). These results
agree with our previous observations that tenuazonic acid is a good
inhibitor of peptide bond formation by human tonsil ribosomes but
has a low activity on yeast ribosomes (Carrasco & Vazquez, 1973).

Binding and competition experiments demonstrated that there are
at least two rather independent areas of antibiotic interaction on

the peptidyl transferase centre as shown schematically in Figs. 4 and 5. One of these areas appears to be common to the larger subunit of both prokaryotic and eukaryotic ribosomes (the *gougerotin-sparsomycin area*) whereas the other one has a higher specificity. Thus the *chloramphenicol area* can be distinguished in the peptidyl transferase centre of bacterial ribosomes (Fig. 4) but is absent in eukaryotic ribosomes. Conversely the *anisomycin area* is present in eukaryotic (Fig. 5) but not in prokaryotic ribosomes. However a number of antibiotics of these different areas have in common their inhibitory effect on binding of puromycin (Fernandez-Muñoz & Vazquez, 1973a) and acceptor substrate (Celma *et al.*, 1970, 1971) explaining their inhibitory effect on the fragment reaction assay. A detailed model of the interaction sites of antibiotics on the peptidyl transferase centre has recently been proposed (Harris & Symons, 1973b).

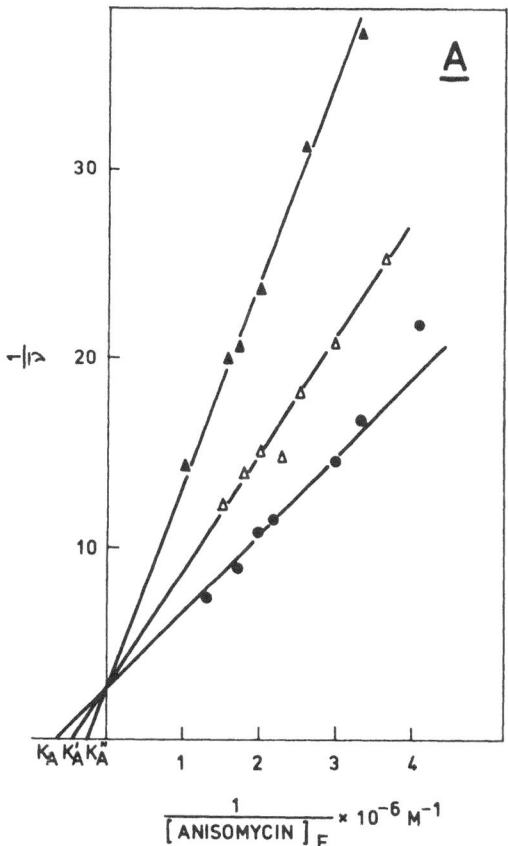

Fig. 3A. Calculation of the affinity constant of tenuazonic acid for human tonsil ribosomes. (●—●) Klotz plot for [^{3}H]anisomycin binding in the absence of tenuazonic acid (K_D = 1.7 x 10^{-6} M); (△—△) Klotz plot for [^{3}H]anisomycin binding in the presence of 10^{-5} M tenuazonic acid; (▲—▲) Klotz plot for [^{3}H]anisomycin binding in the presence of 3 x 10^{-5} M tenuazonic acid. Ribosome concentration was 3 x 10^{-6} M. {^{3}H}anisomycin concentration was ranging from 0.5 to 1.5 x 10^{-6} M. The experiment was carried out at 0°C following the sedimentation method in the absence of ethanol.

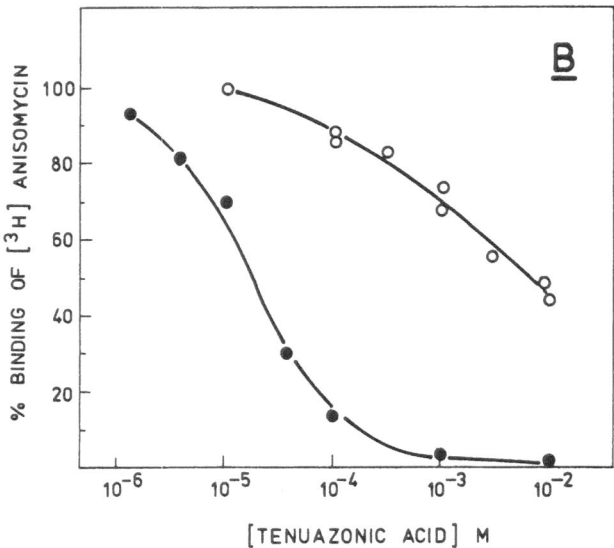

Fig. 3B. Effect of tenuazonic acid on [³H]anisomycin binding to ribosomes.
(O—O) Yeast ribosomes and (●—●) human tonsil ribosomes. Data were taken
from an assay following the sedimentation method in the absence of
ethanol. Yeast ribosome concentration was 2.5×10^{-6} M. Human tonsil
ribosome concentration was 3.5×10^{-6} M. [³H]anisomycin concentration
was in all cases 10^{-6} M (Barbacid and Vazquez, 1974b).

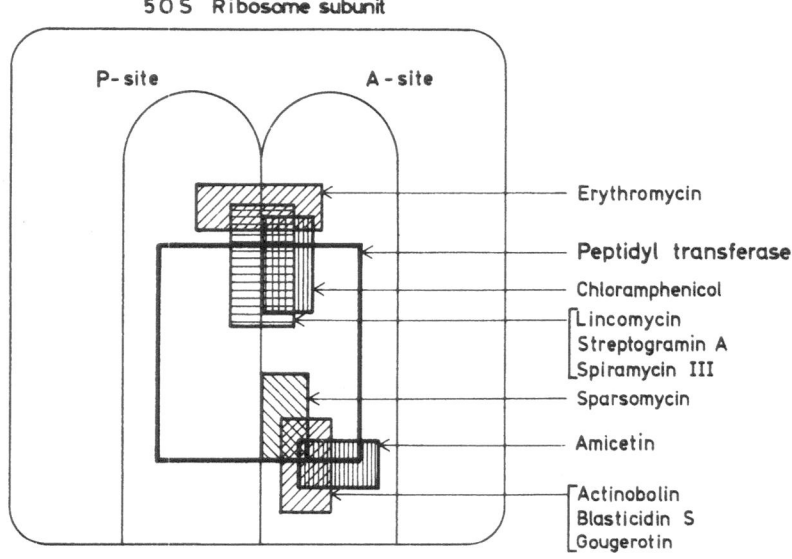

Fig. 4. Antibiotic binding sites on the peptidyl transferase centre
of the larger subunit of bacterial ribosomes.

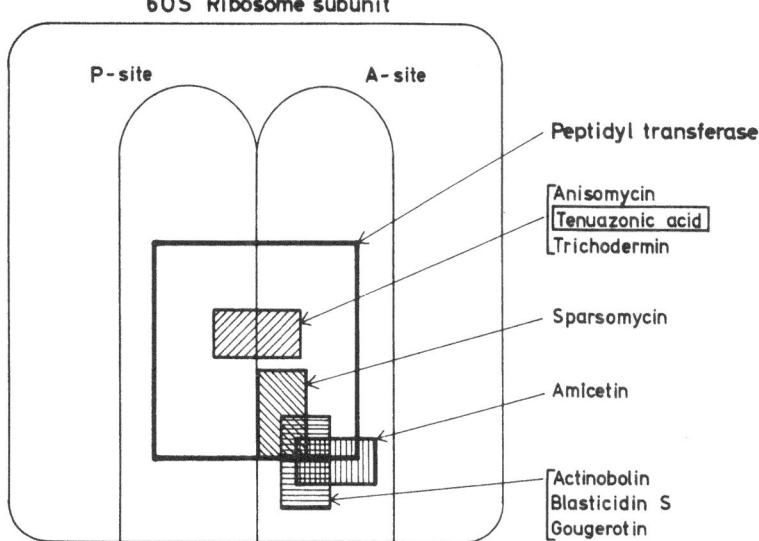

Fig. 5. Antibiotic binding sites on the peptidyl transferase centre of the larger subunit of ribosomes from eukaryotic cells.

The ribosomal components implicated in the different areas of the peptidyl transferase centre are not defined at the present time. It is interesting to quote that non identity of all the *E. coli* and eukaryotic ribosomal proteins has been reported although the gougero-tin-sparsomycin area of the peptidyl transferase centre can be considered by antibiotic binding and competition studies as a common area of prokaryotic and eukaryotic ribosomes. However different ribosomal proteins might have similar functions and properties in various types of ribosomes as it has been shown with proteins L7 and L12 of *E. coli* ribosomes which have similar properties and functions to proteins L40 and L41 of rat liver ribosomes (I.G. Wool, personal communication).

No ribosomal component can be active for peptidyl transferase activity or antibiotic interaction, when dissociated from the ribosomal structure. Therefore a number of different indirect methods have been used to identify the ribosomal components implicated in the peptidyl transferase activity and antibiotic interaction. Thus proteins L11 (Nierhaus & Montejo, 1973) and L15 (Ballesta *et al.*, 1974) have been proposed as implicated in the peptidyl transferase activity. However ribosomal cores deprived of proteins L11 and L15 still bind puromycin (Table 1) and CACCA-Leu-Ac (Nierhaus & Montejo, 1973) and affinity labelling experiments suggest that puromycin interacts with the RNA of the larger ribosome subunit (Harris *et al.*, 1973). Studies on affinity labelling have suggested proteins L2 and L27 (Sonenberg *et al.*, 1973; Pellegrini *et al.*, 1973), L16 and L24 (Pongs *et al.*, 1973), L13, L14, L15, L16 and L27 (Czernilofsky and Kuechler, 1972; Czernilofsky *et al.*, 1973) as involved in the binding of substrates to the peptidyl transferase centre on *E. coli* ribosomes.

Spiramycin-resistant mutants do not bind the antibiotic (Shimizu *et al.*, 1970) and have an altered protein L4 (Tanaka *et al.*, 1971).

Some erythromycin-resistant mutants have an altered L4 protein and do not bind the antibiotic (Otaka et al., 1970; Otaka et al., 1971; Dekio et al., 1971), whereas in some others protein L22 is altered and yet erythromycin binds to the ribosome (Wittman et al., 1973).

Induced and constitutive resistance to erythromycin has been associated with the modification of 23S RNA in which formation of dimethyladenine has been observed (Lai & Weisblum, 1971; Lai et al., 1973).

Antibiotic effects on polysomal systems

Experiments with polysomal systems led to the proposal that many of the antibiotics presented in Table 2 are not inhibitors of peptide bond formation in protein synthesis by intact cells. Thus streptogramin A antibiotics, lincomycin and spiramycin cause polysome breakdown and therefore might act by specifically inhibiting the initiation phase of protein synthesis (Cundliffe, 1969; Ennis, 1972). Furthermore streptogramin A antibiotics, lincomycin and macrolide antibiotics do not inhibit peptidyl-puromycin formation in polysomal systems (Pestka, 1972).

Table 3

Peptidyl-[^3H]puromycin formation by translocated yeast polysomes

Antibiotic conc.	Peptidyl-[^3H]puromycin formation	
	(% Inhibition)	
	Assay A	Assay B
Anisomycin	99	--
Tenuazonic acid	--	0
Trichodermin	75	99
Trichodermol	74	75
Trichothecin	51	99
Fusarenon X	15	89
Verrucarin A	0	0
Sparsomycin	99	100
Blasticidin S	11	73
Cycloheximide	5	0

Yeast polysomes were initially preincubated for 7 min in the presence of the supernatant fraction to translocate the peptidyl-tRNA in the absence of any inhibitor and different conditions were then followed in Assays A and B. In the Assay A the required inhibitors and [^3H] puromycin were simultaneously added at the end of the translocation period. In the Assay B the required inhibitors were added at the end of the translocation period and incubation continued for 3 min more prior to the final reaction with [^3H]puromycin. In both Assays the incubation with [^3H]puromycin was continued for 1 min, stopped by addition of 1 ml of 10% trichloroacetic acid and samples collected by filtration through GF/C glass fiber Whatman filtres. The symbol (--) denotes that the corresponding experiment was not performed.

Hence we have studied the effect of different antibiotics on a polysomal system from yeast showing that anisomycin, trichodermin, trichodermol, trichothecin, fusarenon X, sparsomycin and blasticidin S are effective inhibitors of peptidyl-puromycin formation whereas verrucarin A and cycloheximide do not inhibit the reaction (Table 3).

Most of the results in Table 3 agree with previous studies on the effects of the inhibitors in other experimental systems (Vazquez, 1974; Gale *et al.*, 1972; reviews) although there are some discrepancies. Thus verrucarin A is an effective inhibitor of peptide bond formation in the fragment reaction assay (Carrasco *et al.*, 1973) but not in our polysomal system (Table 3). Trichothecin and fusarenon X have to be added prior to [³H]puromycin (Assay B, Table 3) to clearly observe their inhibitory effect on peptidyl-[³H]puromycin formation. Verrucarin A appears to act on eukaryotic systems similarly to streptogramin A in bacterial systems; indeed verrucarin A has been reported to act as an inhibitor of the initiation phase on protein synthesis (Cundliffe *et al.*, 1974).

Cycloheximide has been reported to inhibit peptide bond formation in a rat liver polysomal system at O.8 M K^+ concentration (Pestka *et al.*, 1972b). We have confirmed this result in a polysomal system from yeast in the presence of O.8 M K^+ (Barbacid & Vazquez, unpublished results) but certainly cycloheximide has no effect in peptide bond formation under more physiological K^+ concentrations (Table 3) (Vazquez, 1974; review). Since cycloheximide has been repeatedly reported to inhibit translocation (Vazquez, 1974; review) the inhibition by the antibiotic at high K^+ concentrations of peptidyl-puromycin formation should be due to blocking the non-enzymic translocation which takes place in eukaryotic ribosomes under these ionic conditions (Blobel & Sabatini, 1971; Baliga *et al.*, 1973), as we have recently observed (Barbacid & Vazquez, unpublished results).

Binding of [³H]anisomycin to polysomes

[³H]anisomycin has the ability to distinguish different ribosomal structures as shown in our studies on [³H]anisomycin binding to standard high salt washed ribosomes from yeast and human tonsils (Barbacid & Vazquez, 1974b). Taking advantage of this property of [³H]anisomycin we have studied [³H]anisomycin binding to yeast polysomes in order to know the conformational changes occurring on the ribosome during the ribosomal cycle and to explain the reasons for the observed heterogeneity of eukaryotic ribosomes washed in high salts. For these purposes we have developed a method to obtain, on a preparative scale, polysome preparations without free ribosomes. These polysomes were blocked in different steps of the elongation cycle by using certain translation inhibitors. The binding of [³H]anisomycin to the polysomes homogeneously blocked in different steps was studied. Thus run-off ribosomes were obtained by either sodium azide treatment or incubation of the polysomes at 8°C; cycloheximide, diphtheria toxin, fusidic acid and doxycycline were used to obtain polysomes blocked at different steps of the elongation as shown in control experiments. In other control polysomal preparations about 2/3 of the peptidyl-tRNA was bound to the A-site and 1/3 was associated with the P-site. The results obtained show that there are drastic conformational or/and structural changes of polysomes and ribosomes during protein synthesis defined by the parameters of the [³H]anisomycin interaction. Furthermore we have shown that heterogeneity of high salt washed ribosomes for [³H]anisomycin binding is due to the washing procedure.

The results obtained can be summarized as indicated in Fig. 6. The dissociation constants for [³H]anisomycin binding corresponding to the different conformational and/or structural states of the ribosomes are (a) free ribosomes (K_d^{R-off} = 3.5 µM), (b) posttranslocated ribosomes (K_{d1}^{DC} = 0.8 µM), (c) pretranslocated ribosomes (K_d^{CHX} = 12 µM), (d) polysomes with EF-2 bound (K_d^{DT} or K_d^{FA} = 1.8 - 1.5 µM) and (e) standard salt washed ribosomes: K_{d1}^{HSW} = 0.5 µM (for approximately 30 % of the ribosomes) and K_{d2}^{HSW} = 5 µM (for 70 % of the ribosomes).

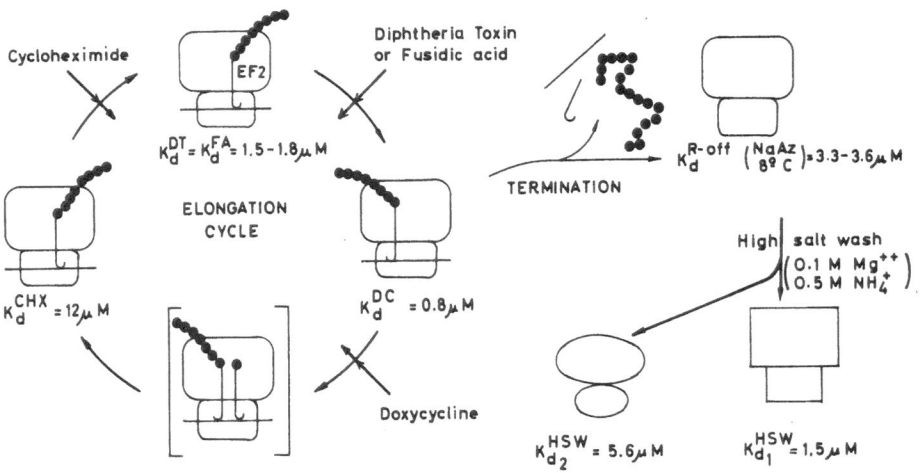

Fig. 6. The dissociation constant for [³H]anisomycin binding to the different conformational states of yeast ribosomes.

Discussion

There is strong evidence supporting the interaction of chloramphenicol and its analogues D-AMP-3, thiamphenicol and D-Win-5094 with the acceptor site of the peptidyl transferase. Although there are no data available on the binding of althiomycin to the ribosome the results presented by different workers strongly support the inhibitory effect of this antibiotic on peptide bond formation (Vazquez, 1974; review).

Antibiotics of the lincomycin and streptogramin A groups bind to the peptidyl transferase centre and are strong inhibitors of peptide bond formation in different cell-free systems when added prior to the binding of the substrate to the donor site of the peptidyl transferase centre. However these antibiotics do not inhibit peptidyl-puromycin formation by polysomal systems (Pestka, 1972) and cause polysome breakdown suggesting that they might act as inhibitors of initiation (Cundliffe, 1969). An inhibitory effect of the lincomycin and streptogramin A antibiotics on the initiation phase can be explained by the inhibition by the antibiotics of the interaction of the 3' terminal end of the initiator substrate (fMet-tRNA$_F$) with the donor site of the peptidyl transferase, when the 50S ribosome subunit joins the initiation complex formed on the 30S subunit. The lack of effect of these antibiotics on peptidyl-puromycin formation in a polysomal system suggest that they only bind to free ribosomes but cannot bind to the ribosomes during the elongation cycle. This is not surprising considering the strong differences in affinity observed in the case of [³H]anisomycin interaction with polysomes at different stages of the cycle (Fig. 6).

Concerning the macrolide antibiotics it appears that erythromycin, oleandomycin, neospiramycins, forocidins, methymycin and lancamycin are not inhibitors of peptide bond formation, although their site of binding on the ribosome can be closely connected or overlapping the binding site of antibiotics acting on the chloramphenicol area of peptidyl transferase. However carbomycins, spiramycins, leucomycins, niddamycin and tylosin bind to the peptidyl transferase centre in salt washed ribosomes and appear to behave similarly to the lincomycin and streptogramin A antibiotics blocking peptide bond formation in model systems but not in polysomal systems. Also these antibiotics induce polysome breakdown in intact bacteria. The macrolides carbomycin, spiramycins, leucomycins, niddamycin and tylosin are similar in having a -mycaminose-mycarose residue linked to the central ring of the antibiotics (Fig. 7). On the contrary the neospiramycins only differ from the spiramycins in lacking the -mycarose residue (Fig. 7). However the mode of action of neospiramycins is similar to that of erythromycin. Therefore an attractive hypothesis for the mode of action of the macrolide antibiotics is that all of them have a common binding site (determined by the macrolide ring) outside the peptidyl transferase but their interaction with this site and the chloramphenicol binding site is mutually exclusive. However only those macrolides having the -mycaminose-mycarose residue directly interact with the peptidyl transferase centre due to this sugar moiety and therefore block peptide bond formation in model systems and possibly initiation in intact cells. This interaction with peptidyl transferase does not take place in the case of neospiramycins, forocidins, erythromycin, oleandomycin, methymycin and lancamycin all of which are lacking of the dissacharide moiety linked to the central ring. The non inhibitory effect of the -mycaminose-mycarose macrolides on polysomal systems appears to be due to lack of interaction of these antibiotics with the polysomes.

All the antibiotics of the gougerotin-sparsomycin area interact on the acceptor site of the peptidyl transferase centre of ribosomes (bacterial and eukaryotic) at mutually exclusive sites. These antibiotics are inhibitors of peptide bond formation in the different systems studied.

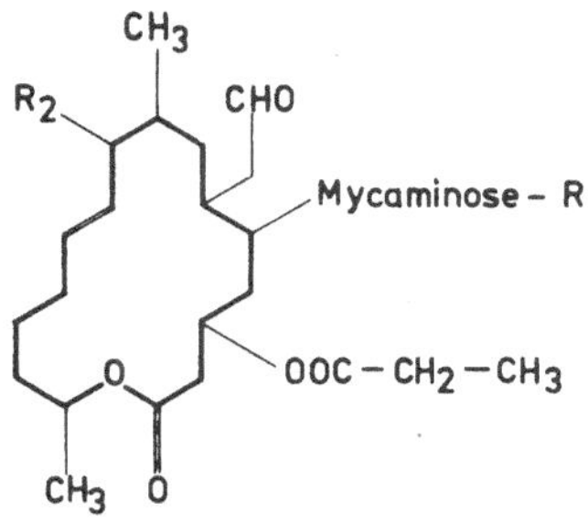

	-R$_1$	-R$_2$
Spiramycin III	Mycarose	Forosamine
Neospiramycin III	H	Forosamine
Forocidin III	H	H

Fig. 7. Chemical structure of spiramycin III, neospiramycin III and forocidin III.

Anisomycin, tenuazonic acid, trichodermin, fusarenon X, trichodermol and trichothecin bind to the anisomycin area of the peptidyl
transferase centre of eukaryotic ribosomes at mutually exclusive
sites. Tenuazonic acid has a striking selectivity since it is active
on mammalian ribosomes but not in yeast ribosomes. All these antibiotics inhibit peptide bond formation in the different experimental
systems in which they have been assayed.

On the other hand the sesquiterpene antibiotic verrucarin A only
partially inhibits [^{14}C]trichodermin binding to the ribosome (Barbacid
& Vazquez, 1974), has no effect on peptidyl-puromycin by yeast polysomes (Table 3) and causes polysome breakdown (Cundliffe *et al.*, 1974).
Therefore verrucarin A has been proposed as an inhibitor of initiation.
Besides inhibiting peptide bond formation (Table 3) the sesquiterpene
fusarenon X might also inhibit initiation since it also causes polysome breakdown (Ueno *et al.*, 1973; Ohtaubo *et al.*, 1972).

Concluding remarks

We should emphasise at this point that interaction of an antibiotic
with the peptidyl transferase centre does not necessarily imply only
inhibition of peptide bond formation. Since peptidyl transferase is
implicated in the peptidyl-tRNA hydrolysis in the termination phase,
all the peptidyl transferase inhibitors which have been tested block
termination in bacterial and in mammalian systems with the same specificity shown in peptide bond formation (Vazquez, 1974; review).

Furthermore, a number of antibiotics interacting with the peptidyl
transferase centre interfere with the attachment of the 3' terminal
end of peptidyl-tRNA and fMet-tRNA acting therefore as inhibitors of
termination. Antibiotics of the lincomycin and streptogramin A groups
and macrolides with the -mycaminose-mycarose moiety behave in this
manner in bacterial systems and verrucarin A is probably the counter-
part antibiotic in eukaryotic systems. Antibiotics of these groups do
not appear to be able to interact with polysomes since they do not
inhibit peptidyl-puromycin formation in polysomal systems. However
fusarenon X appears to behave as verrucarin A in causing breakdown of
polysomes, suggesting its inhibition on initiation, but unlike verrucarin A, also inhibits peptide bond formation in polysomal systems
(Talbe 3).

The results presented above clearly demonstrate the importance of
complementing the results obtained in model systems with the use of
polysomal systems. There are strong changes in the ribosomal structure
which can be shown by [^{3}H]anisomycin binding studies. These differences might be shown more drastically in the case of some other antibiotics which appear to interact with free ribosomes but not with
polysomes in any step of elongation. However, the results on the effect of antibiotics on amino acid incorporation by polysomes can differ from those obtained on cell-free system. Thus some antibiotics,
which do not bind to the peptidyl transferase in polysomal systems,
might inhibit peptide bond formation in intact cells by interacting
with free ribosomes and remaining bound to the peptidyl transferase
when the polysomes are formed.

References

BALIGA, B.S., M.G.SCHECHTMAN, R.D.NOLAN, and H.N.MUNRO: Influence of temperature and monovalent cations on the reactivity of the donor and acceptor sites on mammalian ribosomes. Biochim.Biophys.Acta 312, 349-357 (1973).

BALLESTA, J.P.G., V.MONTEJO, F.HERNANDEZ, and D.VAZQUEZ: Alteration of ribosomal proteins and functions by 2-methoxy-5-nitrotropone. Eur.J.Biochem. 42, 167-175 (1974).

BALLESTA, J.P.G., V.MONTEJO, and D.VAZQUEZ: Reconstitution of the 50S ribosome subunit. Localization of activities related to the peptidyl transferase centre. FEBS Letters 19, 75-78 (1971).

BARBACID, M., and D.VAZQUEZ: Binding of acetyl-[^{14}C]trichodermin to the peptidyl transferase centre of eukaryotic ribosomes. Eur.J. Biochem. 44, 437-444 (1974c).

BARBACID, M., and D.VAZQUEZ: [G-^{3}H]Gougerotin binding to ribosomes. Heterogeneity of eukaryotic ribosomes. Eur.J.Biochem. 44, 445-453 (1974a).

BARBACID, M., and D.VAZQUEZ: [^{3}H]Anisomycin binding to eukaryotic ribosomes. J.Mol.Biol. 84, 603-623 (1974b).

BATTANER, E., and D.VAZQUEZ: Inhibitors of protein synthesis by ribosomes of the 80S type. Biochim.Biophys.Acta 154, 316-330 (1971).

BEAUDET, A.L., and C.T.CASKEY: Polypeptide chain termination. In: The mechanism of protein synthesis and its regulation, ed. L. Bosch, p. 133-172. Amsterdam-London: North Holland Publishing Company (1972).

BERMAN, M.L., and R.MONIER: Influence of the 30S ribosomal subunit on the peptidyl transferase activity of the 50S ribosomal subunit from *Escherichia coli.* Biochimie 53, 233-242 (1971).

BLCBEL, G., and D.SABATINI: Dissociation of mammalian polyribosomes into subunits by puromycin. Proc.Natl.Acad.Sci. U.S. 68, 390-394 (1971).

BRETSCHER, M.S., and K.A.MARCKER: Polypeptidyl-sribonucleic acid and amino-acyl-sribonucleic acid binding sites on ribosomes. Nature 211, 380-384 (1966).

CAPECCHI, M.R., and H.A.KLEIN: Characterization of three proteins involved in peptide chain termination. Cold Spring Harb.Symp. Quant.Biol. 34, 469-477 (1969).

CARRASCO, L., M.BARBACID, and D.VAZQUEZ: The trichodermin group of antibiotics, inhibitors of peptide bond formation by eukaryotic ribosomes. Biochim.Biophys.Acta 312, 368-376 (1973).

CARRASCO, L., and D.VAZQUEZ: Differences in eukaryotic ribosomes detected by the selective action of an antibiotic. Biochim. Biophys.Acta 319, 209-215 (1973).

CASKEY, T., E.SCOLNICK, R.TOMPKINS, J.GOLDSTEIN, and G.MILMAN: Peptide chain termination, codon, protein factor and ribosomal requirements. Cold Spring Harb.Symp.Quant.Biol. 34, 479-488 (1969).

CELMA, M.L., R.E.MONRO, and D.VAZQUEZ: Substrate and antibiotic binding sites at the peptidyl transferase centre of *Escherichia coli* ribosomes. FEBS Letters 6, 273-277 (1970).

CELMA, M.L., R.E.MONRO, and D.VAZQUEZ: Substrate and antibiotic binding sites at the peptidyl transferase center of *Escherichia coli* ribosomes: Binding of UACCA-Leu to 50S subunits. FEBS Letters 13, 247-251 (1971).

CERNA, J., I.RYCHLIK, and J.JONAK: Peptidyl transferase activity of *Escherichia coli* ribosomes digested by ribonuclease T$_1$. Eur.J. Biochem. 34, 551-556 (973b).

CERNA, J., I.RYCHLIK, A.A.KRAYEVSKY, and B.P.GOTTIKH: pA-fMet, a new donor substrate for ribosomal peptidyl transferase. In: Ribosomes and RNA metabolism, ed. J.Zelinka and J.Balan, p. 285-295. Bratislava: Publishing House of the Slovak Academy of Sciences (1973a).

CERNA, J., I.RYCHLIK, J.ZEMLICKA, and S.CHLALEK: Substrate specificity of ribosomal peptidyl transferase. II. 2'(3')-o-aminoacyl nucleosides as acceptors of the peptide chain in the fragment reaction. Biochim.Biophys.Acta 204, 203-209 (1970).

CONTRERAS, A., M.BARBACID, and D.VAZQUEZ: Binding to ribosomes and mode of action of chloramphenicol analogues. Biochim.Biophys. Acta 349, 376-388 (1974).

CUNDLIFFE, E.: Antibiotics and polyribosomes. II. Some effects of lincomycin, spiramycin, and streptogramin A in vivo. Biochemistry 8, 2063-2066 (1969).

CUNDLIFFE, E., M.CANNON, and J.DAVIES: Mechanism of inhibition of eukaryotic protein synthesis by trichothecene fungal toxins. Proc.Natl.Acad.Sci. U.S. 71, 30-34 (1974).

CZERNILOFSKY, A.P., and E.KUECHLER: Affinity label for the tRNA binding site on the Escherichia coli ribosome. Biochim.Biophys.Acta 272, 667-671 (1972).

CZERNILOFSKY, A.P., E.COLLATZ, G.STOFFLER, and E.KUECHLER: Proteins at the tRNA binding sites of Escherichia coli ribosomes. Proc. Natl.Acad.Sci. U.S. 71, 230-234 (1974).

DEKIO, S., R.TAKATA, S.OSAWA, K.TANAKA, and M.TAMAKI: Genetic studies of the ribosomal proteins in Escherichia coli. IV. Pattern of the alteration of ribosomal protein components in mutants resistant to spectinomycin or erythromycin in different strains of Escherichia coli. Mol.Gen.Genet. 107, 39-49 (1970).

ENNIS, H.L.: Polysome metabolism in Escherichia coli: Effect of antibiotics on polysome stability. Antim.Agents Chemother. 1, 197-203 (1972).

ERDMANN, V.A., H.G.DOBERER, and M.SPRINZL: Structure and function of 5S RNA: The role of the 3' terminus in 5S RNA function. Mol.Gen. Genet. 114, 89-94 (1971b).

ERDMANN, V.A., S.FAHNESTOCK, K.HIGO, and M.NOMURA: Role of 5S RNA in the functions of 50S ribosomal subunits. Proc.Natl.Acad.Sci. U.S. 68, 2932-2936 (1971a).

FAHNESTOCK, S.R., and M.NOMURA: Activity of ribosomes containing 5S RNA with a chemically modified 3' terminus. Proc.Natl.Acad.Sci. U.S. 69, 363-365 (1972).

FERNANDEZ-MUÑOZ, R., R.E.MONRO, R.TORRES-PINEDO, and D.VAZQUEZ: Substrate- and antibiotic-binding sites on the peptidyl transferase centre of Escherichia coli ribosomes. Eur.J.Biochem. 23, 185-193 (1971).

FERNANDEZ-MUÑOZ, R., and D.VAZQUEZ: Binding of puromycin to Escherichia coli ribosomes. Effects of puromycin analogues and peptide bond formation inhibitors. Molec.Biol.Reports 1, 27-32 (1973a).

FERNANDEZ-MUÑOZ, R., and D.VAZQUEZ: Kinetic studies of peptide bond formation. Effect of chloramphenicol. Molec.Biol.Reports 1, 75-79 (1973b).

FERNANDEZ-MUÑOZ, R., and D.VAZQUEZ: Quantitative binding of [^{14}C] erythromycin to Escherichia coli ribosomes. J.Antibiotics 26, 107-108 (1973c).

GALE, E.F., E.CUNDLIFFE, P.E.REYNOLDS, M.H.RICHMOND, and M.J.WARING: In: The Molecular Basis of Antibiotic Action, ed.John Wiley and Sons. London-New York (1972).

GOTTESMAN, M.E.: Ribosome peptidyl transferase. In. Methods in Enzymology, vol. XX, ed. K.Moldave and L.Grossman, p. 490-494. New York-London: Academic Press (1971).

GOTTIKH, B.P., L.V.NIKOLAYEVA, A.A.KRAYEVSKI, and L.L.KISSELEV: 3'(2')-o-aminoacyl nucleotides as polypeptide acceptors at the ribosomal peptidyl transferase center. FEBS Letters 7, 112-113 (1970).

HAENNI, A.L., and J.LUCAS-LENARD: Stepwise synthesis of a tripeptide. Proc.Natl.Acad.Sci. U.S. 61, 1363-1369 (1968).

HARBON, S., and F.CHAPEVILLE: Inhibition of protein synthesis in the reticulocytes by aminoacyl adenosine. Eur. J.Biochem. 13, 375-383 (1970).

HARRIS, R.J., P.GREENWELL, and R.H.SYMONS: Affinity labelling of ribosomal peptidyl transferase by a puromycin analogue.Biochem. Biophys.Res.Commun. 55, 117-124 (1973).

HARRIS, R.J., J.E.HANLON, and R.H.SYMONS: Peptide bond formation on the ribosome. Structural requirements for inhibition of protein synthesis and of release of peptides from peptidyl-tRNA on bacterial and mammalian ribosomes by aminoacyl and nucleotidyl analogues of puromycin. Biochim.Biophys.Acta 240, 244-262 (1971).

HARRIS, R.J., and R.H.SYMONS: A detailed model of the active centre of Escherichia coli peptidyl transferase. Bioorganic Chemistry 2, 286-292 (1973a).

HARRIS, R.J., and R.H.SYMONS: On the molecular mechanism of action of ribosomal peptidyl transferase. Bioorganic Chemistry 2, 266-285 (1973b).

HENGESH, E.J., and A.J.MORRIS: Inhibition of peptide bond formation by cytidyl derivatives of puromycin. Biochim.Biophys.Acta 299, 654-661 (1973).

HISHIZAWA, T., and S.PESTKA: Studies on the formation of transfer ribonucleic acid-ribosome complexes. XVII. The effect of tRNA on aminoacyl-oligonucleotide binding to ribosomes. Arch.Biochem. Biophys. 147, 624-631 (1971).

HOMAN, H.E., and K.H.NIERHAUS: Ribosomal proteins. Protein compositions of biosynthetic precursors and artifical subparticles from ribosomal subunits in Escherichia coli K12. Eur.J.Biochem. 20, 249-257 (1971).

HUSSAIN, Z., and J.OFENGAND: Effect of increasing chain length of AA-oligonucleotide acceptors on their reactivity at the peptidyl transferase center in ribosomes and polysomes. Biochem.Biophys. Res.Commun. 49, 1588-1597 (1972).

HUSSAIN, Z., and J.OFENGAND: Terminal oxidation-reduction of yeast phenylalanine tRNA prevents donor and acceptor function at the peptidyl transferase center. Biochem.Biophys.Res.Commun. 50, 1143-1151 (1973).

LAI, C.J., and B.WEISBLUM: Altered methylation of ribosomal RNA in an erythromycin-resistant strain of Staphylococcus aureus. Proc.Natl. Acad.Sci. U.S. 68, 856-860 (1971).

LAI, C.J., B.WEISBLUM, S.R.FAHNESTOCK, and M.NOMURA: Alteration of 23S ribosomal RNA and erythromycin-induced resistance to lincomycin and spiramycin in Staphylococcus aureus . J.Mol.Biol. 74, 67-72 (1973).

LEICK, V., I.VOTRIN, B.S. COOPERMAN, and A.RICH: Affinity labeling of Escherichia coli peptidyl transferase by antibiotic affinity labels. Abstr. 9th Int.Congress Biochem., p. 191 (1973).

LESSARD, J.L., and S.PESTKA: Studies on the formation of transfer ribonucleic acid-ribosome complexes. XXII. Binding of aminoacyl-oligonucleotides to ribosomes. J.Biol.Chem. 247, 6901-6908 (1972).

MADEN, B.E.H., and R.E.MONRO: Ribosome-catalyzed peptidyl transfer. Effects of cations and pH value. Eur.J.Biochem. 6, 309-316 (1968).

MADEN, B.E.H., R.R.TRAUT, and R.E.MONRO: Ribosome-catalysed peptidyl transfer: The polyphenylalanine system. J.Mol.Biol. 35, 333-345 (1968).

MAO, J.C.H.: Substrate specificity of *Escherichia coli* peptidyl transferase at the donor site. Biochem.Biophys.Res.Commun. 52, 595-600
(1973).

MERCER, J.F.B., and R.H.SYMONS: Peptidyl-donor substrates for ribosomal
peptidyl transferase. Chemical synthesis and biological activity
of N-acetyl aminoacyl Di- and Tri-nucleotides. Eur.J.Biochem. 28,
38-45 (1972).

MONRO, R.E.: Catalysis of peptide bond formation by 50S ribosomal
subunits from *Escherichia coli*. J.Mol.Biol. 26, 147-151 (1967).

MONRO, R.E., J.CERNA, and K.A.MARCKER: Ribosome-catalyzed peptidyl
transfer: Substrate specificity at the P-site. Proc.Natl.Acad.Sci.
U.S. 61, 1042-1049 (1968).

MONRO, R.E., R.FERNANDEZ-MUÑOZ, M.L.CELMA, and D.VAZQUEZ: Mode of action
of lincomycin and related antibiotics. In: Drug action and drug
resistance in bacteria. 1. Macrolide antibiotics and lincomycin,
ed. S.Mitsuhashi, p. 305-336. Tokyo: University of Tokyo Press
(1971).

MONRO, R.E., B.E.H.MADEN, and R.R.TRAUT: The mechanism of peptide bond
formation in protein synthesis. In: The genetic elements, ed. D.
Shugar, p. 179-203. London: Academic Press (1967).

MONRO, R.E., T.STAEHELIN, M.L.CELMA, and D.VAZQUEZ: The peptidyl transferase activity of ribosomes. Cold Spring Harb.Symp.Quant.Biol.34,
357-368 (1969).

MONRO, R.E., and D.VAZQUEZ: Ribosome-catalyzed peptidyl transfer:Effects
of some inhibitors of protein synthesis. J.Mol.Biol. 28, 161-165
(1967).

NATHANS, D., and A.NEIDLE: Structural requirements for puromycin inhibition
of protein synthesis. Nature 197, 1076-1077 (1963).

NIERHAUS, D., and K.H.NIERHAUS: Identification of the chloramphenicol-
binding protein in *Escherichia coli* ribosomes by partial reconstitution. Proc.Natl.Acad.Sci. U.S. 70, 2224-2228 (1973).

NIERHAUS, K.H., and V.MONTEJO: A protein involved in the peptidyl
transferase activity of *Escherichia coli* ribosomes. Proc.Natl.Acad.
Sci. U.S. 70, 1931-1935 (1973).

OHTSUBO, K., P.KADEN, and C.MITTERMAYER: Polyribosomal breakdown in
mouse fibroblasts (L-cells) by fusarenon X, a toxic principle
isolated from *Fusarium nivale*. Biochim.Biophys.Acta 287, 520-525
(1972).

OTAKA, E., T.ITOH, S.OSAWA, K.TANAKA, and M.TAMAKI: Peptide analyses
of a protein component, 50-8, of 50S ribosomal subunit from
erythromycin resistant mutants of *Escherichia coli* and *Escherichia
freundii*. Mol.Gen.Genet. 114, 14-22 (1971).

OTAKA, E., H.TERAOKA, M.TAMAKI, K.TANAKA, and S.OSAWA: Ribosomes from
erythromycin-resistant mutants of *Escherichia coli* Q13. J.Mol.
Biol. 48, 499-510 (1970).

PELLEGRINI, M., H.OEN, and C.R.CANTOR: Covalent attachment of a
peptidyl transfer RNA analog to the 50S subunit of *Escherichia
coli* ribosomes. Proc.Natl.Acad.Sci. U.S. 69, 837-841 (1972).

PESTKA, S.: Studies on the formation of transfer ribonucleic acid-
ribosome complexes. X. Phenylalanyl-oligonucleotide binding to
ribosomes and the mechanism of chloramphenicol action. Biochem.
Biophys.Res.Commun. 36, 589-595 (1969).

PESTKA, S.: Inhibitors of ribosome functions. In: Molecular mechanisms
of antibiotic action on protein biosynthesis and membranes, eds.
E.Muñoz, F.Garcia-Ferrandiz and D.Vazquez, p. 160-187. Amsterdam:
Elsevier (1972).

PESTKA, S.: Peptidyl-puromycin synthesis on polyribosomes from *Escherichia
coli*. Proc.Natl.Acad.Sci. U.S. 69, 624-628 (1972).

PESTKA, S., R.GOORHA, H.ROSENFELD, C.NEURATH, and H.HINTIKKA:Studies
on transfer ribonucleic acid-ribosome complexes. XX. Peptidyl-
puromycin synthesis on mammalian polyribosomes. J.Biol.Chem.
247, 4258-4263 (1972a).

PESTKA, S., H.ROSENFELD, R.HARRIS, and H.HINTIKKA: Studies on transfer
    ribonucleic acid-ribosome complex. XXI. Effect of antibiotics on
    peptidyl-puromycin synthesis by mammalian polyribosomes. J.Biol.
    Chem. 247, 6895-6900 (1972b).
PONGS, O., R.BALD, and V.A.ERDMANN: Identification of chloramphenicol-
    binding protein in *Escherichia coli* ribosomes by affinity labeling.
    Proc.Natl.Acad.Sci. U.S. 70, 2229-2233 (1973).
RYCHLIK, I.: Release of lysine peptides by puromycin from polylysyl
    transfer RNA in presence of ribosomes. Biochim.Biophys.Acta 114
    425-427 (1966).
RYCHLIK, I., J.CERNA, S.CHLADEK, P.PULKRABEK, and J.ZENLICKA: Substrate
    specificity of ribosomal peptidyl transferase. The effect of
    the nature of the amino acid side chain on the acceptor activity
    of 2'(3')-o-aminoacyladenosines. Eur.J.Biochem. 16, 136-142 (1970).
RYCHLIK, I., J.CERNA, S.SHLADEK, J.ZEMLICKA, and Z.HALADOVA: Substrate
    specificity of ribosomal peptidyl transferase: 2'(3')-o-aminoacyl
    nucleosides as acceptors of the peptide chain on the amino acid
    site. J.Mol.Biol. 43, 13-24 (1969).
SHIMIZU, M., T.SAITO, and S.MITSUHASHI: Spiramycin resistance in
    Staphylococcus aureus. Decrease in spiramycin-accumulation and
    the ribosomal affinity of spiramycin in resistant staphycococci.
    J.Antibiotics 23, 63-67 (1970).
SKOGERSON, L., and K.MOLDAVE: Evidence for aminoacyl-tRNA binding,
    peptide bond synthesis, and translocase activities in the aminoacyl
    transfer reaction. Arch.Biochem.Biophys. 125, 497-505 (1968a).
SKOGERSON, L., and K.MOLDAVE: Evidence for the role of aminoacyl
    transferase II in peptidyl-transfer ribonucleic acid translocation.
    J.Biol.Chem. 243, 5361 (1968b).
SONENBERG, N., M.WILCHEK, and A.ZAMIR: Mapping of *Escherichia coli*
    ribosomal components involved in peptidyl transferase activity.
    Proc.Natl.Acad.Sci. U.S. 70, 1423-1426 (1973).
TANAKA, K.,M.TAMAKI, I.ITOH, E.OTAKA, and S.OSAWA: Ribosomes from
    spiramycin resistant mutants of *Escherichia coli* Q13. Mol.Gen.
    Genet. 114, 23-30 (1971).
TRAUT, R.R., and R.E.MONRO: The puromycin reaction and its relation
    to protein synthesis. J.Mol.Biol. 10, 63-72 (1964).
UENO, Y., M.NAKAJIMA, K.SAKAI, K.ISHII, N.SATO, and N.SHIMADA:
    Comparative toxicology of trichothec mycotoxins: Inhibition of
    protein synthesis in animal cells. J.Biochem. 74, 285-296 (1973).
VAZQUEZ, D.: The binding of chloramphenicol by ribosomes from *Bacillus
    megaterium.* Biochem.Biophys.Res.Commun. 15, 464-468 (1964).
VAZQUEZ, D.: Binding of chloramphenicol to ribosomes. The effect of
    a number of antibiotics. Biochim.Biophys.Acta 114, 277-288 (1966).
VAZQUEZ, D.: Binding to ribosomes and inhibitory effect on protein
    synthesis of the spiramycin antibiotics. Life Sci. 6, 845-853
    (1967).
VAZQUEZ, D.: Inhibitors of protein synthesis. FEBS Letters 40 Supple-
    ment, 563-584 (1974).
VAZQUEZ, D., E.BATTANER, R.NETH, G.HELLER, and R.E.MONRO:The function
    of 80S ribosomal subunits and effects of some antibiotics. Cold
    Spring Harb.Symp.Quant.Biol. 34, 369-375 (1969).
VOGEL, Z., A.ZAMIR, and D.ELSON: The possible involvement of peptidyl
    transferase in the termination step of protein biosynthesis.
    Biochemistry 8, 5161-5168 (1969).
WALLER, J.P. T.ERDOS, F.LEMOINE, S.GUTTMAN, and E.SANDRIN: Inhibition
    of protein synthesis by aminoacyl 3'(2')-adenosine. Biochim.
    Biophys.Acta 119, 566-580 (1966).
WITTMANN, H.G., G.STOFFLER, D.APIRION, L.ROSEN, K.TANAKA, M.TAMAKI,
    R.TAKATA, S.DEKIO, E.OTAKA, and S.OSAWA: Biochemical and genetic
    studies on two different types of erythromycin resistant mutants
    of *Escherichia coli* with altered ribosomal proteins. Mol.Gen.
    Genet. 127, 175-189 (1973).

ZAMIR, A., P.LEDER, and D.ELSON: A ribosome-catalyzed reaction between N-formylmethionyl-tRNA and puromycin. Proc.Natl.Acad.Sci. U.S. <u>56</u>, 1794-1801 (1966).

Experiments on the Binding Sites and the Action of Some Antibiotics which Inhibit Ribosomal Functions

R. Werner, A. Kollak, D. Nierhaus, G. Schreiner, and K. H. Nierhaus

We describe experiments (A) on an antibiotic which binds to the 50S subunit of procaryotic ribosomes (chloramphenicol), (B) on an antibiotic which binds specifically to the 30S subunit (streptomycin), and (C) on a group of antibiotics whose binding sites are not yet well known (tetracycline and some of its derivatives).

A. CHLORAMPHENICOL

1. *Binding Site*

Binding of $[^{14}C]$chloramphenicol (CAM) to ribosomes or particles was measured by means of equilibrium dialysis. Table 1, Exp. 1, demonstrates that CAM binds to 50S subunits as well as to 70S ribosomes, whereas its binding to 30S subunits is negligible. As show by Scatchard plot (Fernandez-Muñoz *et al.*, 1971b; Nierhaus & Nierhaus, 1973) only one molecule of CAM is bound per ribosome.

Ribosomal proteins can be split off from the 50 S subunits by incubation with LiCl (Homann & Nierhaus, 1971). Incubation of 70S ribosomes with 0.8 LiCl results in the formation of cores (0.8 c cores) and a split protein fraction (SP 0.8). The 0.8c core and the SP 0.4 - 0.8

Table 1

CHLORAMPHENICOL BINDING MEASURED BY EQUILIBRIUM DIALYSIS

Exp.	Particle	$[^{14}C]$Chloramphenicol bound (pM/nM particle)
1	30S	20
	50S	800
	70S	870
2	50S	640
	0.4c	540
	0.8c	49
	SP 0.4-0.8	30
	(0.8c + SP 0.4-0.8)	410

Data are taken from Nierhaus & Nierhaus (1973).

proteins do not bind CAM in contrast to the 0.4c core. The 0.8c core can regain its binding capacity by the addition of the SP 0.4 - 0.8 under reconstitution conditions (see Table 1, Exp. 2). Our strategy was to isolate the split proteins and to determine which protein or proteins are necessary for the 0.8c core particle to regain its CAM binding activity.

The split proteins were passed through a DEAE cellulose column in order to remove the acidic proteins. The basic fraction (as active as the total split proteins with respect to the CAM binding) was subjected to Sephadex G-100 gel filtration. The A $_{235}$ profile is shown in Fig. 1. From each fraction a reconstitution with the non-binding 0.8c core was performed and the binding capacity of the reconstituted particles was measured. As shown in Fig. 1, only the fractions of the third peak were able to restore CAM binding.

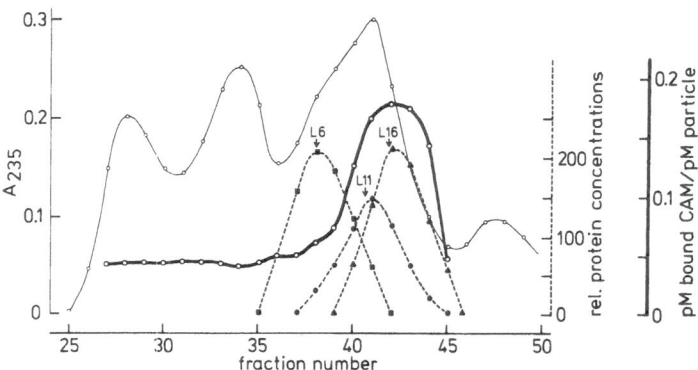

Fig. 1. The gel filtration profile (Sephadex G-100) from the basic fraction of the 50S derived split proteins SP 0.4 - 0.8 (o ――― o). The relative concentration curves of three proteins are included (● -- ●). Each fraction was reconstituted with the non-binding 0.8c core. The reconstituted particles were tested for chloramphenicol binding (o ――― o). For details see Nierhaus & Nierhaus (1973).

The protein content of the third peak was analyzed in the following way: Equal aliquots of each fraction were subjected to acrylamide gel electrophoresis. Density comparisons of the same protein band in different gels were taken to reflect the relative concentrations of this protein in the corresponding fractions. The relative concentration curves are included in Fig. 1. The concentration curve for protein L16 shows the best fit with the curve of binding activity; however, the CAM binding curve also covers the concentration curve of protein L11. The proteins L6, L11 and L16 were purified by successive gel filtration steps and reconstituted in all possible combinations with the 1.0c core (Table 2). When L16 is present, substantial CAM binding can be observed. L11 alone can induce less but significant binding, whereas L6 alone has no effect. The L16 dependent binding can be stimulated by L6. The L11 dependent binding is not enhanced by L6 (Table 2). Thus, L16 and L11 are involved in CAM binding. As there is only one binding site, and as both proteins are part of this site, L16 and L11 should, therefore, be neighbors.

Table 2

CHLORAMPHENICOL BINDING TO RECONSTITUTED PARTICLES

1.0c cores reconstituted with			CAM binding (pM/nM particle)
L6	L11	L16	
–	–	–	4
+	–	–	3
–	+	–	40
–	–	+	78
+	+	–	43
+	–	+	101
–	+	+	98
+	+	+	150
1.0c + all split proteins			156
50S			300

Data are taken from Dietrich *et al.* (1974).

2. *Action of Chloramphenicol*

CAM binds to the A-site moiety of the peptidyltransferase center because it inhibits the binding of either aminoacyl-tRNA fragments or puromycin to the A-site, but it does not interfere with the binding of peptidyl-tRNA fragments to the P-site (Pestka, 1969; Celma *et al.*, 1971; Fernandez-Muñoz *et al.*, 1971a; Lessard & Pestka, 1972; for detailed discussion see Nierhaus & Nierhaus, 1973). In agreement with these reports, we find that the 0.8c core binds the P-site specific fragment C-A-C-C-A-(N-acetyl-Leu) as good as the 50S subunit (Table 3). Thus, the 0.8c core contains the intact P-site moiety of

Table 3

BINDING OF C-A-C-C-A-(Ac[^{3}H]LEU) FRAGMENT

Particle	Cpm of bound fragment
50S	1355
0.8c	1295
30S	322

Data are taken from Nierhaus & Nierhaus (1973).

the peptidyltransferase center. As this core does not bind CAM, the drug cannot bind to the P-site part of the peptidyltransferase center. CAM competes with the aminoacyl-tRNA fragment C-A-C-C-A-Leu for binding to the A-site. Does CAM do so at the aminoacyl end or at the oligonucleotidyl end? We studied the competition of CAM binding with different compounds. Fig. 2 demonstrates that the trinucleotide CpCpA

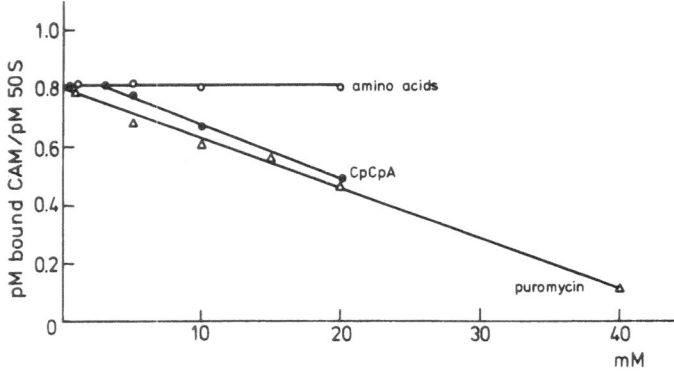

Fig. 2. Inhibition of chloramphenicol binding by increasing amounts of amino acids, puromycin and the trinucleotide CpCpA. The figure is taken from Nierhaus & Nierhaus (1973).

(equivalent to the 3'end of tRNAs) inhibits the CAM binding as efficiently as puromycin. A mixture of 20 different amino acids had no effect. Even the dinucleotide CpA causes significant inhibition of the CAM binding in comparison to the reversed dinucleotide ApC or to the control compound UpU (Table 4). We conclude, that CAM binds specifically to the A-site moiety of the peptidyltransferase center and that it interferes with the attachment of the last two or three nucleotides of the aminoacyl-tRNA. CAM may inhibit directly the peptidyltransferase activity as it binds to L11, since this protein is intimately involved in peptidyltransferase activity (Nierhaus & Montejo, 1973).

Table 4

INHIBITION OF CHLORAMPHENICOL BINDING

Compound added (20 mM)	CAM/nM 50S bound (pM)	% Inhibition
Complete	730	0
+ puromycin	430	41
+ amino acids	720	2
+ CpCpA	470	36
+ CpA	590	19
+ ApC	690	5
+ UpU	700	4

Data are taken from Nierhaus & Nierhaus (1973).

B. STREPTOMYCIN (DIHYDROSTREPTOMYCIN)

1. *Characterization of the Binding*

It was reported that the 16S RNA from the 30S subunit is the target for streptomycin binding and that even the 50S subunits bind 0.7 molecules per subunit (Biswas & Gorini, 1972). We determined the bind-inc of dihydrostreptomycin by a different technique (equilibrium dialysis; Schreiner & Nierhaus, 1973). It was found that the binding of dihydrostreptomycin to 50S subunits, to 16S RNA and to 23S RNA differed considerably depending on the concentrations of ammonium ions (Fig. 3). In contrast, binding to the 30S subunits was not in-

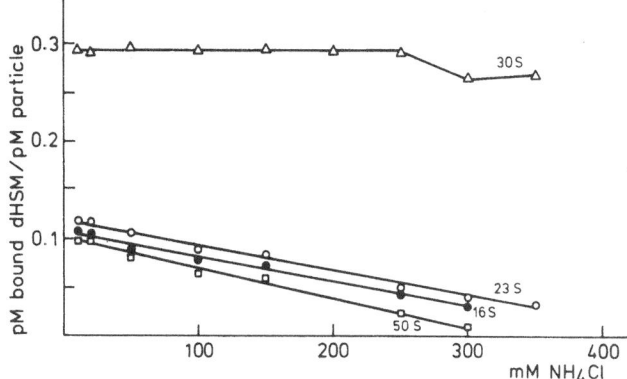

Fig. 3. Binding of dihydrostreptomycin to 30S and 50S subunits and to 16S and 23S RNA at different NH₄Cl concentrations. The figure is taken from Schreiner & Nierhaus (1973).

fluenced up to 250 mM NH_4Cl. The binding to 50S subunits, to 16S RNA and to 23S RNA decreased gradually with increasing NH_4^+ concentrations. We adjusted the NH_4Cl concentration to 250 mM in the following assays. Under these conditions the 30S subunit binds the drug as well as the 70S ribosome, whereas the 50S subunit and 16S RNA show background binding only (Table 5). The streptomycin effects on poly(U) dependent poly(Phe) synthesis are independent of NH_4Cl concentration over a wide range (50 - 250 mM; Schreiner & Nierhaus, unpublished observation). Thus, the binding measured at high NH_4^+ concentration (250 mM) is relevant at least for the *in vitro* effects of the drug. Therefore, the low binding of dihydrostreptomycin to 16S RNA observed under these conditions indicates that the RNA is not a good candidate for forming the binding site.

Table 5

BINDING OF DIHYDROSTREPTOMYCIN TO RIBOSOMES AND RNA

Particle	Dihydrostreptomycin/nM particle bound (pM)
70S ribosomes	240
50S subunits	10
30S subunits	260
23S RNA	14
16S RNA	12

Data are taken from Schreiner & Nierhaus (1973).

To pursue this question, we split off more and more proteins from the 30S subunits by increasing the LiCl concentration and tested the remaining core for its ability to bind dihydrostreptomycin. If RNA is involved directly in the binding, we should expect an increase of dihydrostreptomycin binding with increasing exposure of the RNA. If proteins primarily form the binding site, we should expect a loss of dihydrostreptomycin binding by splitting off the protein(s) responsible for binding. Fig. 4 illustrates the drastic decrease of the binding which is most pronounced during the transition 30S subunit → 1.15c core. In addition to the low binding of dihydrostreptomycin by RNA under our standard conditions, and in addition to the loss of binding by lowering the protein content of the 30S particle, there is a third argument favoring the proteins as the primary target for binding: 16S RNA inside the 30S subunit can be partially digested by RNAse without a remarkable loss of proteins. These particles with the broken RNA backbone showed no activity in the poly(U) system, whereas they bound dihydrostreptomycin to the same extent as intact 30S subunits (Roth & Nierhaus, 1973).

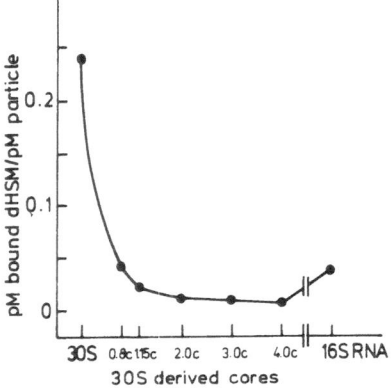

Fig. 4. Binding of dihydrostreptomycin to 30S derived LiCl cores with decreasing protein content and to 16S RNA. Data are taken from Schreiner & Nierhaus (1973).

We conclude that proteins are most likely the primary target for binding the drug.

The Scatchard plot (Fig. 5), determined under standard conditions, revealed not more than one binding site per 30S subunit: 0.8 molecules of dihydrostreptomycin can be attached to each 30S subunit.

2. *Identification of the Proteins Involved in Binding of Dihydro-streptomycin*

When 30S subunits are incubated with 1.15 M LiCl, the resulting 1.15c cores are defective in their capacity to bind dihydrostreptomycin. The activity can be restored by adding the complementary protein fraction SP 1.15 to the 1.15c core under reconstitution conditions. Even the 2.0c core regains activity after reconstitution with the SP 1.15 proteins (Table 6). Since the 2.0c core shows a more defined protein pattern than the 1.15c core (Schreiner & Nierhaus, 1973) we preferred to use the 2.0c core in these reconstitution experiments.

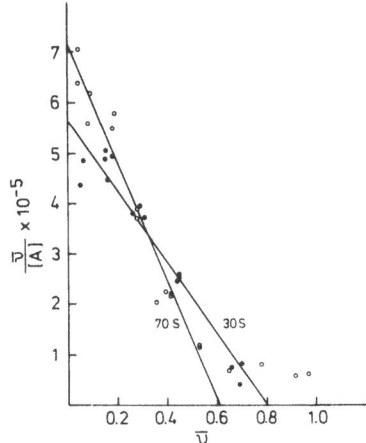

Fig. 5. Scatchard plot of the equilibrium dialysis data from dihydro-streptomycin binding to 30S subunits and 70S ribosomes. The figure is taken from Schreiner & Nierhaus (1973).

The split proteins Sp 1.15 were separated and analyzed in the same way as described above for the 50S-derived fraction: The proteins were chromatographed by a DEAE cellulose column and filtered through a Sephadex G-100 column. The relative concentrations of the proteins were determined in each fraction and the curves of relative concentra-tions were drawn (Fig. 6). Each fraction was reconstituted with the 2.0c core. The binding capacity of the reconstituted particles is also depicted in Fig. 6. It is evident that S5 is the only protein which can convey binding activity to the 1.15c core particle. Sur-prisingly, the S12 region is not able to restore activity (S12 is not present on the 2.0c core). This protein is altered in streptomycin resistant strains. Ribosomes derived from resistant strains do not bind the drug. Maximal binding is seen between the S3 and the S5 peak, whereas S3 alone (fraction 42) has no effect. We cannot expect any effects with S3 alone, since the binding of this protein depends on the presence of S5, S9, S10 and S14 according to the assembly map (Mizushima & Nomura, 1970). The 2.0c core does not contain these proteins. Thus, S3 could stimulate the S5 dependent binding, or, alternatively, could be directly involved in the binding of dihydro-streptomycin in addition to S5.

To clarify the situation we constructed a particle containing S9, S10 and S14 to which S3 should bind to some extent. The particle (2.0c + S9 + S14(S10)) shows only poor binding, whereas the addition of S3 enhances the binding significantly (Table 6). We thus conclude, that both S3 and S5 are part of the one binding site for dihydro-streptomycin and, therefore, must be neighbors. The S5 dependent binding can be stimulated by S9 and S14(S10) (Table 6, for detailed analysis see Schreiner & Nierhaus, 1973).

If S3 and S5 are involved in dihydrostreptomycin binding and S12 in resistant strains can abolish this binding, S3 and S5 should be close to S12. In fact, this was found: S3 and S12 as well as S5 and S12 could be coupled by cross linking reagents (R.R. Traut, personal communication).

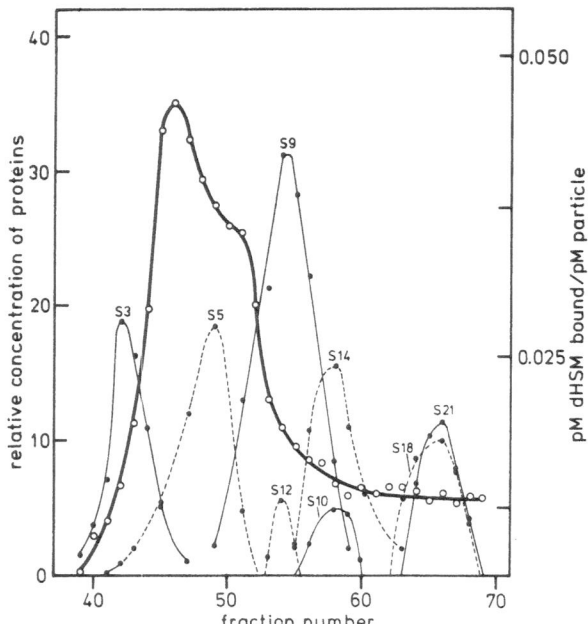

Fig. 6. Sephadex G-100 gel filtration of the basic fraction of the
30S derived split proteins SP 1.15. The relative concentration curves
of the proteins in the eluate is shown (● -- ● and ● —— ●). Each
fraction was reconstituted with the 30S derived 2.0c core. The reconstituted particles were tested for dihydrostreptomycin binding
(o —— o). The figure is taken from Schreiner & Nierhaus (1973).

Table 6

BINDING OF DIHYDROSTREPTOMYCIN TO RECONSTITUTED PARTICLES

Particle	Dihydrostreptomycin/nM particle bound (pM)
2.0c	8
+ S5	31
+ S5 + S3	55
+ S5 + S9	50
+ S5 + S14(S10)	50
+ S5 + S18(S21)	36
+ S3 + S5 + S9 + S14(S10)	124
+ S5 + S9 + S14(S10)	90
+ S9 + S14(S10)	18
+ S3 + S9 + S14(S10)	50
+ SP 1.15	125

Reconstitutions were performed with 2.0c and split protein fractions
from the Sephadex G-100 column. The proteins corresponded to the following fractions of the Sephadex eluate: S3, fraction 42; S5, fraction 49; S9, fraction 56; S14(S10), fraction 59; S18(S21), fraction
66 (Fig. 6).

As mentioned above, a resistant ribosome containing an altered S12 shows poor dihydrostreptomycin binding. It should be possible to construct with components derived from resistant ribosomes a particle which lacks the altered S12 but contains all the proteins important for dihydrostreptomycin binding. This particle should bind significant amounts of dihydrostreptomycin. We performed the experiment and ran through the same analysis as described for the sensitive components. The results are summarized in Table 7: The 2.5c core reconstituted with S3, S5, S9 and S14(S10) bound dihydrostreptomycin significantly (51 nM/pM particles). Both protein and core fractions were derived from resistant ribosomes. Sensitive derived proteins reconstituted with the same core gave the same result (58 nM/pM particle). When protein S12 from a streptomycin resistant mutant (str^r) was added to the 2.5c core and split proteins all derived from a resistant strain the binding of dihydrostreptomycin decreased (35 nM/pM particle). In contrast, the addition of wild type S12 (str^s) lead to a slight stimulation of the binding (65 nM/pM particle). These results confirmed our finding, that S12 modulates the (S3 + S5) dependent binding. It is not yet clear whether S12 from str^r strains impairs the binding by imposing a conformational restriction on the binding site or, alternatively, by simply blocking access to the binding site.

Table 7

BINDING OF DIHYDROSTREPTOMYCIN TO PARTICLES RECONSTITUTED FROM COMPONENTS DERIVED FROM STR^s AND STR^r STRAINS

Particle	Dihydrostreptomycin/pM particle bound (pM)
2.5c	0.006
+ SP 2.5	0.009
SP 2.5	0.110
S12	0.008
S 12	0.008
S3, S5	0.030
S3, S5	0.035
S9, S14(S10)	0.007
S9, S14(S10)	0.008
S9, S14(S10), S3, S5	0.051
S9, S14(S10), S3, S5	0.058
S9, S14(S10), S3, S5, S12	0.035
S9, S14(S10), S3, S5, S12	0.065

Components derived from str^s strains

Components derived from str^r strains

If S3 and S5 are the binding proteins, why do we not observe significant binding of dihydrostreptomycin to the isolated proteins? Two possible explanations may be offered: 1) Two proteins are involved in forming the binding site. Therefore, one protein can carry only a part of the site. 2) The S5 dependent binding can be stimulated by S9 and S14(S10). It is, therefore, obvious that the isolated S5 itself does not have optimal conformation for binding dihydrostreptomycin.

The binding of [^{14}C]streptomycin to some of the reconstituted particles was tested. The results were qualitatively the same as described above with dihydrostreptomycin (Schreiner & Nierhaus, un-published results). Binding to ribosomes derived from streptomycin resistant and sensitive strains is identical for streptomycin and dihydrostreptomycin. Furthermore, the binding of dihydrostreptomycin can be inhibited effectively by streptomycin and *vice versa*. Therefore, streptomycin and dihydrostreptomycin most likely compete for one and the same binding site.

C. TETRACYCLINE AND SOME DERIVATIVES

1. *The Effects of the Tetracyclines in the Poly(U) and Poly(C) Dependent Protein Synthesis System*

The structural formulars of tetracycline and its derivatives and abbreviations used in this study are shown in Fig. 7.

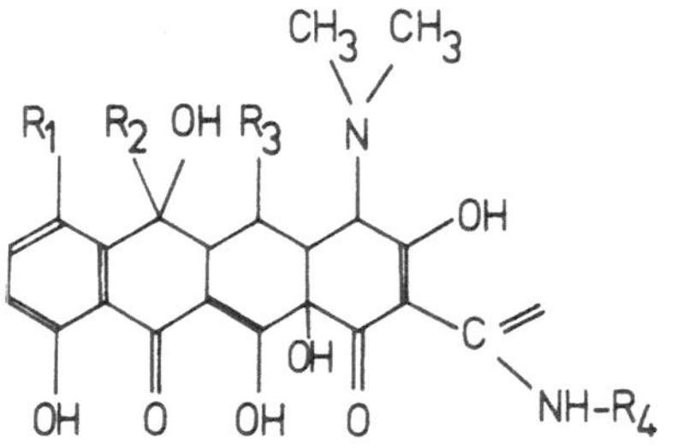

		R_1	R_2	R_3	R_4
Tetracycline	TET	-H	$-CH_3$	-H	-H
Oxytetracycline	OTET	-H	$-CH_3$	-OH	-H
Chlorotetracycline	CTET	-Cl	$-CH_3$	-H	-H
Demethylchloro-tetracycline	DTET	-Cl	-H	-H	-H
Pyrrilidinomethyl-tetracycline	PTET	-H	$-CH_3$	-H	$-CH_2-N$

Fig. 7. Formulas and abbreviations of tetracycline and its derivatives tested.

The inhibitory effects of relatively low concentrations of tetra-cyclines on the poly(U) dependent poly(Phe) synthesis system is dem-onstrated in Fig. 8A. PTET, TET and OTET display about the same gree of inhibition. The strongest inhibitors are DTET and CTET. The same order of inhibitory power is observed in the poly(C) dependent poly(Pro) synthesis system (Fig. 8B). However, the inhibition effects seem to be more pronounced in the poly(C) system than in the poly(U) system.

A

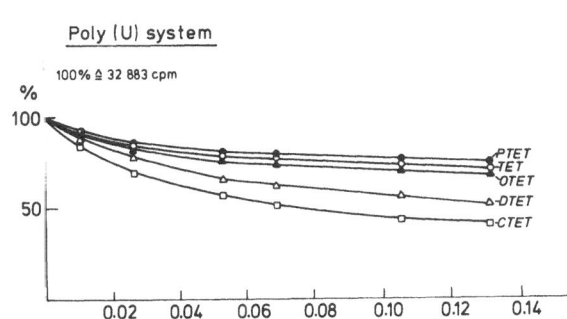

B

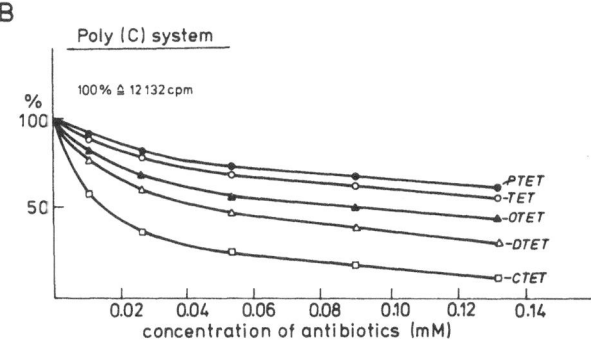

Fiç. 8. Inhibition of the poly(U) (A) and the poly(C) (B) system by increasing concentrations of the drugs.

At first glance, this situation seems to be related to that of chloramphenicol, which inhibits the poly(A) dependent poly(Lys) synthesis stronger than the poly(U) coded synthesis of polyphenylalanine. This different response does not reflect a different sensitivity of the two systems for chloramphenicol but is caused simply by the ability of the filters to retain oligophenylalanines better than oligolysines (Pestka, 1969).

To investigate this possibility in the case of the tetracyclines, the products synthesized in the poly(U) and the poly(C) systems were analyzed by Sephadex G15 gel filtration. The antibiotic oxytetracycline when adjusted to 0.25 mM inhibited the poly(U) system by about 50%. Fig. 9 demonstrates that the depression of the poly(Pro) synthesis (B) by OTET is stronger than the inhibition of the poly(Phe) synthesis (A). Obviously, the poly(C) system is more sensitive to the tetracyclines than the poly(U) system. There is no evident explanation for this finding at the moment.

2. *Experiments on Binding Sites of the Tetracyclines*

Tetracycline binds to RNA and ribonucleoprotein particles (Day, 1966). Up to 300 TET molecules can be bound per ribosome (Maxwell, 1968). Since all of these, except one, can be removed simply by dialysis,

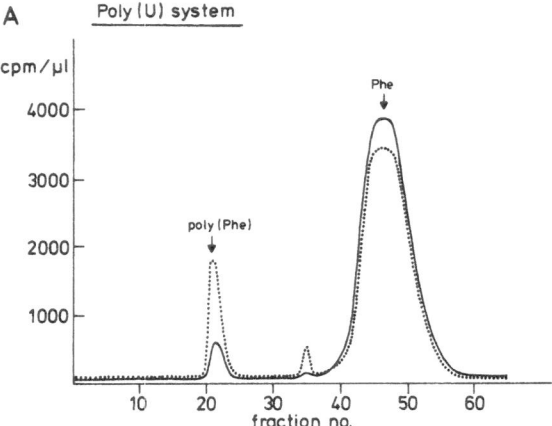

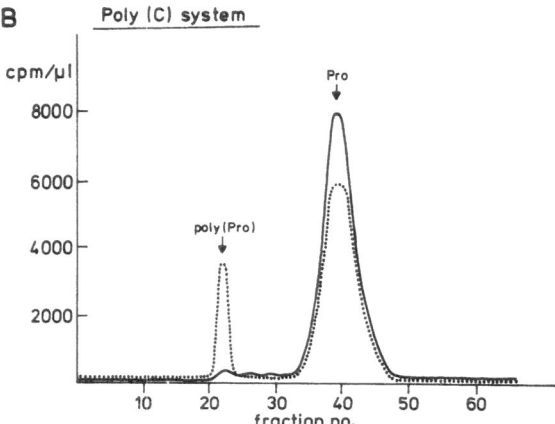

Fig. 9. Sephadex G-15 gel filtration of the products synthesized in the poly(U) system (poly(Phe); (A)) and poly(C) system (poly(Pro); (B)). The synthesis was performed in the absence (.....) and presence (——) of OTET.

one may assume that the binding site relevant for the inhibition effect is a specific one (i.e. a binding site to which the tetracyclines bind with a suitably large association constant). In order to find out which ribosomal subunit is the target for the drug binding, we designed an experiment with the following rationale: A standard poly(U) protein synthesis assay with a drug concentration which inhibits the ribosomal activity by about 50 % is performed. An excess of either the 30S or the 50S ribosomal subunit is then added to the assay. If we assume that the added ribosomal subunit contains the specific binding site relevant for the inhibition effect, the subunit should compete with the 70S ribosomes active in protein synthesis for the tetracycline, and thus the ribosomal activity should increase significantly. On the other hand, if the added subunit does not carry the binding site, we should expect a less drastic alteration of the ribosomal activity. A scheme of the experiment, which we call "dilution of drug binding sites", is presented above Table 8, and the results are summarized in Table 8. Surprisingly, both subunits display

about the same effect. However, the addition of 70S ribosomes causes
an effect much stronger than that of either of the subunits. With
respect to TET, OTET and CTET, the 70S effect is strikingly higher
than the sum of the 30S and 50S effects, whereas for DTET and PTET
the effects of the subunits can be summed up to the stimulation caused
by the 70S ribosomes. Thus, the 70S ribosomes seem to carry the binding site(s) important for the inhibition effect.

Experimental scheme for Table 8:
Activity in the poly(U)-coded cell-free protein synthesizing system.

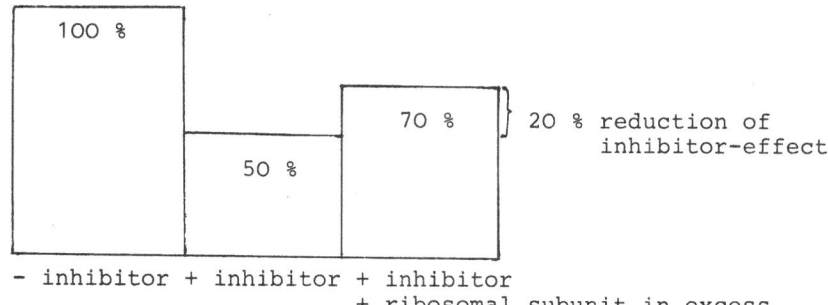

Table 8

DILUTION OF DRUG BINDING SITES

Reduction of inhibitory effects of various tetracyclines on cell-free
protein synthesis by addition of ribosomal particles.

Antibiotic (0.25 mM)	Ribosomes added in excess		
	30S (1000 pM)	50S (500 pM)	70S (500 pM)
TET	4 %	4 %	31 %
OTET	7 %	5 %	22 %
CTET	14 %	9 %	33 %
DTET	21 %	20 %	41 %
PTET	14 %	13 %	28 %

Binding experiments using radioactive labelled tetracyclines were
performed in order to better define the 70S versus subunits effect.
We tritiated oxytetracycline with the NaBH$_4$ method (for details see
Werner, Schreiner & Nierhaus, to be published) and purified the products by Biogel P2 filtration (Fig. 10). In addition to the inclusion
peak, the elution volume contained three peaks which were isolated as
indicated. The inhibitory effect of the three fractions was tested in
a poly(U) system and compared to authentic OTET on a µg per assay
basis. Fig. 11 shows that the inhibition of only fraction 1 was identical to OTET, i.e. fraction 1 contains the intact structure relevant
for the biological activity of OTET. The calculation of the stoichiom-

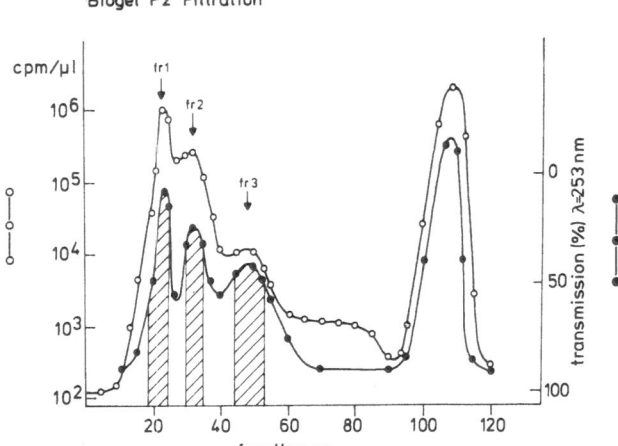

Fig. 10. Analysis of the tritiated products by Biogel P2 gel filtration after tritiating OTET by the NaBH₄ method.

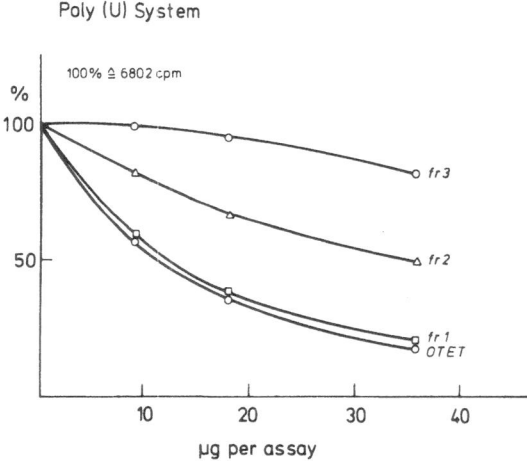

Fig. 11. Inhibition of the poly(U) system by the three fractions isolated after tritiating OTET as demonstrated in Fig. 10. The inhibition is compared to authentic OTET.

etry in the following equilibrium dialysis experiments are based on the assumption that the molecular weight of the compound in fraction 1 was identical to OTET. The results of an equilibrium dialysis experiment with fraction 1 (OTET*) and ribosomes and its subunits are demonstrated in Table 9. The subunits show poor binding, whereas 70S ribosomes bind substantial amounts of the drug. This finding confirms the results of the "dilution of binding sites" experiment (Table 8). One explanation of the dominant role of the 70S ribosome is that the interfaces of both subunits are involved directly in the binding site(s) for tetracyclines. Therefore, one subunit carries only a part of the binding site. Alternatively, one subunit may be involved, and its conformation, important for the optimal configuration of the drug's binding site, is guaranteed only in the 70S couple.

Table 9

BINDING OF TRITIATED OXYTETRACYCLINE TO RIBOSOMES

Particle	Oxytetracycline/nM particle bound (pM)
70S	440
30S	50
50S	30

3. *Inhibition of Some Ribosomal Functions by Tetracycline and Its Derivatives*

A well documented effect of tetracycline is the inhibition of the binding of aminoacyl-tRNA to ribosomes (Hierowsky, 1965; Suarez & Nathans, 1965). TET prevents specifically the binding of aminoacyl-tRNA to the A-site (Gottesman, 1967; Bodley & Zieve, 1969; Cerná *et al.*, 1969; Watanabe, 1972). In similar experiments with tetracycline and its derivatives we found that at low concentration (up to 0.5 mM) all the drugs prevented efficiently, and to about the same extent, the poly(U) dependent binding of Phe-tRNA and ac-Phe-tRNA to the A-site, whereas the binding of ac-Phe-tRNA to the P-site was not impaired (Werner, Schreiner & Nierhaus, to be published).

The effects of the antibiotics on the EF-G dependent GTPase activity is shown in Fig. 12. All the drugs display about the same inhib-

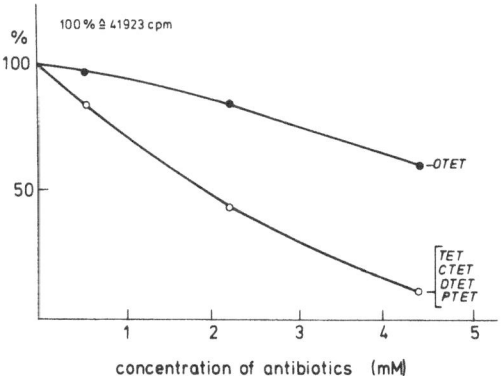

Fig. 12. Inhibition of the uncoupled EF-G dependent GTPase by increasing amounts of the drugs.

itory power except for the weaker OTET. The concentrations used, however, are relatively high. 0.25 mM TET is needed to get a 50 % inhibition in the poly(U) system, whereas this concentration does not
inhibit significantly the EF-G dependent GTPase activity. Therefore,
most probably the inhibition of this GTPase activity does not belong
to the primary effects of the drugs. It may be that the higher concentration necessary for GTPase inhibition allows the binding of the
drugs to secondary binding sites. This would mean that the primary
binding site (or sites) does not overlap appreciably with the GTPase
center.

In contrast to the GTPase activity the peptidyltransferase activity
is affected drastically (Fig. 13). At least for TET, CTET and DTET
the inhibition concentrations are comparable to those of the poly(U)
system (50 % inhibition at about 0.25 mM). Therefore, these three
drugs may act at the peptidyltransferase center in addition to the
inhibition of the aminoacyl-tRNA binding to the A-site. It is not yet
known whether this striking inhibition of the peptidyltransferase is
related to the reported inhibition of the termination reaction (Vogel
et al., 1969; Capecchi & Klein, 1969).

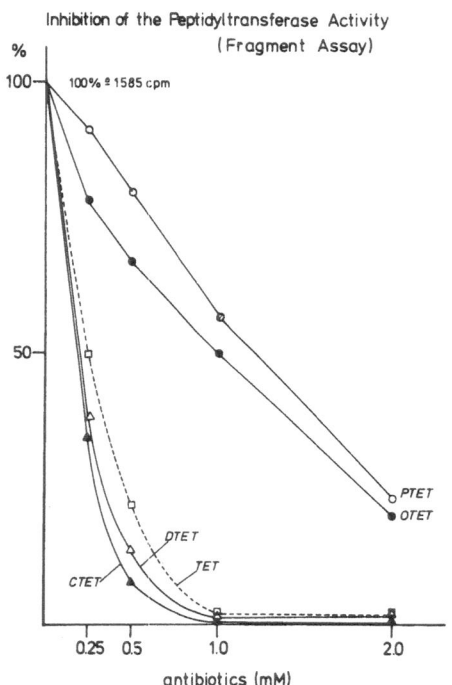

Fig. 13. Inhibition of the peptidyltransferase activity (fragment
assay) by increasing amounts of the drugs.

Acknowledgements

We wish to thank Dr. H.G. Wittman for many helpful criticisms and
discussions. We are grateful to Dr. H. Cronenberger for help and
advice.

REFERENCES

BISWAS, D.K., and L. GORINI: The attachment site of streptomycin to the 30S ribosomal subunit. Proc. Nat. Acad. Sci. USA 69, 2141-2144 (1972).

BODLEY, J.N., and F.J. ZIEVE: On the specificity of the two ribosomal binding sites: studies with tetracycline. Biochem. Biophys. Res. Commun. 36, 463-468 (1969).

CAPECCHI, M.R., and H.A. KLEIN: Characterization of three proteins involved in polypeptide chain termination. Cold Spring Harbor Symp. Quant. Biol. 34, 469-491 (1969).

CELMA, M.L., R.F. MONRO, and D. VAZQUEZ: Substrate and antibiotic binding sites at the peptidyltransferase center of *E. coli* ribosomes: Binding of UACCA-Leu to 50S subunits. FEBS Lett. 13, 247-251 (1971).

CERNÁ, J., I. RYCHLIK, and P. PULKRÁBEK: The effect of antibiotics on the coded binding of peptidyl-tRNA to the ribosome and on the transfer of the peptidylresidue to puromycin. Eur. J. Biochem. 9, 27-35 (1969).

DAY, L.E.: Tetracycline inhibition of cell-free protein synthesis. J. Bacteriol. 92, 197-203 (1966).

DIETRICH, S., I. SCHRANDT, and K.H. NIERHAUS: Interdependence of *E. coli* ribosomal proteins at the peptidyltransferase center. FEBS Letters, in press.

FERNANDEZ-MUNOZ, R., R.E. MONRO, R. TORRES-PINEDO, and D. VAZQUEZ: Substrate- and antibiotic binding sites of the peptidyltransferase center of *Escherichia coli* ribosomes. Eur. J. Biochem. 23, 185-193 (1971a).

FERNANDEZ-MUNOZ, R., R.E. MONRO, and D. VAZQUEZ: Ribosomal peptidyltransferase: Binding of inhibitors. Methods in Enzymology (Academic Press, New York and London), Vol. XX, part C, 481-490 (1971b).

GOTTESMAN, M.E.: Reaction of ribosome-bound peptidyl transfer ribonucleic acid or puromycin. J. Biol. Chem. 242, 5564-5571 (1967).

HIEROWSKI, M.: Inhibition of protein synthesis by chlortetracycline in the *Escherichia coli in vitro* system. Proc. Nat. Acad. Sci. USA 53, 594-599 (1965).

HOMANN, H.E., and K.H. NIERHAUS: Protein compositions of biosynthetic precursors and artificial subparticles from ribosomal subunits in *Escherichia coli* K12. Eur. J. Biochem. 20, 249-257 (1971).

LESSARD, J.L., and PESTKA, S.: Studies on the formation of transfer ribonucleic acid-ribosome complexes. CCIII. Chloramphenicol, aminoacyl oligonucleotides, and *Escherichia coli* ribosomes. J. Biol. Chem. 247, 6909-6912 (1972).

MAXWELL, J.H.: Studies of the binding of tetracycline to ribosomes *in vitro*. Mol. Pharmacol. 4, 25-37 (1968).

MIZUSHIMA, S., and M. NOMURA: Assembly mapping of 30S ribosomal proteins from *E. coli*. Nature (London) 226, 1214-1218 (1970).

NIERHAUS, K.H., and V. MONTEJO: A protein involved in the peptidyltransferase activity of *Escherichia coli* ribosomes. Proc. Nat. Acad. Sci. USA 70, 1931-1935 (1973).

NIERHAUS, D., and K.H. NIERHAUS: Identification of the chloramphenicol-binding protein in *Escherichia coli* ribosomes by partial reconstitution. Proc. Nat. Acad. Sci. USA 70, 2224-2228 (1973).

PESTKA, S.: Studies on the formation of transfer ribonucleic acid-ribosome complexes. XI. Antibiotic effects on phenyl alanyl-oligonucleotide binding to ribosomes. Proc. Nat. Acad. Sci. USA 64, 709-714 (1969).

ROTH, H.E., and K.H. NIERHAUS: Isolation of four ribonucleoprotein fragments from the 30S subunit of *E. coli* ribosomes. FEBS Lett. 31, 35-38 (1973).

SCHREINER, G., and K.H. NIERHAUS: Protein involved in the binding of dihydrostreptomycin to ribosomes of *Escherichia coli*. J. Mol. Biol. 81, 71-82 (1973).

SUAREZ, G., and D. NATHANS: Inhibition of aminoacyl-sRNA binding to ribosomes by tetracycline. Biochem. Biophys. Res. Commun. 18, 743-750 (1965).

VOGEL, Z., A. ZAMIR, and D. ELSON: The possible involvement of peptidyltransferase in the termination step of protein biosynthesis. Biochemistry 8, 5161 (1969).

WATANABE, S.: Interaction of siomycin with the acceptor site of *Escherichia coli* ribosomes. J. Mol. Biol. 67, 443-457 (1972).

The Mode of Action of Pleuromutilin as Compared to Chloramphenicol

Gregor Högenauer

The basidomycete *Pleurotus mutilis* produces a substance, called pleuromutilin, which was found to be effectively inhibiting bacterial growth, mainly that of gram-positive organisms (Kavanagh *et al.*, 1951). The structure of this compound which is an ester of glycolic acid with a tricyclic diterpene moiety, termed mutilin, had been elucidated by Arigoni's group (Naegeli, 1961; Arigoni, 1962) and is depicted in Fig. 1,a. The antibiotic, which loses its activity if the keto group in position 3 or the hydroxy group at the carbon atom 11 are modified remains as effective as the parent compound if the exocyclic vinyl group is saturated. Moreover, if the glycolic acid side chain is substituted with thio ether derivatives the antibiotic activity can be increased by one or two orders of magnitude (Egger and Reinshagen, 1973). The water soluble derivative with the highest effect (Fig. 1,b) was used for most of the experiments reported in this article. The antibacterial spectrum of the compound extends into the gram-negative side as well. The most interesting feature of the drug is, however, its strong effect against infections by mycoplasms.

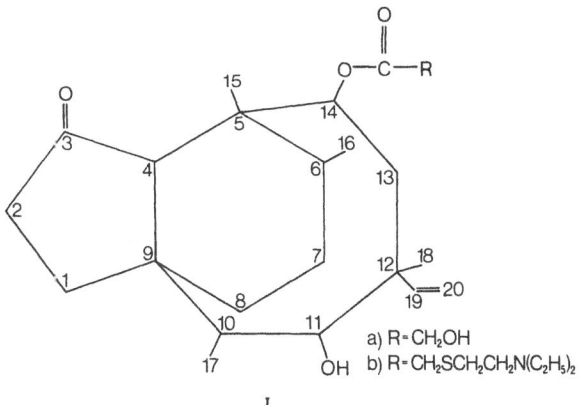

Fig. 1. Structure of pleuromutilin and its derivative. I a = pleuromutilin, I b = 14-deoxy-14-([2-diethylaminoethyl)-mercaptoacetoxy]-mutilin.

Abbreviations used: EF-T, elongation factor T; EF-G, elongation factor G.

When substance I b was added to a poly U-dependent polyphenylalanine synthesizing system containing salt washed ribosomes from *E. coli*
D 10, the elongation factors EF-T and EF-G, poly U and Phe-tRNA, strong
inhibition occurred. At an antibiotic concentration of 1 μM 50 % inhibition of the polyphenylalanine synthesis was observed (Fig. 2 A).
It must be concluded from this observation that protein biosynthesis
is the target of this drug. Like the poly U-dependent polyphenylalanine synthesis, the formation of fMet-puromycin, which occurred in a
reaction mixture of fMet-tRNA$_f^{Met}$, salt washed ribosomes, crude initiation factors, AUG and puromycin, was arrested by compound I b. From
this experiment it may be inferred that the ribosome is the sensitive
component of the polypeptide synthesizing system (Fig. 2 B).

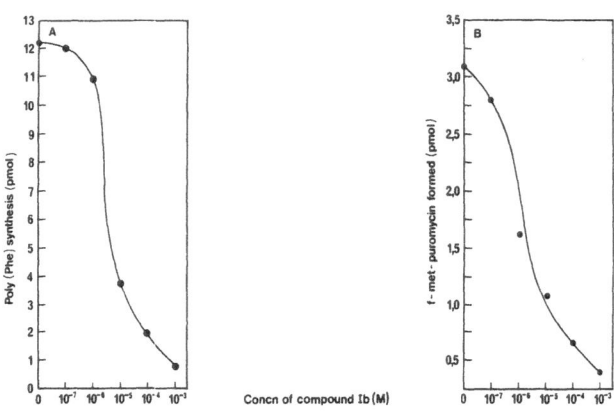

Fig. 2, A and B. (A) Poly(U)-directed polyphenylalanine synthesis in
the presence of compound I b. 100 μl incubation mixtures containing
32 μl of Nirenberg's Mix II without amino acids (Nirenberg, 1963),
2 A$_{260}$ units of salt washed *E. coli* D 10 ribosomes, 10 μg of poly(U),
5.2 μg each of EF-T and EF-G, 60 pmol of Phe-tRNA and various amounts
of compound I b were incubated at 37°C for 15 min. The reaction was
stopped by addition of ice cold washing buffer (0.1 M Tris-HCl, pH
7.2, 0.0075 M MgCl$_2$, 0.05 M NH$_4$Cl), filtered over Millipore filters
and washed with the above mentioned buffer. (B) Influence of compound
II on the fMet release by puromycin. The incubation mixtures containing 66 mM Hepes, pH 7.5, 33 mM NH$_4$Cl, 6.8 mM MgCl$_2$, 0.13 mM GTP, 2
A$_{260}$ units of *E. coli* D 10 ribosomes, 35 μg of crude initiation factor,
0.53 A$_{260}$ units of ApUpG, 10 μl of stock solutions of compound II,
20 pmol of fMet-tRNA$_f^{Met}$ and water, to give 75 μl, were incubated 5 min
at 23°C. Subsequently 5 μl of a 50 mM puromycin solution was added
and the incubation continued for another 15 min. After addition of
1 ml of 0.1 M sodium acetate, pH 5, the fMet puromycin was extracted
with 1 ml of ethylacetate. An aliquot of the organic phase was counted.

Initiation factor catalyzed and AUG-directed binding of fMet-tRNA$_f^{Met}$
remained uninfluenced by compound Ib up to concentrations of 1 mM which
suggests that the ribosomal P-site is unimpaired by pleuromutilin and
that either the catalytic center of the peptidyl-transferase or the
attachment of puromycin to the A-site are perturbed (Fig. 3).

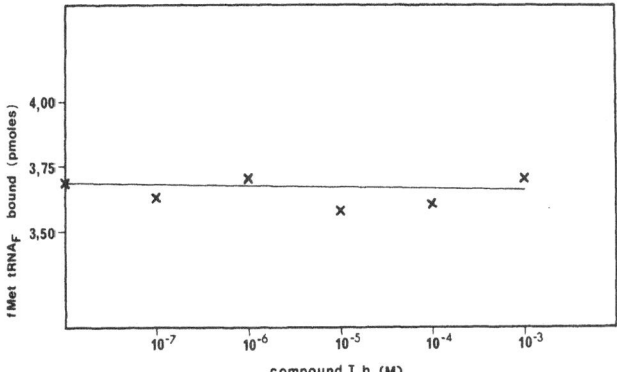

Fig. 3. Influence of compound I b on fMet-tRNA binding. Mixtures containing 2 A_{260} units of *E. coli* D 10 ribosomes, 35 µg of crude initiation factor, 0.265 A_{260} units of ApUpG, 10 pmol [^{35}S]fMet-tRNA$_f^{Met}$ and compound I b at various concentrations were incubated in a medium consisting of 100 mM Hepes, pH 7, 50 mM NH_4Cl, 5.8 mM $MgCl_2$ and 0.2 mM GTP at 23°C. Filtration and washing were performed as described in Fig. 2 (B).

The mode of action of pleuromutilin is different from that of fusidic acid, an inhibitor of the elongation step, because compound I b failed to inhibit the uncoupled EF-G specific GTPase reaction. Fusidic acid, added in a series of control experiments, interfered with that reaction as expected (data not shown).

In order to distinguish between the possible perturbation of the peptidyl transferase and an inhibition of the A-site, the effect of compound Ib on the *in vitro* formation of the bacteriophage R 17-RNA coded dipeptide fMet-Ala was tested. The reaction was limited to the dipeptide level by addition of fMet-tRNA$_f^{Met}$ and Ala-tRNA^{Ala} only. The reaction product, which was still ribosome-bound, was filtered and the filters were counted. From the result which is presented in Table 1 it follows that, even at high concentrations, compound I b does not affect tRNA$_f^{Met}$ binding, a conclusion which was already reached from the AUG-directed binding reaction. Ala-tRNA binding, however, was severely impeded. Surprisingly, little effect was observed in the presence of high concentrations of chloramphenicol while thiostrepton showed the expected and already well described inhibition of A-site binding. This experiment still allows no definite conclusion if compound I b also acts on the catalytic center of the peptidyl-transferase in addition to the inhibition of A-site binding. An impairment of this enzyme activity could be deduced if fMet-Ala formation were completely blocked. In order to test this possibility, both the peptide and unreacted amino acids were hydrolyzed off the filters and separated by high voltage electrophoresis into fMet, the fastest moving component, fMet-Ala which migrates slower and alanine, remaining at the origin. The radioactivity of the first two spots was plotted versus the concentration of compound I b, which initially was present in the reaction mixture (Fig. 4). An analysis of the diagram shows that fMet-Ala is formed in the presence of the pleuromutilin derivative, provided an Ala-tRNA is attached to the A-site which occurs more frequently at low concentrations of the drug. Thus, the only inhibition exerted by this antibiotic appears to be A-site binding.

Table 1. *R 17 phage-RNA directed binding of fMet-tRNA and of Ala-tRNA to E. coli ribosomes*

Antibiotic added	pmol bound	
	fMet-tRNA$_f^{Met}$	Ala-tRNA^{Ala}
Control - no antibiotic	8.1	7.7
Compound I b 1 μM	6.8	2.0
10 μM	6.5	1.2
100 μM	6.7	0.9
1 mM	6.3	0.8
Chloramphenicol 1 mM	7.2	6.5
Thiostrepton 10 μM	5.2	0.3

2 A_{260} units of salt washed *E. coli* D 10 ribosomes were incubated for 15 min at 30°C with 2.7 A_{260} units of R 17 phage-RNA, 66 μg of initiation factor protein, 53.4 pmol of [^{35}S]fMet-tRNA$_f^{Met}$ and various antibiotics at the given concentration in a mixture containing in 100 μl: 17 mM Tris-HCl, pH 7.5, 106 mM NH$_4$Cl, 5.1 mM magnesium acetate, 1 mM glutathione, 0.9 mM 2-mercaptoethanol and 1 mM GTP. After addition of 11.2 μg of EF-T and 60.5 pmol of [^{3}H]Ala-tRNA the incubation was continued for another 15 min at 30°C. The samples were filtered as described in Fig. 2 (A).

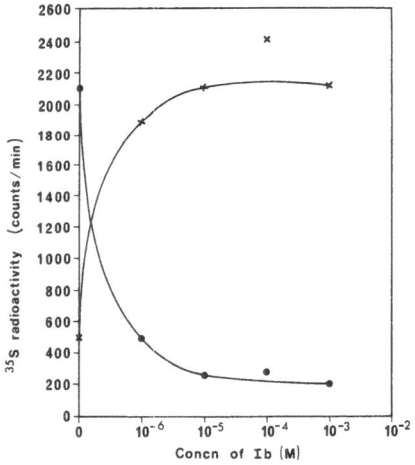

Fig. 4. Degree of fMet-Ala synthesis in the presence of compound I b. The dipeptide fMet-Ala and the free amino acids were hydrolyzed off the filters with NH$_4$OH, pH 10.6. The solutions were dried and the residue dissolved in small volumes of water, containing 7.5 μg each of fMet, fMet-Ala and Ala as carrier. The samples were applied to Whatman 3 MM paper and subjected to high voltage electrophoresis in a pyridine acetate buffer, pH 4.8 (6.25 ml pyridine, 7 ml acetic acid, 1 l of water). The radioactive products, identified by counting 1 cm wide strips in toluene scintillation fluid, migrated the same distances as the nonradioactive standards.

An unexpected and surprising result was, however, obtained from poly(U)-directed, EF-T catalyzed binding of Phe-tRNA to empty ribosomes. As shown in Fig. 5, binding of Phe-tRNA, measured at various concentrations of compound I b, was refractory to this drug at least at low concentrations which already influences Ala-tRNA binding in the above mentioned experiment very strongly. The fact that Ala-tRNA attachment to the A-site of initiation complexes is affected by the pleuromutilin derivative, while binding of Phe-tRNA to the A-site of empty ribosomes is not inhibited suggests that an occupied P-site is the prerequisite for the activity of the drug. The aminoacyl-tRNA, when binding to the A-site, may be able to displace compound I b provided it can leave through the empty P-site. If the P-site is blocked, a steric hindrance by the bound fMet-tRNA may not allow this displacement. As a consequence, binding of the aminoacyl-tRNA to the A-site may not occur.

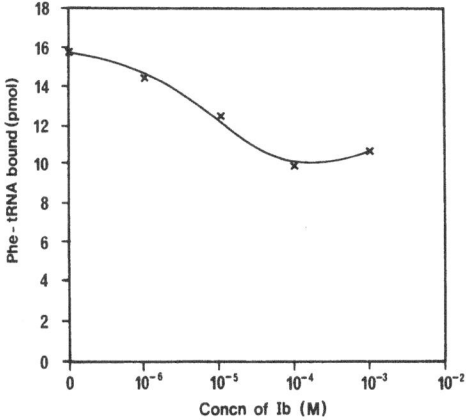

Fig. 5. Effect of compound I b on EF-T-catalyzed, poly(U)-directed binding of Phe-tRNA. Reaction mixtures of 100 µl, which contained 2 A_{260} units of *E. coli* D 10 ribosomes, 44.4 pmol of [^{14}C]Phe-tRNA, 16.8 µg EF-T, 10 µg poly(U), 50 mM Tris-HCl, pH 7.8, 80 mM NH_4Cl, 5 mM magnesium acetate, 6 mM 2-mercapto-ethanol and 0.4 mM GTP were incubated for 15 min at 37°C. The reaction mixtures were filtered as described in Fig. 2 (A).

These effects on bacterial protein biosynthesis are strong and well defined and therefore ought to be generated by a pleuromutilin molecule which is specifically attached to a ribosomal receptor. This concept was tested using a tritium-labelled derivative of compound I b with a saturated exocyclic vinyl group at positions 19 and 20 (compound II). When binding of this derivative to ribosomes was assayed using the equilibrium dialysis technique at varying ligand concentrations, data were obtained which could be fitted into a linear Scatchard plot (Fig. 6). The intersection with the abscissa reveals the presence of one specific binding site per ribosome to which the drug is attached with an association constant $K_{ass} = 1.3 \times 10^7$ 1/mole. For chloramphenicol an association constant $K_{ass} = 3 \times 10^5$ 1/mole was determined. As shown in Fig. 7 the binding of compound II was reduced if chloramphenicol was present in the equilibrium dialysis cell. In the reverse experiment binding of [^{14}C]chloramphenicol was affected by the presence of nonradioactive compound II (Fig. 8). The binding sites for pleuromutilin and chloramphenicol thus appear to be partially overlapping.

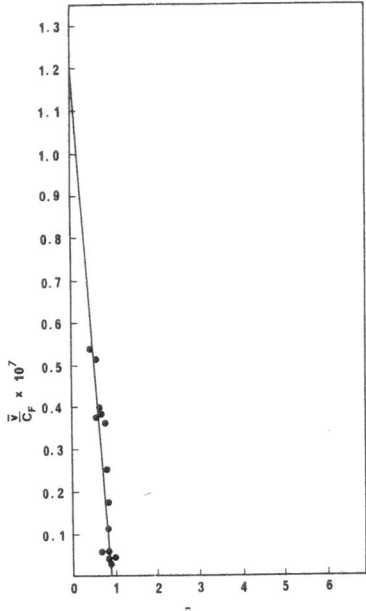

Fig. 6. Scatchard plot of binding of ^{3}H-labelled compound II to ribosomes. Binding of the drug was determined by equilibrium dialysis
using 1 ml cells. One chamber of the dialysis cell was filled with a
solution of salt washed *E. coli* D 10 ribosomes at a concentration of
202 A_{260} units/ml. The other with solutions of ^{3}H-labelled compound II
of various concentrations. Both the ribosomes and the pleuromutilin
derivative were dissolved in 10 mM Tris-HCl, pH 7.8, 10 mM magnesium
acetate, 60 mM KCl and 6 mM 2-mercaptoethanol. The cells were rotated
at 2°C for 3 hours. Aliquots of the cells were removed and their radioactivity was determined.

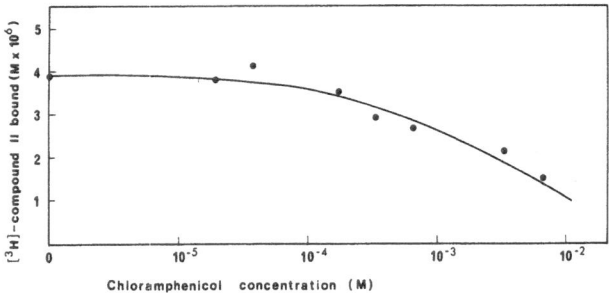

Fig. 7. Displacement of ^{3}H-labelled compound II by chloramphenicol in
ribosomal binding. Solutions of ^{3}H-labelled compound II (6 µM) containing various concentrations of chloramphenicol, as indicated on the
abscissa, were dialyzed to equilibrium against salt washed *E. coli*
D 10 ribosomes (203 A_{260} units/ml) as described in Fig. 6.

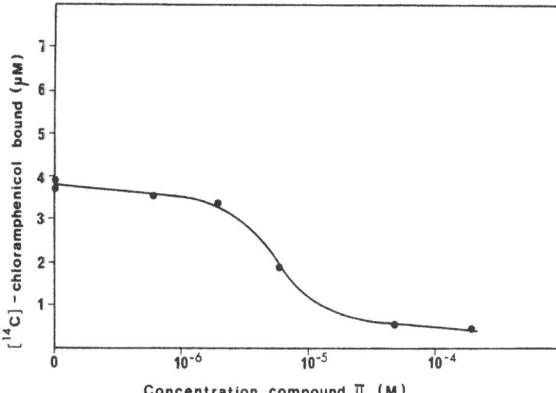

Fig. 8. Displacement of [^{14}C]chloramphenicol by compound II in ribosome binding. Solutions of [^{14}C]chloramphenicol (15.6 µM) containing various concentrations of compound II were dialyzed to equilibrium against salt washed *E. coli* D 10 ribosomes (203 A$_{260}$ units/ml) as described in Fig. 6.

Ribosome-bound compound II was not displaced by lincomycin and by erythromycin while they were reported to influence chloramphenicol attachment (data not shown)(Fernandez-Muñoz *et al.*, 1971). The area of the chloramphenicol binding site which overlaps with that for lincomycin and erythromycin seems, therefore, to be not influenced by pleuromutilin.

Puromycin also effectively displaced the pleuromutilin derivative II from its ribosomal binding region although, owing to the low affinity of puromycin to its ribosomal binding site (Lessard and Pestka, 1972), the effect was detectable only at high concentrations of puromycin (Fig. 9). Since puromycin acts as structural analogue to the amino-

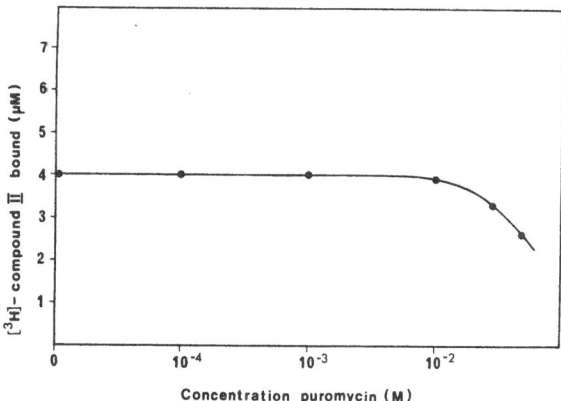

Fig. 9. Displacement of ^{3}H-labelled compound II by puromycin in ribosome binding. Solutions of ^{3}H-labelled compound II (5 µM) were dialyzed to equilibrium against salt washed *E. coli* D 10 ribosomes in the presence of various initial concentrations of puromycin as described in Fig. 6.

acyl terminus of a tRNA, interfering with the attachment of this moiety, it might be concluded that pleuromutilin derivatives also perturb the forces which are involved with the binding of the 3'-terminus of a tRNA. This idea receives support from the above described competition experiments with chloramphenicol because chloramphenicol was also shown to inhibit the attachment of the 3'-terminus of a tRNA (Nierhaus and Nierhaus, 1973). Direct evidence, however, was obtained from experiments with nucleotides which are sequence analogues of the 3'-terminal region of a tRNA as competitors of pleuromutilin binding. The nucleotides employed were CpA and CpCpA. As shown in Table 2, the dinucleotide, at an initial concentration of 40 mM in one dialysis compartment, produced a 54 % reduction of compound II binding while 10 mM CpCpA caused an effect of similar magnitude (47 %). The effect exerted by the trinucleotide is stronger because it occurs at a lower concentration. This is not surprising since, as a result of the additional cytidylic residue, the trinucleotide probably exhibits a stronger affinity for the ribosome. The controls with the nucleotides UpU and UpUpU gave a slight depression of the binding of compound II only. This suggests that the displacement of the drug by CpA and CpCpA is specific.

An interesting feature of pleuromutilin compounds is their complete loss of antibacterial activity as well as the inhibitory effect on cell-free protein biosynthesis after oxydation of the hydroxy group in position 11. The keto derivative of compound I b will be called compound III. When present at a concentration of 10^{-5} in a poly(U)-directed, polyphenylalanine synthesizing system, containing an $E.\ coli$ S 30-extract, compound III produced only a 6 % reduction of synthesis while compound I b at the same concentration blocked 64 % of the reaction. Compound III, however, was still able to bind to the ribosomal attachment site, although with a slightly reduced affinity, as competition experiments with labelled compound II indicate. In a similar way, this substance effectively displaced chloramphenicol as shown by a series of dialysis experiments in Fig. 10. These data may indicate

Table 2. *Displacement of compound I b by various nucleotides in ribosome binding*

40 mM dinucleotide added	10 mM trinucleotide added	Compound I b bound (μM)
no addition	---	3.7
CpA	---	1.7
UpU	---	3.2
---	no addition	3.7
---	CpCpA	1.95
---	UpUpU	3.1

5 μM solutions of ^{3}H-labelled compound I b were dialyzed against salt washed $E.\ coli$ D 10 ribosomes (202 A_{260} units/ml) in a micro dialysis cell containing 20 μl of liquid in each chamber. Di- or trinucleotides at an initial concentration as indicated were added. The cells were slowly rotated at 2°C for 3 hours. 10 μl aliquots were withdrawn from each chamber, mixed first with 1 ml of water, then with 9 ml Instagel and counted.

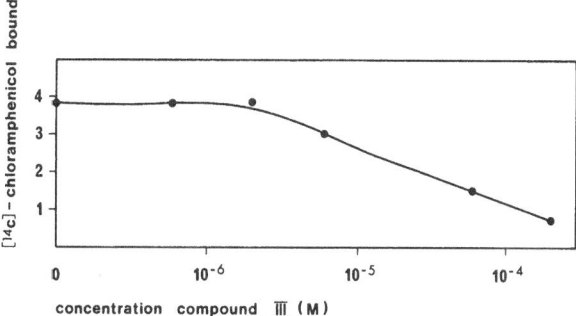

concentration compound III (M)

Fig. 10. Displacement of [^{14}C]chloramphenicol by compound III in ribosomal binding. Solutions of [^{14}C]chloramphenicol (15.6 μM containing
compound III at various initial concentrations were dialyzed to equilibrium against salt washed *E. coli* D 10 ribosomes as described in
Fig. 6.

that tight binding of a molecule to the chloramphenicol- and pleuro-
mutilin-specific receptor is not necessarily followed by an inactivation of the ribosomal A-site. A simple model of steric hindrance cannot explain sufficiently the failure of compound III to inhibit polypeptide synthesis. Active drugs, in addition to their ability to attach
to a specific receptor, are probably also capable to distort in a specific way the region to which the 3'-terminus of a tRNA is bound.
This property but not the binding ability may be lost by oxydizing the
11-OH group in the pleuromutilin derivatives.

In summary, pleuromutilin derivatives have been shown to block bacterial protein biosynthesis by inactivating a portion of the ribosomal
A-site which is close to the peptidyl transferase. The drug exerts its
inhibiting activity only if the P-site is occupied by a tRNA molecule.
One specific binding site per ribosome with a high affinity for pleuromutilin derivatives has been revealed. Binding to this region, which
is partially identical with the chloramphenicol-receptor, seems to
affect the attachment of the terminal nucleotides of a tRNA.

Acknowledgements

The participation of Mrs. G. Hartmann, Miss L.A. Hodgin and Mrs. B.
Stumper in this work is gratefully acknowledged.

References

ARIGONI, D.: La structura di un terpene di nuovo genere. Gazz. chim.
    Ital. 92, 884 - 901 (1962).
EGGER, H., and H. Reinshagen: Neue Pleuromutiline und Verfahren zu
    ihrer Herstellung. Ger. Offen. 2.248,237 (Chem. Abstr. 79, 65901 v)
    (1973).
FERNANDEZ-Muñoz, R., R.E. Monro, R. Torres-Pinedo, and D. Vazquez:
    Substrate- and Antibiotic-Binding Sites at the Peptidyl-Transfer-
    ase Centre of *Escherichia coli* Ribosomes. Eur. J. Biochem. 23,
    '85 - 193 (1971).

KAVANAGH, F., A. Hervey, and W.J. Robbins: Antibiotic Substances from
    Basidomycetes. VIII. Pleurotus Multilus (FR.) Sacc. and Pleurotus
    Sasseckerianus Pilat. Proc. Nat. Acad. Sci. USA 37, 570 - 574 (1951).
LESSARD, J.L., and S. Pestka: Studies on the Formation of Transfer
    Ribonucleic Acid-Ribosome Complexes. J. Biol. Chem. 247, 6909 -
    6912 (1972).
NAEGELI, P.: Zur Kenntnis des Pleuromutilins. Ph. D. thesis, ETH
    Zürich. Juris Verlag, Zürich (1961).
NIERHAUS, D., and K.H. Nierhaus: Identification of the Chloramphenicol-
    Binding Protein in *Escherichia coli* Ribosomes by Partial Reconsti-
    tution. Proc. Nat. Acad. Sci. USA 70, 2224 - 2228 (1973).
NIRENBERG, M.: Cell-free Protein Synthesis Directed by Messenger RNA.
    Methods in Enzymology Vol. VI (Eds. S.P. Colowick and N.O. Kaplan)
    Academic Press, New York and London, pp. 17 - 23 (1963).

A Structural Model of the Chloramphenicol Receptor Site

Fred E. Hahn and Peter Gund

I. INTRODUCTION

Having a relatively simple chemical structure, chloramphenicol became the first antibiotic to be synthesized by organic-chemical methods (Controulis, Rebstock and Crooks, 1949). A large number of chloramphenicol derivatives was subsequently prepared. Kolosov, Shemiakin, Khokhlov and Gurevich tabulated, in 1961, more than 500 such compounds, and the total number of known chloramphenicol derivatives is, by now, much greater.

For many of these substances, data on their growth-inhibitory potencies for bacteria have been reported. Also, after it was recognized that chloramphenicol acts through specific inhibition of bacterial protein biosynthesis (Hahn and Wisseman, 1951; Gale and Folkes, 1953; Wisseman, Smadel, Hahn and Hopps, 1954) and cell-free model systems of protein synthesis were subsequently developed, chloramphenicol derivatives have been tested for inhibitions of such systems. Hence, the chloramphenicol series of compounds appears to be suited to the derivation of structure-activity relationships.

The recent identification of a chloramphenicol binding protein which is a constituent of the 50s subunit of 70s ribosomes (Nierhaus and Nierhaus, 1973; Pongs, Bald and Erdmann, 1973) has renewed our interest in these structure-activity relationships and has encouraged us to analyze them with a view to deriving a structural model of a chloramphenicol receptor site which we infer to be located on the peptidyl transferase which is part of the 50s ribosomal subunit.

II. STRUCTURE-ACTIVITY RELATIONSHIPS WHICH DETERMINE INHIBITION OF BACTERIAL GROWTH

First systematic efforts to derive for chloramphenicol derivatives structure-activity rules for bacterial growth inhibition were made by Hahn (1955), Shemiakin, Kolosov, Levitov, Germanova, Karapetian, Shvetsov and Bamdas (1955, 1956) and Hahn, Hayes, Wisseman, Hopps and Smadel (1956). Both groups of workers arrived independently at the same conclusions; reviews of these conclusions represented the state of the art for several years (Kolosov et al., 1961; Hahn, 1967a). Both groups also called attention to the fact that data on growth inhibitions by chloramphenicol derivatives had been obtained in many laboratories using varieties of methods and test organisms and could not be considered to be better than semi-quantitative approximations which did not lend themselves to the derivation of quantitative structure-activity relationships.

In 1966, Garrett, Wright, Miller and Smith determined the antibacterial potencies of chloramphenicol and nine derivatives with variations in the para-substituent of the phenyl residue by measuring decreases in exponential growth rates of Escherichia coli caused by graded concentrations of the test compounds. The same procedure was subsequently applied (Hansch, Nakamoto, Gorin, Denisevich, Garrett, Heman-Ackah and Won, 1973) to 37 chloramphenicol derivatives with variations of either the para-substituent or the acyl moiety. A third study, employing recording of growth curves and comparing 16 derivatives of chloramphenicol with different structural variations, was reported by Kono, O'Hara, Honda and Mitsuhashi (1969).

Multiple regression analyses of structure-activity data (Hansch, Muir, Fujita, Maloney, Geiger and Streich, 1963; Cammarata, 1967; Hansch, Kutter and Leo, 1969; Hansch et al., 1973) have focused on resolving the electronic and penetration properties which are conferred upon the chloramphenicol molecule by derivatization. Specifically, this approach was intended to design derivatives "better" than the antibiotic itself (Hansch et al., 1973). However, the resolution into different contributions to antibacterial activity was not persuasively accomplished, and the empirical discovery of two derivatives with greatly superior antibacterial properties (Kono et al., 1969) was not forecast by theoretical considerations which failed to address themselves to the steric specificities of chloramphenicol. We consider it sufficient, therefore, to summarize factually the apparent structure-activity relationships without attempting to improve on their theoretical treatment.

The molecule of chloramphenicol can be subdivided (Fig. 1) into three parts: I. The substituted aromatic ring system, II. The acyl side chain, and III. The propanediol moiety. We shall consider, in turn, structure-activity relationships for these three portions of the molecule.

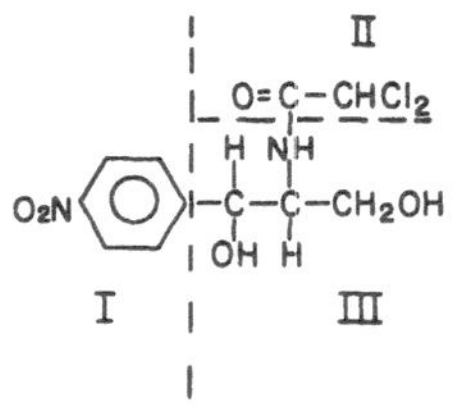

CHLORAMPHENICOL

Fig. 1. Structure of chloramphenicol, partitioned into three major portions.

I. The aromatic ring system permits of considerable variations with respect to the ring structure itself and to its substituents, resulting in compounds whose antibacterial activities are modified rather than abolished. The p-nitrophenyl group can be replaced by biphenyl, 4'-bromobiphenyl or 4'-methylbiphenyl without significant loss (and for Sarcina lutea even a gain up to 2.8 times) in antibacterial potency (Rebstock, Stratton and Bambas, 1955). The p-nitroazobenzene derivative of chloramphenicol approaches the antibacterial potency of the antibiotic itself (Shemiakin et al., 1956). The p-SCH$_3$ derivative, also has high antibacterial activity (Hansch et al., 1973). Replacing p-nitrophenyl by 5-nitro-2-thienyl, 5-nitro-1-naphthyl or 4-pyridyl results in compounds with significant antibacterial activities (revs: Hahn et al., 1956; Kolosov et al., 1961). Evidently, the steric properties of the aromatic system are not of critical importance for the antibacterial action of chloramphenicols, except that ortho or meta substitution appears substantially to reduce potency.

Originally, one of us (FEH) speculated from scattered growth inhibition data (Hahn et al., 1956) that the antibacterial potency of chloramphenicols was a function of the relative electronegativity of the para substituent. While the electronic properties of the substituents might be determinants of the antibacterial potencies of these derivatives, one should not exclude additional contributions from hydrophobic effects which may play a role in the penetration of the compounds into the bacterial cells and especially in the attachment to their site of action: Shemiakin et al. (1956) reported that substitution in the para position of six ionogenic and, hence, hydrophilic groups abolished antibacterial activity.

II. The acyl side chain is essential for antibacterial potency: the deacylated chloramphenicol base is almost devoid of activity (Rebstock, Crooks, Controulis and Bartz, 1949). Variations of the acyl substituent have been the most frequently introduced alterations of the chloramphenicol molecule; in 1961, Kolosov et al. listed 123 such derivatives. On the basis of insufficient growth inhibition data, Hahn et al. (1956) had speculated that the electronegativities of the acyl substituent were determinants of antibacterial potency. When this idea was reexamined, using the inhibition data of Hansch et al. (1973), no satisfactory correlation was obtained. For example, chloramphenicol itself had a log k of 2.00 with dichloroacetic acid having a K_α of 3.32 x 10^{-2} and a pK of 1.48, while the trichloroacetyl derivative had a log k of 0.75 with trichloroacetic acid having a K_α of 2 x 10^{-1} and a pK of 0.70. It should be noted that the electronic Hammett constants σ^* for 20 chloramphenicol derivatives with different acyl residues, R, showed marginally significant correlation with the antibacterial potencies of these compounds (Hansch et al., 1973). Moreover, the charges of O, C, N and H for the acylamino side-chains of 11 chloramphenicol derivatives have been calculated (Höltje and Kier, 1974) and reveal no detectable relationship to the antibacterial activities of these compounds. Shemiakin et al. (1956) have proposed that not only the polarity but the polarizing action of the acyl substituent is important for antibacterial activity, and Hansch et al. (1973) conjectured that the acyl substituent affects the acidity of the amide nitrogen proton. In fact, substitution of the amide H with methyl abolishes antibacterial activity (Collins, Ellis, Hansen, Mackenzie, Moualin and Petrow, 1952).

Many workers agree (Hahn et al., 1956; Shemiakin et al., 1956; Hansch et al., 1973) that the steric properties of the acyl moiety limit the antibacterial action of chloramphenicol derivatives and that increases in the size of this substituent decrease potency. "Bulky substituents are undesirable (Hansch et al., 1973)."

III. The propanediol moiety possesses two asymmetric carbon atoms which give rise to four stereoisomers. Two of these, the D-threo (chloramphenicol) and the L-threo enantiomers, carry the amide side chain and the hydroxyl on carbon 1 on opposite sides of the plane of the two asymmetric centers, while the other two enantiomers, the L-erythro and D-erythro stereoisomers, carry the two substituents on the same side of this plane. Only chloramphenicol itself, the D-threo isomer, has strong antibacterial properties (Maxwell and Nickel, 1954). Methyl substitution for the H on carbon atom 2 abolishes antibacterial activity (Huebner and Scholz, 1951). The absolute stereospecificity of chloramphenicol's action also applies to active derivatives of the antibiotic.

Substitutions of the two hydroxyls, exchanging them for H atoms or suppression or extension of the terminal -CH_2OH result in non-active compounds (rev: Hahn et al., 1956). Diacetylation of the hydroxyls is the phenotypic expression of R-factor determined resistance to chloramphenicol (Shaw, 1967; Suzuki and Okamoto, 1967).

An x-ray diffraction analysis of the dibromoacetyl derivative of chloramphenicol (Dunitz, 1952) had shown that the two hydroxyls approach each other closely in the crystalline compound and suggested the formation of a hydrogen bond which closed a five-membered ring structure. Nuclear magnetic resonance spectroscopy seemed initially to support the same conclusion for chloramphenicol in partially aqueous solutions (Jardetzky, 1963). However, when the conformation of chloramphenicol was reinvestigated by NMR and infrared spectroscopy (Bustard, Egan and Perun, 1973), no evidence of hydrogen bonding in solution was obtained.

The earlier view of chloramphenicol as forming a hydrogen-bonded five-membered ring structure in solution led to speculations that the drug was alternately an analog of uridylic acid (Jardetzky, 1963; Jardetzky and Julian, 1964) or of an amino-acylated nucleoside, resembling puromycin (Coutsogeorgopoulos, 1966, 1967). Both speculations had in common that they regarded the assumed hydrogen-bonded five-membered ring structure in chloramphenicol to be analogous to ribose.

The structural variations which are permissible for the aryl moiety of active chloramphenicol derivatives collectively weaken analogies of this aryl to uracil or dimethyl adenine. Observations on growth-inhibitory activities of several chloramphenicol derivatives with covalently closed six-membered alicyclic systems were ambiguous (rev: Hahn et al., 1956). The analogy of the putative ring system to ribose has, however, been tested directly through the synthesis of the ribosyl derivative of chloramphenicol, Fig. 2 (Klein, Lotick, Watanabe and Fox, 1971). This compound was totally non-active against 10 different bacterial strains and showed only insignificant effects on the growth of E. coli on plates (R.S. Klein, personal communication).

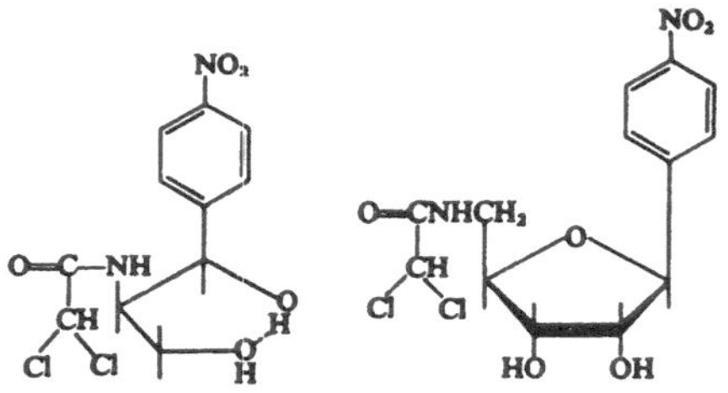

Fig. 2. Conjectural hydrogen-bonded ring structure in the chloramphenicol molecule at left and structure of a ribosyl derivative of chloramphenicol at right (Klein et al., 1971).

Intromolecular hydrogen bonding as a determinant of antimicrobial activity had already become doubtful after it was shown that replacement of the hydroxyl of carbon atom 1 by Cl (Farkaš and Sicher, 1953) or conversion of the 1-hydroxy into the 1-keto compound (Long and Troutman, 1951) produced substances with appreciable antimicrobial activity. A tabulation of >40 derivatives having the 1-keto group (Kolosov et al., 1961) listed several actively antibacterial compounds. Most important, Fig. 3 shows two chloramphenicol 1-keto derivatives which are molecule for molecule 60 and 38 times more active than chloramphenicol itself in inhibiting the growth of Staphylococcus aureus (Kono et al., 1969). Intramolecular hydrogen bonding is excluded for both derivatives.

III. STRUCTURE-ACTIVITY RELATIONSHIPS WHICH DETERMINE INHIBITIONS OF CELL-FREE SYSTEMS

A first indication of an effect of chloramphenicol on cell-free model protein synthesis in a system of bacterial origin (Lamborg and Zamecnik, 1960) was followed by studies of inhibitions of more defined systems which employed synthetic

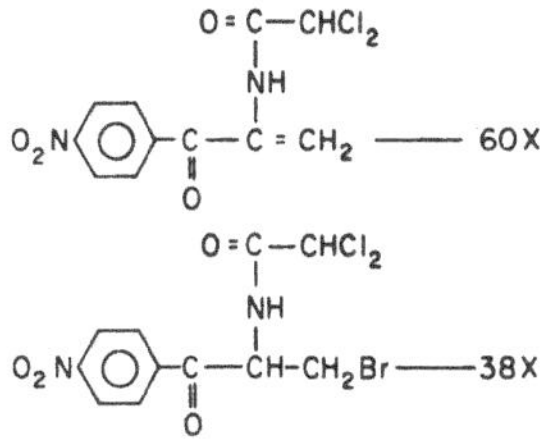

SUPERIOR CHLORAMPHENICOL DERIVATIVES

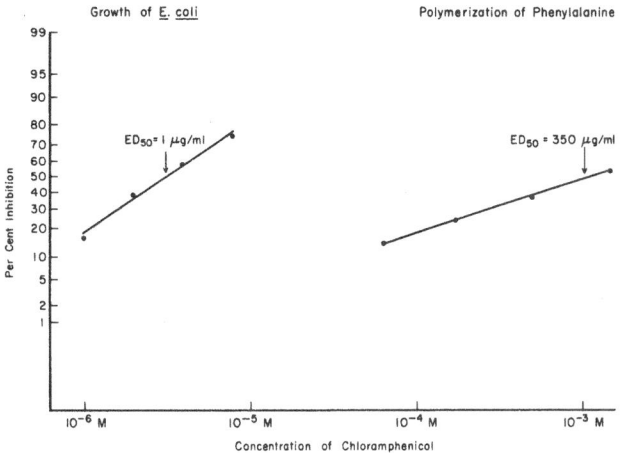

Fig. 3. Structures of chloramphenicol derivatives with superior antibacterial
activities (Kono et al., 1969).

Fig. 4. Dosage-response correlation for the inhibition of growth of E. coli at
left and for the inhibition of an E. coli ribosome-poly U system,
polymerizing phenylalanine, at right.

polynucleotides as messenger RNA (Nirenberg and Matthaei, 1961; Kućan and Lipmann, 1964; Vazquez, 1966). Disadvantages of working with such systems are illustrated in Figs. 4 and 5 (Hahn, 1967b). Fig. 4 presents dosage response correlations for the inhibitions of growth of E. coli and of the cell-free E. coli ribosome-poly U system which polymerizes phenylalanine. The 50 per cent effective concentrations of chloramphenicol differ by a factor of 350; it is practically impossible to obtain more than 60 per cent inhibition of the poly U system with chloramphenicol. Fig. 5 shows inhibitions by chloramphenicol of poly UC systems polymerizing proline. The relative potency of 3×10^{-5} M chloramphenicol is directly proportional to the cytidylic acid content of a series of poly UCs. The sensitivity of such cell-free systems is not a function of the amino acid which is polymerized but rather of the base composition of the synthetic messenger (Speyer, Lengyel, Basilio, Wahba, Gardner and Ochoa, 1963; Kućan and Lipmann, 1964). Since, additionally, chloramphenicol analogs produce different responses in poly U, poly A and poly C systems (Vazquez, 1966), such systems are not well suited for a comparative study of structure-activity relationships.

Consequently, messenger-free systems for the assay of the formation of single peptide bonds have been employed in the study of chloramphenicol analogs; these systems used puromycin as the peptidyl acceptor and either an N-formyl-methionyl-hexanucleotide fragment (Monro and Vazquez, 1967), polylysyl-tRNA (Coutsogeorgopoulos, 1967) or acetyl-phenylalanyl-tRNA (Pestka, 1970) as peptidyl donors.

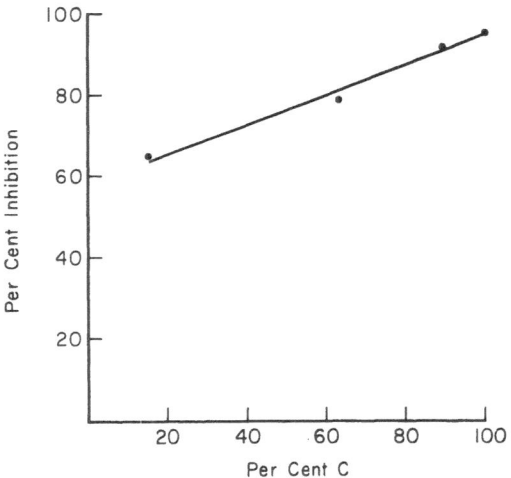

Fig. 5. Correlation between the inhibition by 3×10^{-5} M chloramphenicol of ribosome-poly UC systems, polymerizing proline, and the cytidylic acid content of a series of poly UCs.

I. The aromatic ring system has been phenyl in all chloramphenicol derivatives studied in cell-free systems. Para-substituents were $-SCH_3$, $-SO_2CH_3$, $-SO_2NH_2$ and $-NHCOCH_3$. At concentrations between 3.13×10^{-6} M and 4×10^{-4} M, compounds inhibited a variety of amino acid polymerization systems with (Vazquez, 1966) or without (Telesnina, Novikova, Zhdanov, Kolosov and Shemiakin, 1967) added messengers. The p-amino reduction product of chloramphenicol is devoid of activity (Coutsogeorgopoulos, 1966). The N-formyl-methionyl "fragment reaction" was inhibited to the same extent by chloramphenicol and its methylsulfonyl and aminosulfonyl derivatives, while the thiomethyl derivative was about half as active (Monro and Vazquez, 1967). Displacement of ^{14}C-chloramphenicol from bacterial ribosomes was 99 per cent for ^{12}C-chloramphenicol, and 98 per cent for the methylsulfonyl, 96 per cent for the aminosulfonyl and 94 per cent for the thiomethyl derivatives (Vazquez, 1966). Binding of the ^{14}C-labeled thiomethyl derivative of chloramphenicol to E. coli ribosomes has recently been measured; the apparent association constant for this reaction is identical to that for chloramphenicol binding (Contreras, Barbacid and Vazquez, 1974). These few data on cell-free actions of p-substitution variants of chloramphenicol do not lend themselves to a derivation of structure-activity relationships; all substances showed appreciable activity with the exception of the p-amino compound.

II. The acyl side chain is essential for in vitro activity: the deacylated chloramphenicol base has only ∿6 per cent of the activity of chloramphenicol in a poly UC (1:1) system which polymerizes phenylalanine (Coutsogeorgopoulos, 1966). At 4×10^{-4} M, the dibromoacetyl, monochloroacetyl, trichloroacetyl, acetyl and dichlorocrotonyl derivatives were as active as chloramphenicol itself in an incorporation system without added messenger RNA (Telesnina et al., 1967). The monobromo- and monoiodoacetyl derivatives of chloramphenicol bind irreversibly to the ribosomal site of action of the antibiotic, probably by reacting with a strategically placed amino acid functional group; therefore, these derivatives inhibit model protein synthesis irreversibly (Bald, Erdmann and Pongs, 1972).

Interestingly, the glycyl, leucyl, phenylalanyl and p-methoxyphenylalanyl derivatives of chloramphenicol show considerable activities in a poly UC system, polymerizing phenylalanine (Coutsogeorgopoulos, 1966) and also in a system which synthesizes puromycyl-polylysine without added messenger RNA (Coutsogeorgopoulos, 1967). Data from these studies are reproduced in Table I.

TABLE I

INHIBITIONS OF CELL-FREE MODEL PROTEIN SYNTHESES BY CHLORAMPHENICOL ANALOGS

(COUTSOGEORGOPOULOS, 1966, 1967)

Compounds at 10^{-3} M	Inhibition of phenyl- alanine polymerization in a poly (UC) system		Inhibition of polylysyl transfer to puromycin	
	% Actual	Relative	% Actual	Relative
dichloroacetyl- (chloramphenicol)	88	(100)	90	(100)
p-methoxyphenylalanyl-	55	(62)	92	(102)
glycyl-	70	(80)	83	(92)
leucyl-	52	(59)	60	(67)
phenylalanyl-	53	(60)	56	(62)

III. The propanediol moiety in the D-threo configuration is important for inhibition of cell-free protein synthesis. Rendi and Ochoa (1962) found in an E. coli ribosome system without extraneous messenger that the L-threo enantiomer and the L-erythro isomer had much less inhibitory activity than chloramphenicol itself. All three stereoisomers of chloramphenicol are incapable of displacing the antibiotic from bacterial ribosomes as are also the enantiomers of the methyl-sulfonyl and thiomethyl para-substituted derivatives (Vazquez, 1966). Aminoacyl-oligonucleotide fragments of aminoacyl tRNA are bound to bacterial ribosomes in the absence of messenger RNAs. Examples of such compounds are phenylalanyl-A-C-C, lysyl-A-C-C and leucyl-A-C-C. Chloramphenicol at 3×10^{-5} M inhibits this reaction but its three stereoisomers, even at 33 times higher concentrations, fail to inhibit ribosomal binding of these aminoacyl-nucleotide fragments (Pestka, rev. 1974).

IV. COMPARISON OF IN VIVO AND IN VITRO STRUCTURE-ACTIVITY RULES

A comparison of the structure-activity relationships for bacterial growth inhibition with those for inhibitions of cell-free processes related to protein biosynthesis may lead to the recognition of those structural features which are necessary for the inhibition of protein biosynthesis per se, i.e. to the binding of chloramphenicol to its receptor site, in contrast to other properties which are requirements for the penetration of the drug into bacterial cells. The only work which has compared in vivo and in vitro effects of chloramphenicol derivatives side by side is that of Telesnina et al. (1967) whose stated objective was to bring "the structure-activity study closer to the molecular level."

I. The aromatic ring system is conducive to both in vivo and in vitro activities. Telesnina et al. (1967) found for two para-substituted variants of chloramphenicol that they were less active on model protein synthesis than on growth of E. coli as, indeed, chloramphenicol itself typically is. However, the p-NHCOCH₃ derivative inhibited growth to only 0.2 per cent of the activity of chloramphenicol at 1.5 and 2.6×10^{-7} M, while inhibiting model protein synthesis by >40 per cent relative to the antibiotic over a thousandfold concentration range. The p-amino derivative has low activities on bacterial growth (Garrett et al., 1966) and on the polymerization of phenylalanine in a ribosome-poly UC system (Coutsogeorgopoulos, 1966).

II. The acyl side chain is necessary for both in vivo and in vitro activity: the free chloramphenicol base exhibits low activity in both instances. However, while strong electronegativity and, also, lipophilic properties of the acyl substituents are requirements for bacterial growth inhibition in addition to restrictions of the size of this substituent, no such requirements appear to exist for the inhibition of model protein synthesis in vitro. For five acyl derivatives of chloramphenicol, Telesnina et al. (1967) found superior in vitro activities on model protein synthesis when compared to bacterial growth inhibition and concluded that the most important function of the acyl substituent is "in the penetration of the antibiotic into the bacterial cell."

It is most important that amino acyl derivatives of the drug possess high in vitro activity (Table I); the glycyl derivative inhibits model protein syntheses to 80-90 per cent of the activity of chloramphenicol itself but has an ED₅₀ on the growth of Streptococcus faecalis of 2×10^{-4} M, while this ED₅₀ for chloramphenicol is 4×10^{-7} M (Coutsogeorgopoulos, personal communication). We assume that the fivehundredfold difference between the two ED₅₀s reflects differences in the uptake of the glycyl and dichloroacetyl compounds into bacteria. Earlier (Rebstock and Stratton, 1955), the glycyl, phenylalanyl and alanyl derivatives of chloramphenicol had been reported to "exhibit a low order of antibacterial activity." We conclude that the electronic and steric requirements of the acyl side chain for antibacterial activity are determinants of permeation into bacteria but represent only a sub-set of less stringent requirements for inhibition of protein synthesis.

III. The propanediol moiety when present in compounds of the chloramphenicol series must be in the D-threo configuration for both in vivo and in vitro action. The remaining three stereoisomers are devoid of antibacterial properties (Maxwell and Nickel, 1954), do not displace chloramphenicol from ribosomes (Vazquez, 1966), do not inhibit ribosomal binding of aminoacyl trinucleotide fragments (Pestka, rev: 1974) and are poor inhibitors of model protein synthesis (Rendi and Ochoa, 1962). Observations (Hahn, Wisseman and Hopps, 1954) that the L-erythro stereoisomer of chloramphenicol inhibits the formation of γ-D-glutamyl polypeptide in Bacillus subtilis (now classified as B. lichenoformis) suggest that this isomer acts on a peptide-forming enzyme which processes a D-amino acid and must, therefore, possess a stereochemical configuration different from that of ribosomal peptidyl transferase which operates on L-amino acids and is inhibited by chloramphenicol itself. The most highly active of the two derivatives in Fig. 3 indicates that the propane moiety can be altered to eliminate stereoisomerism altogether. Evidently, the stereochemistry of chloramphenicol is an incidental property of a natural product rather than an absolute requirement to be met by all active members of the synthetic chloramphenicol series.

IV. Features which are necessary for penetration of chloramphenicol into bacterial cells must be considered in the light of the kinetics of entry. These have been measured for ¹⁴C-chloramphenicol with cells of E. coli at 0°, i.e. under physical conditions in which any active transport was minimized (Das, Goldstein and Kanner, 1966). During the first minute, 75 per cent of the total entry was effected; by a second and slower process, the remaining 25 per cent were taken up within 10 minutes. The first entry process was not subject to isotopic competition with ¹²C-chloramphenicol and, hence, represented an equilibration of the drug between extracellular and intracellular water rather than binding to the cell surface or to intracellular ribosomes. These observations strongly argue against active transport, requiring the expenditure of metabolic energy, as the means by which chloramphenicol enters bacteria.

It also is unlikely that chloramphenicol permeates into bacteria as a result of an exchange in the lipid constituents of the membrane. The log P (octanol/water) for chloramphenicol is 1.14 (Leo, Hansch and Elkins, 1971). Multiple regression analysis for 37 chloramphenicol derivatives gave an optimal log P of 1.3 - 1.5 which contains a receptor-substrate hydrophobic binding contribution of at least 0.5 (Hansch et al., 1973). By comparison, a regression analysis study on numerous toxic chemicals has shown that the optimal log P for Gram-positive bacteria is about 6 and for Gram-negative bacteria about 4 (Lien, Hansch and Anderson, 1968). These log P values have been attributed to the permeation characteristics of compounds through bacterial envelopes of lesser (Gram-positive) or greater (Gram-negative) lipid contents. The log P values of chloramphenicol and of its most active derivatives fall far outside this optimal numerical range.

We speculate that the drug enters bacteria by facilitated diffusion which involves a carrier or channel with steric and electronic specificities which favor the permeation of compounds of the chloramphenicol series when the acyl residue is not larger than acetyl, is hydrophobic and is substituted with halogen atoms. This view is supported by a recently constructed model of a lipoprotein of the outer membrane of E. coli (Inouye, 1974). This model allows for hydrophilic channels which are acidic, owing to their lining with glutamic and aspartic acid residues; the diameters of the channels vary between 12.5 to 35.8 Å and their numbers per cell from 1.25×10^5 to 0.63×10^5, depending upon the number of lipoproteins per assembly. These channels occupy from 35 to 46 per cent of the cell surface.

The hypothesis of facilitated diffusion of chloramphenicol can be tested by the isotope counter transport assay (Wilbrandt and Rosenberg, 1961). Such experiments will be undertaken in the laboratory of one of these authors (FEH).

V. A STRUCTURAL MODEL OF THE CHLORAMPHENICOL RECEPTOR

On the basis of the empirical structure-activity relationships analyzed above, it might be possible to derive, in abstraction, a model of a chloramphenicol-binding site by proper placement of surfaces, cavities and stereoelectronic requirements. However, such an abstract model would be difficult to relate to the mechanism of action of chloramphenicol although it might be useful in the consideration of the reactivity of chloramphenicol derivatives with chloramphenicol-specific antibodies (Hamburger and Douglass, 1969): deletion of the two chlorine atoms causes a large decrease in the haptene inhibition of the chloramphenicol-antibody reaction.

Chloramphenicol inhibits the formation of single peptide bonds on the 50s subunit of 70s prokaryotic ribosomes (rev: Hahn, 1967a; Pestka, 1974). This reaction is catalyzed by the enzyme peptidyl transferase which is an integral part of the 50s particle. A two-site substrate-binding model is conventionally assumed in which a P (peptidyl) site accommodates the binding of peptidyl-tRNA and an A (amino acyl) site the binding of amino acyl-tRNA. Peptidyl transferase is thought to be located between the two substrate-binding sites.

Peptidyltransferase can, in fact, act as a straightforward transesterification enzyme by transferring N-formylmethionine in the "fragment reaction" to the α-hydroxyl group of the phenyl-lactic acid amide of the puromycin base (Fahnestock, Naumann, Shashous and Rich, 1970) or synthesizing poly-phenyl-lactic acid from phenyl-lactyl-tRNA[phe] (Fahnestock and Rich, 1971). Both transesterification reactions are inhibited by chloramphenicol.

Numerous authors, however, consider chloramphenicol an inhibitor of peptidyl transfer. The drug has been alternately regarded as an antagonist of the acceptor (amino acyl) or of the donor (peptidyl) in this reaction scheme. An inhibition of the binding of a leucyl-pentanucleotide to 50s ribosomes by 10^{-3} M chloramphenicol as well as a slight stimulation of the binding of acetyl-leucyl-pentapeptide (Celma, Monro and Vazquez, 1971) is difficult to evaluate in terms of these two alternatives. The concentration of chloramphenicol was excessive in these experiments and 50 per cent ethanol in the experimental medium is likely to have caused surface perturbations of the 50s binding sites.

Antagonism of the amino acyl reactant was postulated on the basis of results which suggested a competition between chloramphenicol and puromycin, an established antagonist of the amino acyl partner in the reaction on the A-site (Coutsogeorgopoulos, 1966; Pestka, 1970). The inhibition of the puromycin reaction by chloramphenicol is, however, not unambiguously competitive with puromycin (Goldberg and Mitsugi, 1967; Pestka, 1972) and others (Das et al., 1966; Hahn, 1968; Harris and Symons, 1973; Cheney, 1974) have proposed that chloramphenicol acts as an antagonist of the peptidyl donor. This is consistent with observations that the drug inhibits peptide bond formation much more strongly when the P site is occupied by amino acyl amides such as N-formyl-methionine (Monro and Vazquez, 1967) and acetylphenyl-alanine (Pestka, 1970) or by actual peptides (Coutsogeorgopoulos, 1967) than in those instances in which (such as in the poly U system, Fig. 5) amino acyl-tRNA is erroneously forced into the P site by excessive concentrations of Mg^{++}. The alternatives of chloramphenicol acting as an antagonist of the peptidyl acceptor or of the peptidyl donor have been tested conclusively through an analysis of the reaction products of an E. coli ribosome-poly A system which synthesizes oligolysine (Julian, 1965). Chloramphenicol does not interfere with the formation of lysyl-lysine from two molecules of lysyl-tRNA and, in fact, causes an accumulation of this dipeptide. The drug does, however, inhibit the elongation of the dipeptide which in uninhibited control systems, leads to the preferential synthesis of hexa-, hepta-, and octapeptides.

Finally, when sparsomycin was used to stabilize the complexes of ribosomes with either phenylalanyl-tRNA or acetyl-phenylalanyl-tRNA, the subsequent binding of chloramphenicol to these complexes was forestalled when acetyl-phenylalanyl-tRNA was locked in place but was appreciable for the ribosome complex with phenylalanyl-tRNA. Hence, occupancy of the peptidyl site (P) prevented subsequent binding of the drug while occupancy of the amino acyl (A) site permitted of considerable chloramphenicol binding (Yukioka and Morisawa, 1972).

A view of chloramphenicol as an antimetabolite of either of the two substrates of peptidyl transferase must be entertained with some reservations. Protein biosynthesis by 70s ribosomes of procaryotic cells and by 80s ribosomes of eucaryotic cells, operates with the same reactants, especially puromycin. Yet, only 70s ribosome-based protein synthesis is susceptible to chloramphenicol inhibition. This difference may reside in structural differences between peptidyltransferase isoenzymes. If this were the case, mutations to high-level chloramphenicol resistance should occur which would be phenotypically expressed by an altered peptidyltransferase.

The first genetic analysis of high-level chloramphenicol resistant mutants of E. coli K12 (Cavalli and Maccacaro, 1952) showed, however, that this resistance was a cooperative polygenic phenomenon and that the individual resistance markers were located in different cistrons. More recently, one E. coli mutant, selected for resistance to erythromycin (Cerná and Rychlik, 1968), was cross-resistant to chloramphenicol. Oligolysyl transfer to puromycin by ribosomes of the parent and mutant strains was inhibited 50 per cent by 10^{-4} and 10^{-3} M chloramphenicol, respectively; this illustrates the limited extent to which genetic restructuring of the enzyme has produced chloramphenicol resistance at the site of action.

Affinity-labeling experiments with monoiodochloramphenicol (Pongs et al., 1973) have not only implicated the protein L16 in the 50s subunit but also the protein S3 in the 30s subunit as binding this chloramphenicol analog. S3 is involved in transfer RNA binding to ribosomes. If, indeed, chloramphenicol's site of action were to extend over both ribosomal subunits, such a two-site model would explain failures to isolate one-step mutants with high-level resistance to chloramphenicol; it might also explain the peculiar dependence of the relative inhibition of model protein synthesis upon the cytidylic acid abundance in synthetic poly UC messengers (Fig. 5).

However, chloramphenicol (Monro and Marcker, 1967) and some of its anti-bacterial analogs (Monro and Vazquez, 1967) do inhibit the "fragment reaction" which assays for the synthesis of one peptide bond by peptidyl transferase at 50 per cent inhibitory concentrations which range from 8×10^{-6} to 5×10^{-5} M (Monro and Vazquez, 1967); the reaction requires neither 30s ribosomes nor transfer RNA, nor messenger RNA.

This susceptibility to chloramphenicol and to some of its derivatives of the transfer of N-formylmethionine to puromycin suggests a single receptor site model on 50s rather than one with dual binding of the antibiotic to L16 and S3 across the subunital interface of 70s ribosomes.

The wide structural variations which are permitted for the aryl moiety of chloramphenicol analogs as well as the evident absence of an intramolecularly hydrogen bonded 5-membered ring structure (Bustard, Egan and Perun, 1973), eliminate from consideration the idea that the drug is an analog of uridylic acid (Jardetzky, 1963) or of puromycin (Coutsogeorgopoulos, 1966, 1967). Chloramphen-icol was early considered (Molho and Molho-Lacroix, 1952) an analog of a dipeptide, a view which was later adopted by investigators (Das et al., 1966; Hahn, 1968; Harris and Symons, 1973; Cheney, 1974) who regard the antibiotic as an antagonist of the peptidyl substrate of peptidyl transferase. Dichloroacetyl-serine (Zygmunt, 1961) has no significant antibacterial activity.

In cell-free models of peptide bond synthesis, puromycin analogs in which the O-methyl tyrosine portion is replaced by other amino acids show no stringent amino acid specificity of their peptidyl acceptor activities, except for the need of a cyclic amino acyl moiety which is considered necessary for binding to peptidyl transferase (Eckermann, Greenwell and Symons, 1974). Analogously, one might speculate that chloramphenicol is not an antagonist of any specific donor peptide and that the nonspecific need for a hydrophobic aryl moiety, likewise, reflects a requirement for binding to the enzyme.

Candidates for such planar and hydrophobic receptor surfaces to which the aryl moiety of chloramphenicol and its active derivatives might bind are, of course, the ring systems of cyclic amino acids in the receptor protein such as phenyl, p-hydroxyphenyl or indolyl. Höltje and Kier (1974) have found the best correlation between antibacterial activity and the energies of interaction with a flat receptor surface for para-substituted chloramphenicol congeners when the receptor surface was the indole ring system (of tryptophan) and the drug-receptor distance was 4.5 Å. Fig. 6 shows the correlation between the antibacterial activity and the calculated interaction energy with tryptophan of 14 para-substi-tuted chloramphenicol derivatives (Höltje and Kier, 1974).

VI. COMPUTER MODELING OF CHLORAMPHENICOL BOUND TO RIBOSOME

The antibacterial effect of chloramphenicol may only be fully understood in terms of the three-dimensional structures of drug and receptor site, and in terms of the energetics of their interaction. Although we are still a long way from knowing the detailed molecular structure of the ribosome, nevertheless, if we can determine the conformation of agents which complex to the ribosome by complemen-

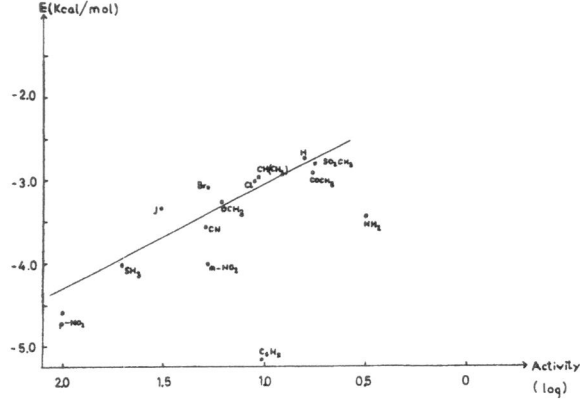

Calculated interaction energy *vs.* biological activity for a separation distance of 4.5 Å.

Fig. 6.   Correlation between antibacterial activities of p-substituted
          chloramphenicol derivatives and the calculated energies of interaction
          of the corresponding p-phenyl residues with indole (Höltje and Kier,
          1974).

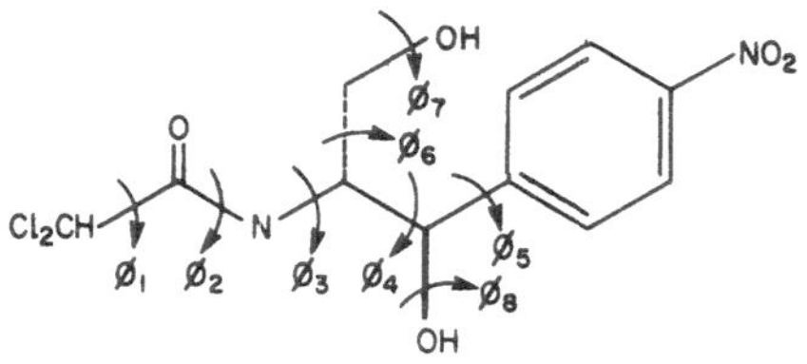

Fig. 7.   Rotatable bonds in chloramphenicol.

tarity, we may infer major features of the topography of the active site. In an
effort to derive a workable model which could serve as the basis for further work
in designing improved antibiotic agents, we have attempted to determine the likely
conformations of chloramphenicol, both as free drug and when bound to the transpeptidase active site.

     In principle, chloramphenicol has eight rotatable single bonds (Fig. 7).
The amide bond (ϕ_2) is usually fixed as trans-planar, while rotation of hydroxy
hydrogens (ϕ_7 and ϕ_8) should be facile. Rotation about the acetamide (ϕ_1) and
aryl (ϕ_5) bonds should also be relatively easy. Of the remaining three axes, the
C-C bonds (ϕ_4 and ϕ_6) have been assigned a rotation barrier of 2.7 kcal/mole by
Bustard et al. (1973), while the C-N bond (ϕ_3) barrier is only 0.6 kcal.

     Despite the many degrees of conformational freedom, chloramphenicol was found
by Dunitz (1952) to exist primarily in one conformation in the crystal (Fig. 8);
the proximity of the alcohol groups suggested that an intramolecular hydrogen bond
stabilized the structure. While Jardetzky (1963) had inferred from the NMR
spectrum that the same conformation was favored in solution, Bustard, Egan and
Perun (1973) have recently reached a different conclusion. They proposed from
potential energy calculations that a similar, but non-hydrogen bonded, conformation prevailed (Fig. 9); a second conformer was less than 1 kcal. higher in

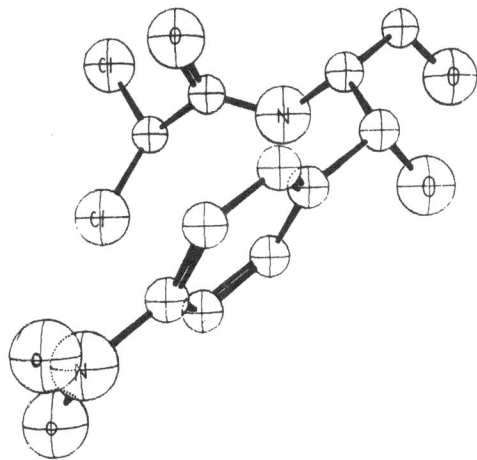

Fig. 8. Chloramphenicol, crystalline conformation (Dunitz, 1952).

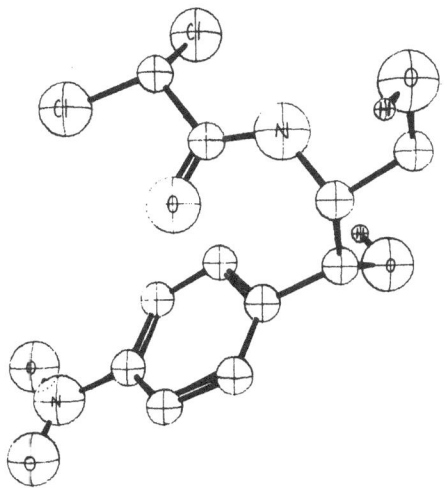

Fig. 9. Chloramphenicol, calculated ground state conformation (Bustard et al.,
1973).

energy, and many others were energetically accessible. Furthermore, they demonstrated the absence of an intramolecular hydrogen bond by high dilution IR
spectroscopy, and by the observation that the NMR of chloramphenicol phenyl-
boronate (which contains a 6-membered ring) exhibited substantially different
proton couplings. Consideration of solvent polarity effects suggested that the
non-hydrogen bonded conformation was even more highly favored. One may speculate
that, while solvation stabilizes an extended conformation, crystal forces favor
the more compact, hydrogen bonded conformation.

Bustard's conformational calculations were based on nonbonded and torsional
potential energy functions, and did not explicitly consider energetic effects of

hydrogen bonding or partial charge interactions. Furthermore, no full geometry search was attempted, so that those results must be considered as suggestive rather than rigorous. Höltje and Kier (1974) have recently investigated chloramphenicol conformations using quantum mechanical methods; two isoenergetic conformations -- one essentially identical to Bustard's first conformer, and one corresponding to his second conformer -- were calculated to be equally favored. Despite this essential confirmation of Bustard's results, extended Hückel calculations are known to be somewhat unreliable in determining preferred conformations (for example, Ajo et al., 1973) and a definitive study remains to be done.

There thus appears to be no reason to expect that the conformation which chloramphenicol assumes in the crystal state is the same as obtains on the active site. There is also little evidence to suggest that Bustard's calculated minimum conformation is the active form; in fact, the higher activity of Kono's analogs (Fig. 3), which have reduced stereoisomeric possibilities, may be interpreted to suggest that chloramphenicol is not most strongly bound in its ground state conformation. Similarly, Cheney (1974) has suggested that peptidyl tRNA exists in a bound conformation which is different from its form in solution.

One approach to determining the conformation of bound chloramphenicol is to compare the structure of various conformers with that of the natural substrate, or with that of antibiotics which are chloramphenicol antagonists, looking for similarities in the three-dimensional structure. Unfortunately, the structure of peptidyl-tRNA on the active site is unknown. However, Shipman, Christoffersen and Cheney (1974) have modeled lincomycin free base by an ab initio molecular fragment technique, and obtained a structure which they believe corresponds to the biologically active conformation; Cheney (1974) has used this structure and model calculations to propose a conformation for the natural peptidyl substrate when bound to the enzyme surface. Despite the rather tentative string of assumptions on which this line of reasoning hangs, the resulting model is fairly appealing.

We therefore searched for conformations of chloramphenicol which could be superimposed (utilizing interactive computer graphics) with the three-dimensional

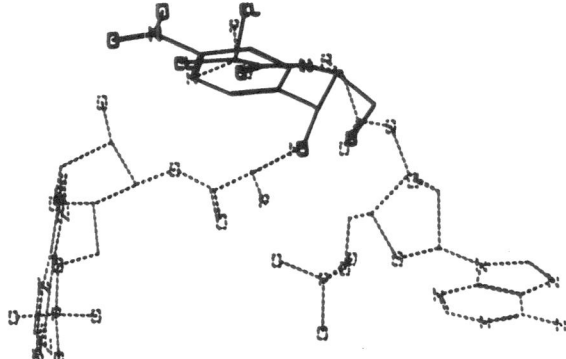

Fig. 10. Superposition of chloramphenicol (solid lines) and bound transpeptidase substrates (dotted lines). Substrate coordinates are from Cheney (1974) except that peptide side chains are represented by R-groups. Peptidyl-tRNA is at the top, aminoacyl-tRNA at lower left. Chloramphenicol is in the best conformation which we could find for superposition according to the proposal of Harris and Symons (1973). This and Fig. 11 were photographed directly from the Princeton Computer Graphics Laboratories PDP 10/LDS1 display.

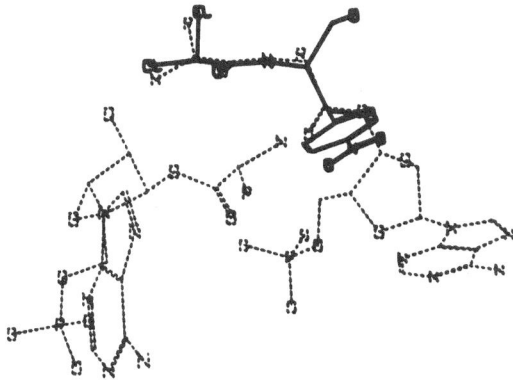

Fig. 11. Superposition of chloramphenicol (solid lines) and bound peptidyl
transferase substrates (dotted lines) according to the model proposed
by Cheney (1974).

structure of lincomycin (Shipman, Christoffersen and Cheney, 1974) and/or the
substrate model for peptide bond formation proposed by Cheney (1974). We found
several well-matching conformations, of which the two most likely are shown in
Figs. 10 and 11. The first model is similar to one proposed by Harris and Symons
(1973) on the basis of examining Dreiding models of various transpeptidase
substrates, while the second model is essentially the same as one proposed by
Cheney (1974) by comparison of chloramphenicol crystal structure with his models
of lincomycin and bound peptidyl-tRNA. We discuss the advantages and disadvantages
of these viewpoints in the next section.

VII. MODEL FOR CHLORAMPHENICOL INHIBITION OF TRANSPEPTIDATION

We suppose that the transpeptidation active site of the ribosome possesses
an acceptor (aminoacyl or "A") site and a donor (peptidyl or "P") site according
to the classical view. In the elongation step of protein synthesis, the growing
peptide chain is attached to the free amine of aminoacyl-tRNA, leaving the P-site
momentarily empty. Normally, the uncharged tRNA is then eliminated from the 30s
ribosomal P'-anticodon binding site, and the elongated peptidyl-tRNA becomes
transferred back to the P-site in a translocation step. We suggest that chloramphenicol preferentially attaches itself to the newly abandoned P-site, trapping
the nascent peptide on the A-site and preventing translocation. This mechanism
explains why the drug leads to the formation of dipeptide in an isolated system
which normally synthesizes up to octapeptides (Julian, 1965).

It appears to be important to determine whether chloramphenicol binds
preferentially to the A-site or the P-site: the L16 ribosomal protein has been
assigned to the A-site, partly on the basis of its chloramphenicol binding ability
(review: Pongs et al., 1974). The difficulty is that the sites must be extremely
similar, since the A-site must bind the peptidyl-tRNA temporarily after the
elongation step and before translocation back to the P-site. The de-dichloro-
acetylated derivative of chloramphenicol would be a proper acylamino-tRNA analog,
but is nonactive; the dichloroacetyl group would appear to have no analogy in the
normal A-site substrate. Nevertheless, because of site similarities and since
the ethanol required for the "fragment reaction" must somewhat perturb the enzyme
conformation, it is possible that chloramphenicol actually does bind to the A-site
in isolated cell-free systems.

According to our mechanism, chloramphenicol mimics a dipeptide and attaches itself to the amide recognition site of the P-receptor, then orients itself so that secondary interactions are maximized. The resulting complex appears to be quite strong, but without any covalent bonds. We now examine the source of these secondary interactions in terms of the Harris-Symons and Cheny models (Figs. 10 and 11).

In both models the dichloroacetyl group occupies the position reserved for the penultimate peptide moiety in the natural substrate. This view is supported by the binding ability of Coutsogeorgopoulos' aminoacylated analogs (Table I) and by the inactivity of the deacetylated drug. The tolerance of some bulk at this position for in vitro binding activity is reasonable in view of the large bulk of polypeptide chain in the natural substrate (lack of in vivo activity appears to be due to transport problems). The amide recognition site may involve bonding to the hydrogen on the amide nitrogen. Although this might explain the σ^* contribution of acetyl substituents to activity observed by Hansch et al. (1973), CNDO/2-calculated charge densities of 11 acylated derivatives (Höltje and Kier, 1974) failed to confirm the existence of this effect.

In the Harris-Symons model (Fig. 10), the chloramphenicol CH_2OH group occupies the site normally taken by the adenine singly bonded ester oxygen, while ArCHOH takes the terminal peptide side chain position (R in Fig. 10). This arrangement places the aryl group into a groove which is adaptable enough to accommodate all 20 amino acid side chains, partly rationalizing the activity of bulky para-substituted derivatives. Nitrophenyl would correspond to the natural phenylalanine substrate, and, indeed, it has been pointed out that chloramphenicol arises from an offshoot of the same metabolic pathway as phenylalanine (Harris and Symons, 1973). On the other hand, chloramphenicol should bind more strongly than the natural substrates, or else enzyme inhibition would be temporary. Höltje and Kier's calculated interaction energies (Fig. 6) suggest that nitrophenyl is almost 2 kcal/mole more strongly bound than phenyl and these results are consistent with occurrence of a charge-transfer interaction at the active site (review: Shifrin, 1973). There is also a hydrophobic component to the aryl binding, as shown by dependence on log P and polarizability (Hansch et al., 1973; Cammarata, 1967). The benzylic alcohol oxygen is either an analog of a serine hydroxymethyl side chain, or it may impinge on the active site where the free amine of aminoacyl-tRNA is bound to the A-site according to the mechanism of Cheney (1974). Interestingly, this conformation of chloramphenicol differs from the crystal conformation largely by rotation about the acetyl and aryl groups; an intramolecular hydrogen bond could still form. However, this model for binding suffers from the disadvantages that chloramphenicol does not appear to show preferential antagonism towards any particular amino acids (Speyer et al., 1963; Kućan and Lipmann, 1964), and that the CH_2OH group does not seem to be necessary for activity (Kono, 1969).

In the Cheney model (Fig. 11), on the other hand, the benzylic alcohol oxygen occupies the adenyl ester oxygen binding site, while the aryl group extends away from the transpeptidase receptor site; an alternative conformation (not shown) places the benzylic oxygen at the ester carbonyl oxygen position, and the nitrophenyl group onto the receptor A-site. (The former conformation is similar to the chloramphenicol crystal structure, the latter is not). A serious problem with this model is that the CH_2OH group now does not correspond to the R-group of the terminal peptide. It could act by stabilizing the active conformation by a hydrogen bond (for the conformation shown), or it could have no real importance since it is missing in some more active derivatives (Kono, 1969). Interestingly, the L(+) erythro isomer of chloramphenicol has the proper configuration for CH_2OH to simulate a peptide side chain, and this isomer does have some antibacterial activity -- but only 1-2% of that of chloramphenicol. If a tryptophan residue is involved in proton transfer at the active site during transpeptidation, its complexation with nitrophenyl of chloramphenicol would explain the drug's effectiveness. A disadvantage of this model, besides the inverted configuration at C1, is that the aryl group no longer has structural analogy in the natural substrate and the steric requirements of aryl substituents are not easily derived.

SUMMARY

The preceding examination of the relationship between structure and activity among chloramphenicol derivatives encourages us to propose a prototypical structure of compounds which interact with peptidyl transferase in the manner in which chloramphenicol does (Fig. 12). The propane chain with its amide group, -NH-CO-, binds to the peptidyl recognition site of peptidyl transferase. An acyl (or aminoacyl) residue is necessary for activity but its steric and electronic requirements for inhibition of peptidyl transferase are not very stringent. Of the two propane chain functional groups, one hydroxyl is accepted by the enzyme at the adenyl ester oxygen site. Depending on which alcohol is thus bound, the nitrophenyl group binds hydrophobically to either the peptidyl side chain accommodating groove, or to the transpeptidase active site. We hope that further experimentation will offer greater insight into the mechanism of binding of this old and useful drug whose deceptively simple structure doubtless still holds a few surprises.

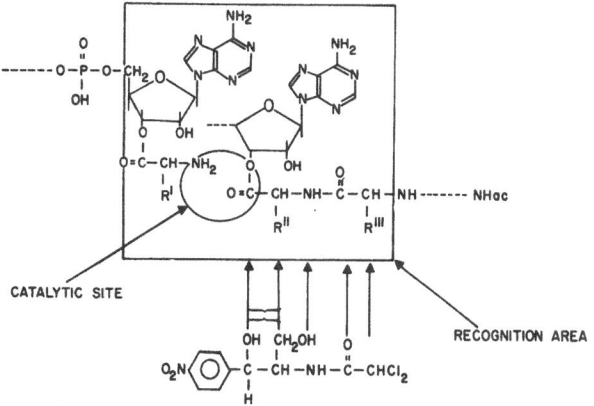

Fig. 12. Correspondence of chloramphenicol and peptidyl transferase structural features.

Acknowledgment. We thank Dr. B.V. Cheney for supplying us with coordinates of his models of lincomycin and the transpeptidase bound substrates. The Princeton Computer Graphics Laboratory is supported by the National Institutes of Health.

ADDENDUM IN PROOF

After submission of this article, the authors received a personal communication from Dr. Albert J. Leo who since had the opportunity of examining original experimental data of Sankyo Co., Tokyo, on the two chloramphenicol derivatives of Kono et al. (1969). These data show that the high activity ratios of the two compounds relative to that of chloramphenicol itself were found in a partially chloramphenicol-resistant strain of Staphylococcus aureus. In a sensitive strain, the two compounds were as active as chloramphenicol. For our purpose of modelling the chloramphenicol receptor site, the assumption remains valid that the two derivatives of Kono et al. (1969) interact with this site.

REFERENCES

Ajò, D., M. Bossa, A. Damiani, R. Fidenzi, S. Gigli and G. Ramunni: Conformational Analysis. Quantum-Mechanical and Empirical Methods. In Conformation of
Biological Molecules and Polymers, E.D. Bergmann and B. Pullman, eds., Jerusalem,
1973, p. 571.

Bald, R., V.A. Erdmann and O. Pongs: Irreversible binding of chloramphenicol
analogues to E. coli ribosomes. FEBS Letters 28, 149 (1972).

Bustard, T.M., R.S. Egan and T.J. Perun: Conformational studies on chloramphenicol
and related molecules. Tetrahedron 29, 1961 (1973).

Cammarata, A.: An apparent correlation between the in vitro activity of
chloramphenicol analogs and electronic polarizability. J. Med. Chem. 10, 525
(1967).

Cavalli, L.L. and G.A. Maccacaro: Polygenic inheritance of drug-resistance in
the bacterium Escherichia coli. Heredity 6, 311 (1952).

Celma, M.L., R.E. Monro and D. Vazquez: Substrate and antibiotic binding sites
at the peptidyl transferase centre of E. coli ribosomes: Binding of UACCA-Leu
to 50s subunits. FEBS Letters 13, 247 (1971).

Černá, J. and I. Rychlík: Cross resistance of Escherichia coli B ribosomes to
inhibition of the puromycin reaction by erythromycin, spiramycin and chloramphenicol. Biochim. Biophys. Acta 157, 436 (1968).

Cheney, V.: Ab initio calculations on large molecules using molecular fragments,
structural correlations between natural substrate moieties and some antibiotic
inhibitors of peptidyl transferase. J. Med. Chem. 17, 590 (1974).

Collins, R.J., B. Ellis, S.B. Hansen, H.S. Mackenzie, R.J. Moualim, V. Petrow,
O. Stephenson and B. Sturgeon: Some observations on the structural requirements
for antibiotic action in the chloramphenicol series. Part II. J. Pharm. Pharmacol.
4, 693 (1952).

Contreras, A., M. Barbacid and D. Vazquez: Binding to ribosomes and mode of
action of chloramphenicol analogues. Biochim. Biophys. Acta 349, 376 (1974).

Controulis, M., M.C. Rebstock and H.M. Crooks: Chloramphenicol (Chloromycetin).
V. Synthesis. J. Am. Chem. Soc. 71, 2458 (1949).

Coutsogeorgopoulos, C.: On the mechanism of action of chloramphenicol in protein
synthesis. Biochim. Biophys. Acta 129, 214 (1966).

Coutsogeorgopoulos, C.: Inhibitors of the reaction between puromycin and
polylysyl-RNA in the presence of ribosomes. Biochem. Biophys. Res. Comm. 27,
46 (1967).

Das, H.K., A. Goldstein and L.C. Kanner: Inhibition by chloramphenicol of the
growth of nascent protein chains in Escherichia coli. Mol. Pharmacol. 2, 158
(1966).

Dunitz, J.D.: The crystal structure of chloramphenicol and bromamphenicol.
J. Am. Chem. Soc. 74, 995 (1952).

Eckermann, D.J., P. Greenwell and R.H. Symons: Peptide-bond formation on the
ribosome. A comparison of the acceptor-substrate specificity of peptidyl
transferase in bacterial and mammalian ribosomes using puromycin analogues. Eur.
J. Biochem. 41, 547 (1974).

Fahnestock, S., H. Neumann, V. Shashoua and A. Rich: Ribosome-catalyzed ester formation. Biochemistry 9, 2477 (1970).

Fahnestock, S. and A. Rich: Ribosome-catalyzed polyester formation. Science 173, 340 (1971).

Farkaš, J. and J. Sicher: The chloramphenicol series. V. Analogs containing chlorine in the side chain and oxazolines. Chem. Listy. 47, 552 (1953).

Gale, E.F.: Mechanism of antibiotic action. Pharm. Rev. 15, 481 (1963).

Gale, E.F. and J.P. Folkes: The assimilation of amino acids by bacteria. 15. Actions of antibiotics on nucleic acid and protein synthesis in Staphylococcus aureus. Biochem. J. 53, 493 (1953).

Garrett, E.T., O.K. Wright, G.H. Miller and K.L. Smith: Quantification and prediction of the biological activities of chloramphenicol analogs by microbial kinetics. J. Med. Chem. 9, 203 (1966).

Goldberg, I.H. and K. Mitsugi: Inhibition by sparsomycin and other antibiotics of the puromycin-induced release of polypeptide from ribosomes. Biochemistry 6, 383 (1967).

Hahn, F.E.: Relations between chemical structure and antibiotic action of chloramphenicol. 3ème Congres International de Biochimie, Bruxelles 1955. Résumés des Communications 92.

Hahn, F.E.: Chloramphenicol. In Antibiotics I, Mechanism of Action. Springer, Berlin-Heidelberg-New York, 1967a, p 308.

Hahn, F.E.: Effects of chloramphenicol in cell-free amino-acid polymerizing systems. Proc. 5th Internat. Congr. Chemoth. C 6/5, 387 (1967b).

Hahn, F.E.: Relationship between the structure of chloramphenicol and its action upon peptide synthetase. Experientia 24, 856 (1968).

Hahn, F.E., J.E. Hayes, C.L. Wisseman, H.E. Hopps and J.E. Smadel: Mode of action of chloramphenicol. VI. Relation between structure and activity in the chloramphenicol series. Antibiot. & Chemotherapy 6, 531 (1956).

Hahn, F.E. and C.L. Wisseman: Inhibition of adaptive enzyme formation by antimicrobial agents. Proc. Soc. Exptl. Biol. Med. 76, 533 (1951).

Hahn, F.E., C.L. Wisseman and H.E. Hopps: Mode of action of chloramphenicol. II. Inhibition of bacterial D-polypeptide formation by an L-stereoisomer of chloramphenicol. J. Bact. 67, 674 (1954).

Hamburger, R.N. and J.H. Douglass: Chloramphenicol-specific antibody. II. Reactivity to analogous of chloramphenicol. Immunology 17, 587 (1969).

Hansch, C., E. Kutter and A. Leo: Homolytic constants in the correlation of chloramphenicol structure with activity. J. Med. Chem. 12, 746 (1969).

Hansch, C., R.M. Muir, T. Fujita, P.P. Maloney, F. Geiger and M. Streich: The correlation of biological activity of plant regulators and chloromycetin derivatives with Hammett constants and partition coefficients. J. Am. Chem. Soc. 85, 2817 (1963).

Hansch, C., K. Nakamoto, M. Gorin, P. Denisevich, E.R. Garrett, S.M. Heman-Ackah and C.H. Won: Structure-activity relationship of chloramphenicols. J. Med. Chem. 16, 917 (1973).

Harris, R.J. and R.H. Symons: On the molecular mechanism of action of certain substrates and inhibitors of ribosomal peptidyl transferase. Bioorganic Chem. 2, 266 (1973).

Höltje, H.-D. and L.B. Kier: A theoretical approach to structure-activity relationships of chloramphenicol and congeners. J. Med. Chem. 17, 814 (1974).

Huebner, C.F. and C.R. Scholz: The synthesis of chloramphenicol analogs. J. Am. Chem. Soc. 73, 2089 (1951).

Inouye, M.: A three-dimensional molecular assembly model of a lipoprotein from the Escherichia coli outer membrane. Proc. Nat. Acad. Sci. USA 71, 2396 (1974).

Jardetzky, O.: Studies on the mechanism of action of chloramphenicol. I. The conformation of chloramphenicol in solution. J. Biol. Chem. 238, 2498 (1963).

Jardetzky, O. and G.R. Julian: Chloramphenicol inhibition of polyuridylic acid binding to E. coli ribosomes. Nature 201, 396 (1964).

Julian, G.R.: ^{14}C-Lysine peptides synthesized in an in vitro Escherichia coli system in the presence of chloramphenicol. J. Mol. Biol. 12, 9 (1965).

Klein, R.S., M.P. Kotick, K.A. Watanabe and J.J. Fox: Nucleosides. LXXIII. Ribosyl analogs of chloramphenicol. J. Org. Chem. 36, 4113 (1971).

Kolosov, M.N., M.M. Shemiakin, A.S. Khokhlov and A.I. Gurevich: Chloramphenicol, In Khimia Antibiotikov I, Iedatsto Akademii Nauk USSR, 1961.

Kono, M., K. O'Hara, M. Honda and S. Mitsuhashi: Drug resistance of staphylococci. XI. Induction of chloramphenicol resistance by its derivatives and analogues. J. Antibiot. (Tokyo) 22, 603 (1969).

Kućan, Z. and F. Lipmann: Differences in chloramphenicol sensitivity of cell-free amino acid polymerization systems. J. Biol. Chem. 239, 516 (1964).

Lamborg, M.R. and P.C. Zamecnik: Amino acid incorporation into protein by extracts of E. coli. Biochim. Biophys. Acta 42, 206 (1960).

Leo, A., C. Hansch and D. Elkins: Partition coefficients and their use. Chem. Rev. 71, 525 (1971).

Lien, E.J., C. Hansch and S.M. Anderson: Structure-activity correlations for antibacterial agents on Gram-positive and Gram-negative cells. J. Med. Chem. 11, 430 (1968).

Long, L.M. and H.D. Troutman: Chloromycetin. Synthesis of alpha-dichloracetamido-beta-hydroxy-p-nitropropiophenone. J. Am. Chem. Soc. 73, 481 (1951).

Maxwell, R.E. and V.S. Nickel: The antibacterial activity of the isomers of chloramphenicol. Antib. & Chemotherap. 4, 289 (1954).

Molho, D. and L. Molho-Lacroix: Étude comparée de l'antagonisme entre quelques dérivés de la phénylalanine et la chloromycétine la β_2 thiénylalanine et la β phenylsérine. Bull. Soc. chim. biol. 34, 99 (1952).

Monro, R.E. and K.A. Marcker: Ribosome-catalyzed reaction of puromycin with a formylmethionine-containing oligonucleotide. J. Mol. Biol. 25, 347 (1967).

Monro, R.E. and D. Vazquez: Ribosome-catalyzed peptidyl transfer: Effects of some inhibitors of protein synthesis. J. Mol. Biol. 28, 161 (1967).

Nierhaus, D. and K.N. Nierhaus: Identification of the chloramphenicol-binding protein in Escherichia coli ribosomes by partial reconstitution. Proc. Nat. Acad. Sci. USA 70, 2224 (1973).

Nirenberg, M.W. and J.H. Matthaei: The dependence of cell-free protein synthesis in E. coli upon naturally occurring or synthetic polyribonucleotides. Proc. Nat. Acad. Sci. USA 47, 1588 (1961).

Pestka, S.: Studies on the formation of transfer ribonucleic acid-ribosome complexes. VIII. Survey of the effects of antibiotics on N-acetyl-phenylalanyl-puromycin formation: Possible mechanism of chloramphenicol action. Arch. Biochem. Biophys. 136, 80 (1970).

Pestka, S.: Studies on transfer ribonucleic acid-ribosome complexes. XIX. Effects of antibiotics on peptidyl puromycin synthesis on polyribosomes from Escherichia coli. J. Biol. Chem. 247, 4669 (1972).

Pestka, S.: Chloramphenicol. In Antibiotics III, Corcoran and Hahn, Edts. Springer, Berlin-Heidelberg-New York, 1974, p 370.

Pongs, O., R. Bald and V.A. Erdmann: Identification of chloramphenicol-binding protein in Escherichia coli ribosomes by affinity labeling. Proc. Nat. Acad. Sci. USA 70, 2229 (1973).

Pongs, O., K.H. Nierhaus, V.A. Erdmann and H.G. Wittmann: Active sites in Escherichia coli ribosomes. FEBS Letters 40 Suppl., 28 (1974).

Rebstock, M.C., H.M. Crooks, J. Controulis and Q.R. Bartz: Chloramphenicol (chloromycetin). IV. Chemical studies. J. Am. Chem. Soc. 71, 2458 (1949).

Rebstock, M.C. and C.D. Stratton: Some compounds related to chloromycetin. J. Am. Chem. Soc. 77, 4054 (1955).

Rebstock, M.C., C.D. Stratton and L.L. Bambas: Compounds related to chloromycetin. 1-Biphenyl and ring-substituted 1-biphenyl-2-dichloracetamido-1,3-propanediols. J. Am. Chem. Soc. 77, 24 (1955).

Rendi, R. and S. Ochoa: Effect of chloramphenicol on protein synthesis in cell-free preparations of Escherichia coli. J. Biol. Chem. 237, 3711 (1962).

Shaw, W.V.: The enzymatic acetylation of chloramphenicol by R-factor resistant Escherichia coli. J. Biol. Chem. 242, 687 (1967).

Shemiakin, M.M., M.N. Kolosov, M.M. Levitov, K.I. Germanova, M.G. Karpetian, Iu.B. Svetsov and E.M. Bamdas: Dependency between structure and antimicrobial activity of chloromycetin (Levomycetin) and the mechanism of its effect. Doklady Akademii Nauk USSR 102, 953 (1955).

Shemiakin, M.M., M.N. Kolosov, M.M. Levitov, K.I. Germanova, M.G. Karpetian, Iu.B. Shetsov and E.M. Bamdas: Researches into the chemistry of chloromycetin (Levomycetin). VIII. Dependency of antimicrobial activity of chloromycetin on its structure and the mechanism of effect of chloromycetin. Zhurnal obschei khimii 26, 773 (1956).

Shifrin, S.: The Role of Charge Transfer in Pharmacology. In Structure-Activity Relationships, Vol. 1, C.J. Cavallito, ed., Pergamon Press, Oxford, 1973, p 167.

Shipman, L.L., R.E. Christoffersen and B.V. Cheney: Ab initio calculations on large molecules using molecular fragments. Lincomucin model studies. J. Med. Chem. 17, 583 (1974).

Speyer, J.F., P. Lengyel, C. Basilio, A.J. Wahba, R.S. Gardner and S. Ochoa: Synthetic polynucleotides and the amino acid code. Cold Spring Harb. Symp. Quant. Biol. 28, 559 (1963).

Suzuki, Y. and S. Okamoto: The enzymatic acetylation of chloramphenicol by the multiple drug-resistant Escherichia coli carrying R-factor. J. Biol. Chem. 242, 4722 (1967).

Telesnina, G.N., M.A. Novikova, G.L. Zhdanov, M.N. Kolosov and M.M. Shemiakin: The effect of chloramphenicol analogs on protein biosynthesis in a cell-free Escherichia coli B system. Experientia 23, 427 (1967).

Vazquez, D.: Mode of action of chloramphenicol and related antibiotics. 16. Symp. Soc. Gen. Microbiol. Biochemical Studies of Antimicrobial Drugs, p 169. Cambridge Univ. Press 1966.

Wilbrandt, W. and T. Rosenberg: The concept of carrier transport and its corollaries in pharmacology. Pharm. Rev. 13, 109 (1961).

Wisseman, C.L., J.E. Smadel, F.E. Hahn and H.E. Hopps: Mode of action of chloramphenicol. I. Action of chloramphenicol on assimilation of ammonia and on synthesis of proteins and nucleic acids in Escherichia coli. J. Bact. 67, 662 (1954).

Woolley, D.W.: A study of non-competitive antagonism with chloromycetin and related analogues of phenylalanine. J. Biol. Chem. 185, 293 (1950).

Yukioka, M. and S. Morisawa: Inhibition of the chloramphenicol binding to ribosomes by the sparsomycin-induced binding of aminoacyl-tRNA to ribosomes. Biochem. Biophys. Res. Comm. 48, 1444 (1972).

Zygmunt, W.A.: Studies of chloroacetyl derivatives as bacterial antagonists. Canad. J. Microbiol. 7, 833 (1961).

V. Microbial Enzymes as Drug-Receptors

Spin-Labelled Intermediates as Targets of Antibiotic Action in Peptidoglycan Synthesis

L. S. Johnston, W. P. Hammes, H. A. Lazar, and F. C. Neuhaus

Spin labels provide sensitive probes to study the microenvironments of intermediates in membrane catalyzed reactions. The electron spin resonance (ESR) spectrum of the spin label is a function of the motion that the probe experiences and the polarity of the solvent surrounding the probe. Thus, information about the mobility of the spin label and its microenvironment can be deduced from its spectrum. Indeed, McConnell and other investigators have utilized this technique to analyze lateral diffusion of phospholipids, conformation changes, flip-flop of phospholipids, phase transitions, and fluidity in membranes. It is the purpose of this paper to report some of our observations on spin-labeled intermediates in cell wall biosynthesis and how they may be used as targets of antibiotic action.

The biosynthesis of peptidoglycan, the major cell wall structural polymer, requires two nucleotide activated precursors, UDP-N-acetylglucosamine and UDP-N-acetylmuramyl-pentapeptide. Enzymes intercalated into the membrane matrix utilize these precursors in a cycle of reactions with undecaprenyl-phosphate as the carrier (Figure 1) (Ghuysen and Shockman, 1973). These enzymes catalyze the synthesis of the lipid dimer, undecaprenyl-diphosphate-MurNAc-(-pentapeptide)-GlcNAc.[1] At this stage amino acid residues for interpeptide bridge formation are transferred to the lipid dimer. In addition, amidation of the α-carboxyl group of glutamic acid occurs. Peptidoglycan synthetase utilizes this intermediate for the formation of nascent peptidoglycan. In the extracellular phase, nascent peptidoglycan is transferred to pre-existing peptidoglycan as a result of two enzyme-catalyzed reactions, transglycosylation and transpeptidation. In effect, the biosynthesis of this polymer is represented by three phases: cytoplasmic, membranous, and extracellular. A probe that reflects the microenvironment in each phase will be useful in unraveling this complex biosynthetic system.

---

[1] Unless stated, all abbreviations of amino acid residues denote the L-configuration. The omission of the hyphen, i.e. -DAla- for -D-Ala- conforms with the suggestion cited in Biochemistry 5, 2485 (1966). Although not stated, all D-glutamic acid residues are linked through the γ-carboxyl group to the diamino acid. The abbreviations used are: MurNAc, N-acetylmuramyl; GlcNAc, N-acetylglucosamine; Tempyo, 2, 2, 5, 5-tetramethyl-1-pyrrolin-1-oxyl-3-carbonyl- .

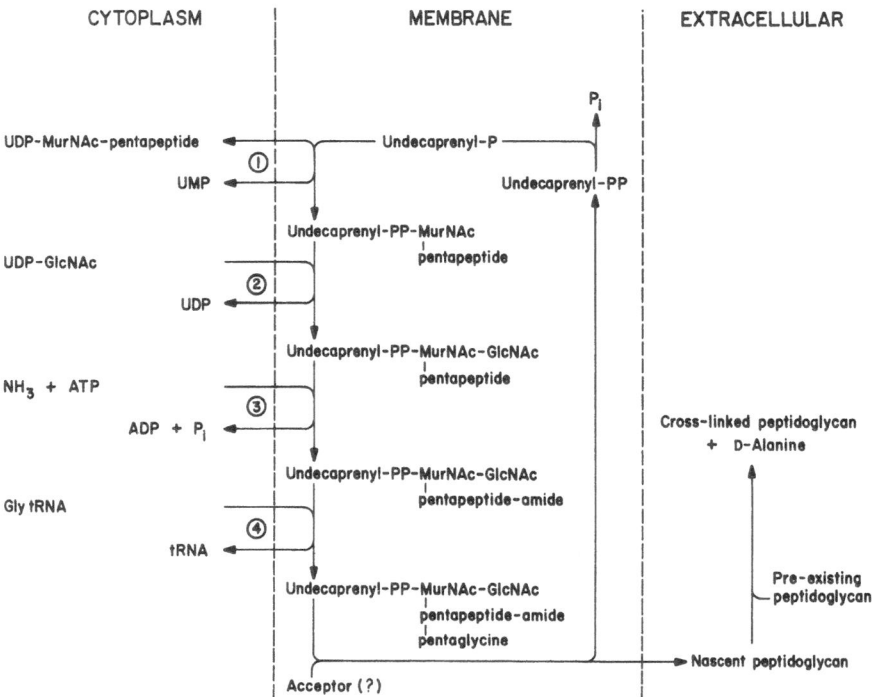

Figure 1. Biosynthesis of peptidoglycan in <u>Staphylococcus</u> <u>aureus</u> Copenhagen (Matsuhashi <u>et</u> <u>al</u>., 1965).

Spin-labeled UDP-MurNAc-pentapeptide

The structure of spin-labeled UDP-MurNAc-pentapeptide is illustrated in Figure 2. As will be shown, attachment of the spin label to amino acid residue 3 of the nucleotide does not exert a major perturbation in the activities catalyzed by phospho-MurNAc-pentapeptide translocase (Reaction 1, Figure 1) and the peptidoglycan synthesizing system. For preparation of this derivative the ε-amino group of the lysine residue was acylated with 2, 2, 5, 5-tetramethyl-1-pyrrolin-1-oxyl-3-carbonyl in a reaction mixture that contained: 3 μmoles of UDP-MurNAc-pentapeptide (salt free) in 0.5 ml of water, 15 μmoles of 2, 2, 5, 5-tetramethyl-1-pyrrolin-1-oxyl-3-carboxylic acid N-hydroxysuccinimide ester, 2 ml of hexamethyl phosphoramide, and 10 μl of triethylamine. The reaction mixture was maintained at 37° for 20 hr. The spin-labeled nucleotide was isolated from the reaction mixture by the procedure of Johnston and Neuhaus (unpublished results). As part of the isolation procedure, the spin-labeled UDP-MurNAc-pentapeptide is readily separated from unreacted nucleotide by virtue of its charge difference (Figure 3). Since the ε-amino group of the lysine residue is unreactive to fluorodinitrobenzene, it is concluded that the spin label is attached to this functional group. Thus, the spin-labeled nucleotide has a net negative charge at pH 8 of -3 in contrast to UDP-MurNAc-pentapeptide (-2).

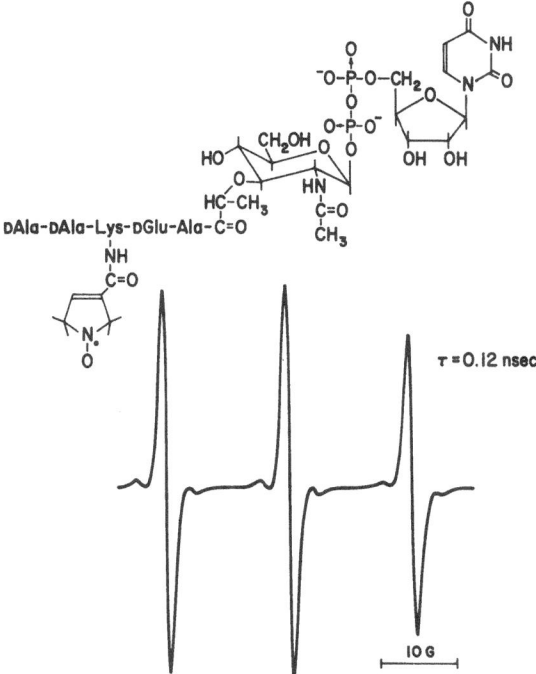

Figure 2.   Spin-labeled UDP-MurNAc-(Tempyo-εN)-pentapeptide and its ESR
spectrum (Johnston and Neuhaus, unpublished observations).   The
rotational correlation time is 0.12 nsec.

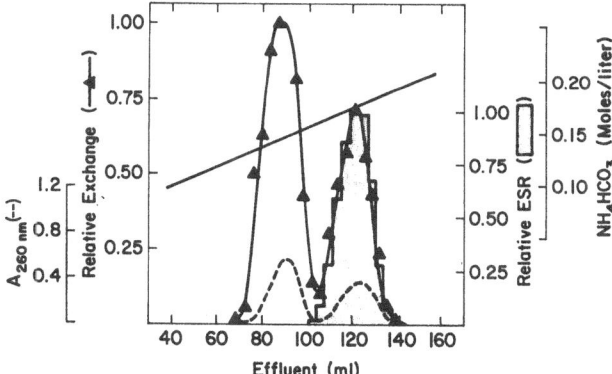

Figure 3.   Separation of spin-labeled UDP-MurNAc-(Tempyo-εN)-pentapeptide
and UDP-MurNAc-pentapeptide on DEAE-cellulose (Johnston and
Neuhaus, unpublished observations).   The relative exchange (▲-▲)
catalyzed by phospho-MurNAc-pentapeptide translocase was
assayed in the exchange assay (Hammes and Neuhaus, 1974).   The
relative ESR▨was quantitated on a Varian E-4 Spectrometer.

The ESR spectrum (Figure 2) of the spin-labeled nucleotide can be characterized by a motion parameter called the rotational correlation time (τ). It is calculated with the expression formulated by Stone et al. (1965). As indicated by Mukai et al. (1972), the value of τ calculated by this method involves certain assumptions and approximations. Thus, although the value may not be absolute, the value provides a useful measure of relative mobility. A simple definition of τ is the average time required for a spin label undergoing Brownian motion to rotate through a significant arc. Large values of τ reflect lower rates of molecular rotation of the spin label. The spin label attached to the nucleotide has a rotational correlation time of 0.12 nsec in contrast to the free spin label that has a correlation time of 0.025 nsec.

Interaction of Vancomycin and Spin-labeled UDP-MurNAc-pentapeptide

As a model for studying immobilization of the spin label, we have examined the complex formed between vancomycin and spin-labeled UDP-MurNAc-pentapeptide. Vancomycin is an inhibitor of the biosynthesis of peptidoglycan (Jordan and Reynolds, 1967). The mechanism of action of this antibiotic is related to its ability to complex with D-alanyl-D-alanine moieties that are present at various phases of polymer synthesis (Perkins and Nieto, 1974). The antibiotic complexes with the terminal D-alanyl-D-alanine moiety of UDP-MurNAc-pentapeptide. UDP-MurNAc-tetrapeptide and UDP-MurNAc-tripeptide do not complex with vancomycin (Perkins, 1969). Recently these specificity studies were correlated with the inhibitory action of vancomycin on in vitro peptidoglycan formation with membrane fragments from Gaffkya homari (Hammes and Neuhaus, submitted). Vancomycin inhibits the synthesis of peptidolgycan with UDP-MurNAc-pentapeptide as the substrate but not with either UDP-MurNAc-tetrapeptide or -tripeptide.

Complexation with the antibiotic (Equation 1) results in isotropic broadening of the nitroxide spectrum (Figure 4). The rotational correlation time

$$\text{UDP-MurNAc-(Tempyo-}\epsilon\text{N)-pentapeptide} + \text{Vancomycin} \quad \rightleftharpoons \quad (1)$$

$$\text{UDP-MurNAc-(Tempyo-}\epsilon\text{N)-pentapeptide} \cdot \text{Vancomycin}$$

increases from 0.13 nsec to 0.35 nsec. Ristocetin, whose mode of action is similar to that of vancomycin (Wallas and Strominger, 1963), results in a similar immobilization of the spin label. Antibiotics such as bacitracin (Sievert and Strominger, 1967) and moenomycin (Hammes and Neuhaus, in press) that inhibit peptidoglycan synthesis by other mechanisms do not complex with the nucleotide and, thus, do not result in the immobilization of the spin label.

Immobilization of the spin-labeled UDP-MurNAc-pentapeptide by vancomycin is a function of the antibiotic concentration (Figure 5). In this graph the abcissa represents the moles of vancomycin per mole of spin-labeled UDP-MurNAc-pentapeptide. The ordinate represents the difference in the rotational correlation time with and without vancomycin. From these data a dissociation constant of 8.8×10^{-6} M was calculated assuming a molecular weight of 1750 and a 1:1 stoichiometry. For comparison, Nieto and Perkins (1971) established the dissociation constant of the vancomycin· UDP-MurNAc-Ala-DGlu-Dap-DAla-DAla complex to be 1.4×10^{-6} M. The reversibility of vancomycin binding to

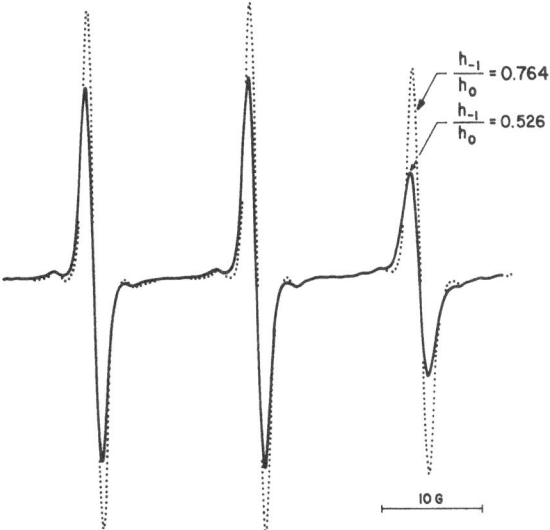

$\dfrac{h_{-1}}{h_0} = 0.764$

$\dfrac{h_{-1}}{h_0} = 0.526$

10 G

Figure 4.   Complex formation between vancomycin and spin-labeled UDP-
             MurNAc-pentapeptide (Johnston and Neuhaus, unpublished observ-
             ations). The spectrum of UDP-MurNAc-(Tempyo-ϵN)-pentapeptide
             is $\cdots\cdots$ and the spectrum for the complex is ———. The ratio,
             moles vancomycin/mole UDP-MurNAc-(Tempyo-ϵN)-pentapeptide
             for ——— is 5 and the concentration of spin-labeled nucleotide is
             2.1 x 10^{-5} M. The ratios of the peak heights and line width ($m = 0$)
             are used to calculate τ by the method of Stone et al. (1965). For
             all comparative spectra the gain and concentration of spin label are
             identical.

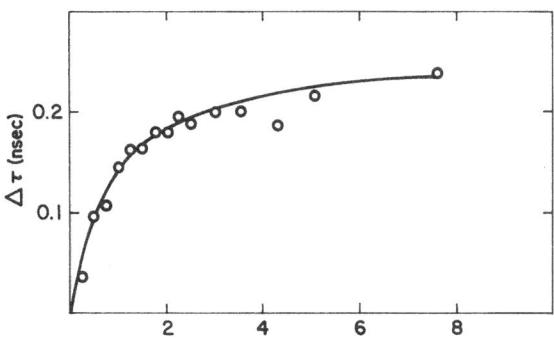

moles Vancomycin/mole UDP-MurNAc-(Tempyo-ϵN)-pentapeptide

Figure 5.   Difference in correlation time as a function of vancomycin concen-
             tration with spin-labeled UDP-MurNAc-(Tempyo-ϵN)-pentapeptide
             (Johnston and Neuhaus, unpublished observations).

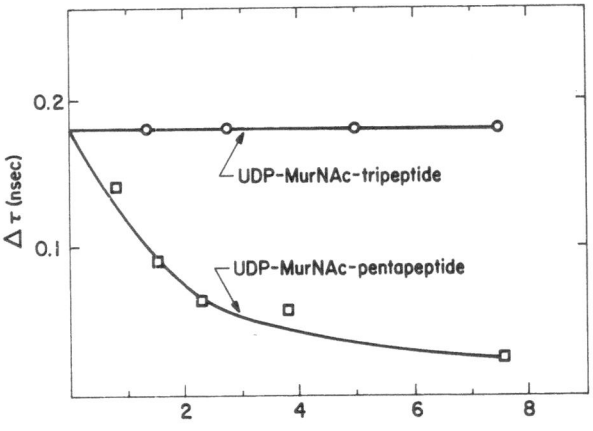

moles UDP-MurNAc-peptide/mole UDP-MurNAc-(Tempyo-εN)-pentapeptide

Figure 6. Reversibility of vancomycin binding to spin-labeled UDP-MurNAc-
pentapeptide (Johnston and Neuhaus, unpublished observations).
Increasing amounts of UDP-MurNAc-peptide were added to a reaction
mixture containing vancomycin and UDP-MurNAc-(Tempyo-εN)-
pentapeptide in a molar ratio of 1.8 to 1.

spin-labeled UDP-MurNAc-pentapeptide is illustrated in Figure 6. In this
experiment varying amounts of UDP-MurNAc-pentapeptide were added to a
solution containing UDP-MurNAc-(Tempyo-εN)-pentapeptide· vancomycin complex. Addition of the unlabeled nucleotide-pentapeptide results in a decrease in
the correlation time whereas addition of the UDP-MurNAc-tripeptide results in
no decrease. Thus, the unlabeled UDP-MurNAc-pentapeptide competes with the
spin-labeled UDP-MurNAc-pentapeptide for the site on vancomycin. The dissociation constant, 5.4×10^{-6} M, for the vancomycin· UDP-MurNAc-pentapeptide
complex was calculated by the competitive displacement technique described by
Klotz (1948).

Interaction of Ristocetin with Spin-labeled UDP-MurNAc-pentapeptide

Ristocetin has a mechanism of action similar to that described for vancomycin (Wallas and Strominger, 1963). There are, however, certain specificity
differences that have been noted (Nieto and Perkins, 1971). For example,
replacement of D-alanine in the C-terminal residue by D-leucine does not result
in a change in the dissociation constant of the diacetyl-Lys-DAla-DAla· ristocetin
complex whereas it has a significant effect on the dissociation of the vancomycin
complex. One of our interests has been concerned with the proposed conformation
of acyl-DAla-DAla as that of penicillin in the reaction catalyzed by the transpeptidase (Tipper and Strominger, 1965). Since vancomycin specifically binds
the acyl-DAla-DAla of the peptide, it is possible that it might also bind penicillin.
As illustrated in Figure 7, however, benzylpenicillin lacks the ability to compete
with the spin-labeled UDP-MurNAc-pentapeptide for the binding site on vancomycin. On the other hand, benzylpenicillin does have the ability to compete with

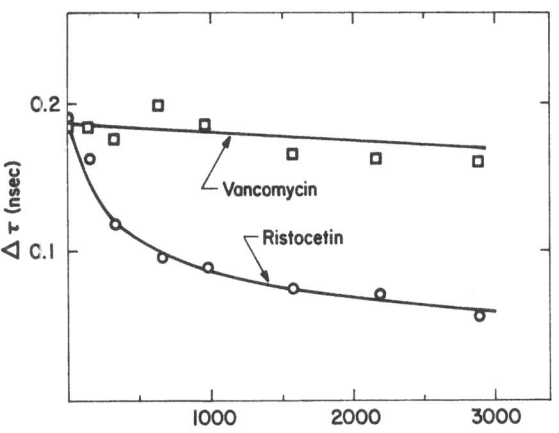

moles Penicillin/mole UDP-MurNAc-(Tempyo-εN)-pentapeptide

Figure 7.   Displacement of the spin-labeled nucleotide from the ristocetin
complex by benzylpenicillin (Johnston and Neuhaus, unpublished
observations). Increasing amounts of benzylpenicillin were added
to the vancomycin complex (□-□) and the ristocetin complex (○-○).
For the ristocetin complex the ratio is 1.8:1 and for the vancomycin complex the ratio is 2:1.

the spin-labeled UDP-MurNAc-pentapeptide for the acyl-DAla-DAla binding site
on ristocetin (Figure 7). The dissociation constant is 3.1×10^{-2} M. For comparison, the dissociation constant of the ristocetin· UDP-MurNAc-(Tempyo-εN)-
pentapeptide complex is 5.1×10^{-5} M. These results are consistent with the
lower specificity for the C-terminal residue observed by Nieto and Perkins (1971)
for ristocetin-peptide complexes. Thus, the methodology described in this section provides a useful probe for further defining the acyl-DAla-DAla binding site
of vancomycin and ristocetin.

Phospho-MurNAc-pentapeptide Translocase

Phospho-MurNAc-pentapeptide translocase (Reaction 1, Figure 1) catalyzes the transfer of phospho-MurNAc-pentapeptide from UDP-MurNAc-pentapeptide to undecaprenyl-phosphate according to Equation 2.

$$\text{UDP-MurNAc-pentapeptide + undecaprenyl-phosphate} \xrightleftharpoons{\text{Mg}^{2+}\ \text{K}^+}$$

(2)

undecaprenyl-diphosphate-MurNAc-pentapeptide + UMP

In addition, the translocase catalyzes the exchange of [^{3}H]UMP with the UMP
moiety of UDP-MurNAc-pentapeptide (Equation 3).

$$\text{UDP-MurNAc-pentapeptide + [}^3\text{H]UMP} \xrightleftharpoons{\text{Mg}^{2+}\ \text{K}^+}$$

(3)

[^{3}H]UDP-MurNAc-pentapeptide + UMP

This enzyme also utilizes the spin-labeled UDP-MurNAc-pentapeptide in the exchange reaction (Table 1). At low substrate concentrations, the apparent first-order rate constant, R_{max}/K_m, for the spin-labeled nucleotide is 0.35 of that for UDP-MurNAc-pentapeptide. At high substrate concentrations, the rate of exchange is virtually identical for the two substrates. Substitutions involving amino acid residue 3 do not markedly affect activity. For example, the substitution of diaminopimelic acid for lysine decreases the maximum rate of exchange by only 28%. As shown by Dr. Swenson in our laboratory, the UDP-MurNAc-hexapeptide has a maximum rate of exchange very similar to that of unmodified UDP-MurNAc-pentapeptide. Thus, acylation of the ϵ-NH$_2$ with L-alanine does not affect the activity. From these results acylation of the ϵ-amino group with the spin label does not perturb the system to a great extent. The transfer of spin-labeled phospho-MurNAc-pentapeptide to undecaprenyl-phosphate results in the formation of spin-labeled undecaprenyl-diphosphate-MurNAc-pentapeptide. The resulting nitroxide spectrum has been isotropically broadened with a corresponding rotational correlation time of 0.54 nsec (Figure 8). The type of broadening is similar to that observed for the vancomycin spin-labeled nucleotide complex. The spin-labeled undecaprenyl-diphosphate-MurNAc-pentapeptide has isotropically broadened spectrum similar to that for spin-labeled UDP-MurNAc-pentapeptide in a 50% glycerol solution.

Incubation of undecaprenyl-diphosphate-MurNAc-pentapeptide associated with membrane fragments with UMP results in the formation of UDP-MurNAc-pentapeptide (Struve et al., 1966). Incubation of the spin-labeled lipid intermediate attached to membranes with UMP results in isotropic sharpening of the spectrum. The value of 0.15 nsec for τ is identical to that observed for spin-labeled UDP-MurNAc-pentapeptide. This is consistent with the reverse transfer reaction.

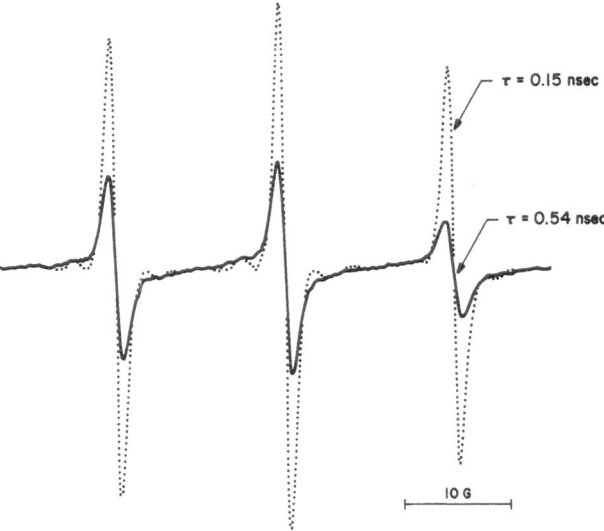

Figure 8.   Spectrum of undecaprenyl-diphosphate-MurNAc-(Tempyo-$\epsilon\underline{N}$)-pentapeptide (——) and reaction mixture after addition of U$\overline{M}$P ($\cdots\cdots$) (Johnston and Neuhaus, unpublished observations).

Table 1

Specificity of phospho-MurNAc-pentapeptide translocase

S. aureus Copenhagen

Substrate	R_{max}	K_m	R_{max}/K_m
		μM	$min^{-1} \times 10^3$
UDP-MurNAc-Ala-DGlu-Lys-DAla-DAla [1]	4.9	20	25
UDP-MurNAc-Ala-DGlu-Lys-DAla [1]	6.0	58	10
UDP-MurNAc-Ala-DGlu-Lys [1]	0.3	180	0.17
UDP-MurNAc-Ala-DGlu-mDap-DAla-DAla [1]	3.6	22	16
UDP-MurNAc-Ala-DGlu-Lys-DAla-DAla [2] NH Ala	4.5	18	25
UDP-MurNAc-Ala-DGlu-Lys-DAla-DAla [3] NH C=O (nitroxide ring structure)	4.6	52	8.8

[1] Hammes and Neuhaus, 1974.

[2] Swenson, 1974.

[3] Johnston and Neuhaus, unpublished results.

Interaction of Vancomycin and Spin-labeled Undecaprenyl-diphosphate-MurNAc-pentapeptide

With the available methodology (Nieto and Perkins, 1971), it has been impossible to study the interaction of undecaprenyl-diphosphate-MurNAc-pentapeptide associated with the membrane and vancomycin. A knowledge of the dissociation constant of this complex may provide a clue to the primary site of action of this antibiotic. Secondly, it is important to know whether the lipid intermediate is accessible to the antibiotic when attached to the membrane. As illustrated in Figure 9, the addition of vancomycin to membranes labeled with phospho-MurNAc-(Tempyo-ϵN)-pentapeptide results in a decrease in the rotational correlation time. From these data a dissociation constant of $6\pm2 \times 10^{-5}$ $\underline{M}$ is estimated. Thus, the spin-labeled intermediate is accessible to vancomycin. For comparison, the dissociation constant of the UDP-MurNAc-(Tempyo-ϵN)-pentapeptide· vancomycin is 8.8×10^{-6} $\underline{M}$.

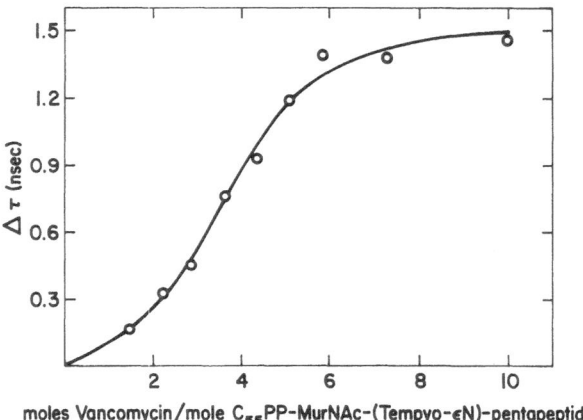

moles Vancomycin/mole C$_{55}$PP-MurNAc-(Tempyo-ϵN)-pentapeptide

Figure 9.   Difference in correlation time as a function of vancomycin concentration with spin-labeled undecaprenyl-diphosphate MurNAc-pentapeptide (Johnston and Neuhaus, unpublished observations).

Biosynthesis of Spin-labeled Peptidoglycan

Since isolated membranes from Staphylococcus aureus Copenhagen do not catalyze a high rate of peptidoglycan synthesis in vitro, the peptidoglycan synthesizing system from Gaffkya homari (Hammes and Neuhaus, 1974) was used to synthesize peptidoglycan. The requirements for glycan synthesis by membrane fragments from G. homari are illustrated in Table 2. The incorporation N-acetyl[^{14}C]glucosamine into peptidoglycan requires UDP-MurNAc-pentapeptide and is stimulated by the addition of NH$_4^+$, Mg^{2+}, and ATP. When UDP-MurNAc-pentapeptide is replaced by spin-labeled UDP-MurNAc-pentapeptide, 128 pmoles of lysozyme sensitive polymer is synthesized in 15 min. The requirement for

Table 2

Requirements for [^{14}C]GlcNAc incorporation into peptidoglycan in G. homari

Additions	Incorporation	
	UDP-MurNAc-pentapeptide [1]	UDP-MurNAc-(Tempyo-εN)-pentapeptide [2]
	pmoles/15 min	
Complete	170	128
-UDP-MurNAc-peptide	6	4
-NH$_4^+$	162	85
-Mg^{2+}	3	2
-ATP	5	2
+Lysozyme	2	4

[1] Hammes and Neuhaus, in press.

[2] Johnston and Neuhaus, unpublished observations.

The reaction mixture contained: 3.0×10^{-5} M UDP-MurNAc-peptide, 3.8×10^{-4} M UDP-[^{14}C]GlcNAc (11.9 cpm/pmole); 0.05 M MgCl$_2$; 8.3×10^{-3} M NH$_4$Cl; 0.21 M KCl; 6.7×10^{-3} M ATP; 0.05 M Tris-HCl; pH 8.0; membrane fragments (94 μg of membrane protein); 250 μg benzylpenicillin per ml in a total volume of 60 μl. Lysozyme (300 μg) was added to a complete reaction mixture after terminating synthesis at 15 min. and incubated for 1 hr. at 37°. The amount of peptidoglycan was determined by the method described by Hammes and Neuhaus (in press).

ATP and the stimulation by ammonium ions is consistent with the amidation of the α-carboxyl group of the glutamic acid residue (Reaction 3, Figure 1). The specificity of peptidoglycan synthesis for six nucleotides is shown in Table 3. At low substrate concentration, the apparent first-order rate constant, V_{max}/K_m of the spin-labeled nucleotide is 0.45 of that for UDP-MurNAc-pentapeptide. At high substrate concentrations the maximum velocity is also 0.45 of that observed for the unmodified nucleotide. As observed for phospho-MurNAc-pentapeptide

Table 3

Specificity of peptidoglycan synthesis

Gaffkya homari

Substrate	V_{max} [4]	K_m	$\dfrac{V_{max}/K_m}{10^6}$
		μM	
UDP-MurNAc-Ala-DGlu-Lys-DAla-DAla[1]	270	57	4.7
UDP-MurNAc-Ala-DGlu-Lys-DAla [1]	200	77	2.6
UDP-MurNAc-Ala-DGlu-Lys [1]	22	74	0.3
UDP-MurNAc-Ala-DGlu-mDap-DAla-DAla [1]	180	67	2.7

UDP-MurNAc-Ala-DGlu-Lys-DAla-DAla [2]
  —NH
   —Ala
	200	55	3.6

UDP-MurNAc-Ala-DGlu-Lys-DAla-DAla [3]
  —NH
   —C=O 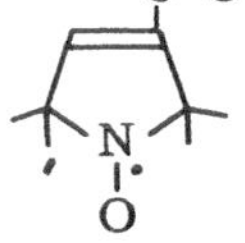
	117	54	2.1

[1] Hammes and Neuhaus, in press.

[2] Swenson, 1974.

[3] Johnston and Neuhaus, unpublished observations.

[4] V_{max} = pmoles/94 μg per min.

translocase (Hammes and Neuhaus, 1974), modifications of amino acid residue 3 do not radically affect the activity of the system. For example, acylation of the ε-amino group of lysine with L-alanine decreases the maximum velocity only 25%. Frequently the introduction of spin labels as a probe in biological systems perturbs the system it is meant to study. However, in the case of both phospho-MurNAc-pentapeptide translocase and the peptidoglycan synthesizing system, the introduction of this bulky substituent does not dramatically affect the system under observation.

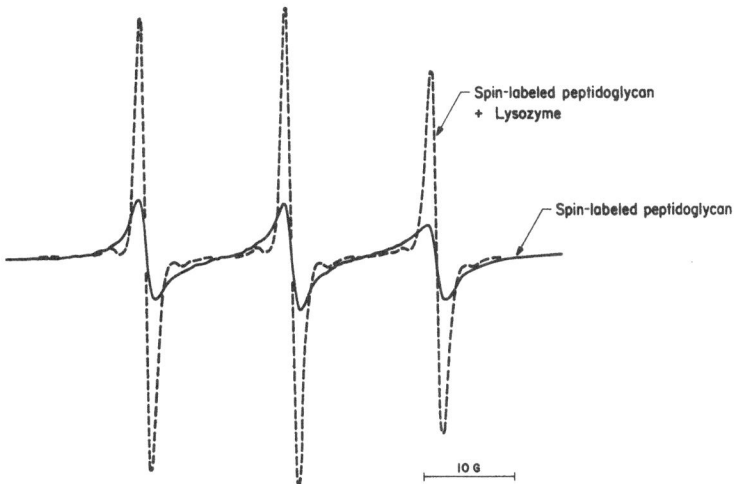

Figure 10.   Spectrum of spin-labeled peptidoglycan (———) and lysozyme degradation products (·····) (Johnston and Neuhaus, unpublished observations). The spin-labeled peptidoglycan (membrane-bound) was synthesized according to procedures similar to those described by Hammes and Neuhaus (in press).

The ESR spectrum of spin-labeled peptidoglycan is shown in Figure 10. This spectrum has a unique line-broadening characteristic of nitroxide-nitroxide interactions. Such a spectrum is frequently observed when there is a high concentration of spin-label (Jost and Griffith, 1972). Since every lysine residue in the in vitro synthesized peptidoglycan is acylated with the spin label, nitroxide-nitroxide interaction would appear to play a role in determining the shape of the spectrum. Because of the complex nature of the spectrum, τ can not be calculated. Further analysis may allow an estimation of the physical separation of the nitroxide labels. Incubation of the spin-labeled peptidoglycan with lysozyme results in marked sharpening of the spectrum (Figure 10). The spin-labeled degradation products have a mobility similar to that for spin-labeled UDP-MurNAc-pentapeptide. In addition, nitroxide-nitroxide interaction can not be observed. Addition of vancomycin to spin-labeled peptidoglycan results in the pronounced immobilization of the nitroxide label (Figure 11). Thus, as in the case of the lipid intermediate, the spin-labeled peptide is accessible to the antibiotic.

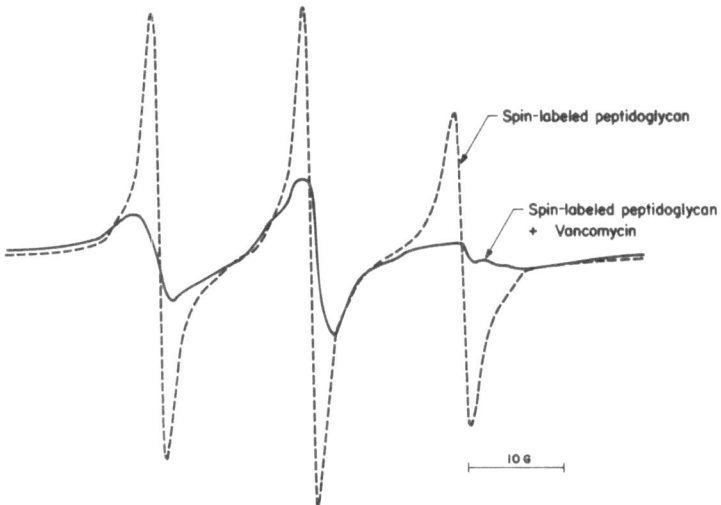

Figure 11.   Complex formation between vancomycin and spin-labeled peptidoglycan (Johnston and Neuhaus, unpublished observations).

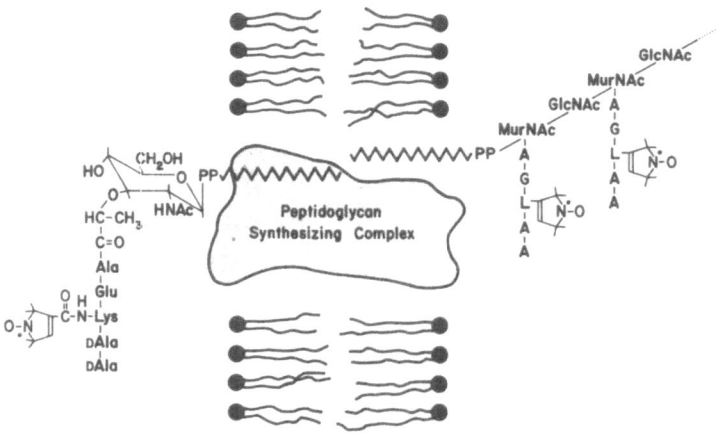

Figure 12.   Schematic representation of peptidoglycan synthesizing complex.

Summary

In conclusion, we have synthesized a spin-labeled precursor that can be used to probe the three phases of peptidoglycan synthesis (Figure 12). The inter-action of spin-labeled UDP-MurNAc-pentapeptide with vancomycin and ristocetin is a model for immobilization of the probe. The transfer of spin-labeled phospho-MurNAc-pentapeptide to membranes resulted in spin-labeled lipid intermediate whose spectrum indicated that it was weakly immobilized relative to spin-labeled UDP-MurNAc-pentapeptide. Interaction of the lipid intermediate with vancomycin indicated the accessibility of the intermediate to the antibiotic. The synthesis of spin-labeled peptidoglycan was accomplished and its interaction with vancomycin was demonstrated. Thus, we have described a highly sensitive probe that can be easily detected in our bacterial membranes. In addition, these enzyme systems will provide a variety of potentially useful substrates. For example, spin-labeled peptidoglycan is an excellent substrate for lysozyme. With this methodology it is felt that we have a probe to analyze some of the dynamics of the translocation processes involved in the synthesis of the extracellular polymer. In particular, the role of the membrane in the assembly process may be better understood.

Acknowledgments

We thank Sue Ellen Goyer for excellent technical assistance and Dr. John C. Swenson for helpful discussions. The research is supported in part by grant AI-04615 from the National Institute of Allergy and Infectious Diseases. We thank Dr. Otto K. Behrens, Lilly Research Laboratories, and Dr. Eugene L. Woroch, Abbott Laboratories, for generous samples of vancomycin and ristocetin, respectively. We thank Professor Brian M. Hoffman for the spin-labeling reagent. W. P. H. was a visiting scholar and recipient of a fellowship from the Deutsche Forschungsgemeinschaft. Present address, Botanisches Institut der Universitat München, München, Germany. H. A. L., present address, Gillette Research Institute, Rockville, Maryland.

References

Ghuysen, J.-M. and G. D. Shockman: Biosynthesis of peptidoglycan, In L. Leive (Editor), Bacterial Membranes and Walls, vol. 1, p. 37-130. Marcel Dekker, Inc., New York (1973).

Hammes, W. P. and F. C. Neuhaus: On the specificity of phospho-$\underline{N}$-acetylmuramyl-pentapeptide translocase: the peptide subunit of uridine diphosphate-$\underline{N}$-acetylmuramyl-pentapeptide. J. Biol. Chem. 249, 3140-3150 (1974).

Hammes, W. P. and F. C. Neuhaus: Biosynthesis of peptidoglycan in Gaffkya homari: role of the peptide subunit of UDP-MurNAc-pentapeptide. J. Bacteriol. in press.

Hammes, W. P. and F. C. Neuhaus: On the mechanism of action of vancomycin: inhibition of peptidoglycan synthesis in Gaffkya homari. Submitted for publication. Antimicrobial Agents and Chemotherapy.

Johnston, L. S. and F. C. Neuhaus, unpublished observations (1974).

Jost, P. and O. H. Griffith: Electron spin resonance and the spin labeling method, In C. Chignell (Editor), Methods in Pharmacology, vol. 2, p. 223-276. Appleton-Century-Crofts, New York (1972).

Jordan, D. C. and P. E. Reynolds: Vancomycin, In D. Gottlieb and P. D. Shaw (Editors), Antibiotics: mechanism of action, vol. 1, p. 102-116. Springer-Verlag, Heidelberg (1967).

Klotz, I. M., H. Triwush, F. M. Walker: The binding of organic ions by proteins. Competition phenomena and denaturation effects. J. Amer. Chem. Soc. 70, 2935-2941 (1948).

Matsuhashi, M., C. P. Dietrich, J. L. Strominger. Incorporation of glycine into the cell wall glycopeptide in Staphylococcus aureus: role of sRNA and lipid intermediates. Proc. Nat. Acad. Sci. U.S.A. 54, 587-594 (1965).

Mukai, K., C. M. Lang, D. B. Chesnut: A spin label investigation of some model membrane systems. Chem. Phys. Lipids 9, 196-216 (1972).

Nieto, M. and H. Perkins: Modifications of the acyl-D-alanyl-D-alanine terminus affecting complex-formation with vancomycin. Biochem. J. 123, 789-803 (1971).

Perkins, H. R.: Specificity of combination between mucopeptide precursors and vancomycin or ristocetin. Biochem. J. 111, 195-205 (1969).

Perkins, H. R. and M. Nieto: The chemical basis for the action of the vancomycin group of antibiotics. Annals of the New York Academy of Science 235, 348-363 (1974).

Siewert, G. and J. L. Strominger: Bacitracin: an inhibitor of the dephosphorylation of lipid pyrophosphate, an intermediate in biosynthesis of the peptidoglycan of bacterial cell walls. Proc. Nat. Acad. Sci. U.S.A. 57, 767-773 (1967).

Stone, T. J., T. Buckman, P. L. Nordio, H. M. McConnell: Spin-labeled biomolecules, Proc. Nat. Acad. Sci. U.S.A. 54, 1010-1017 (1965).

Struve, W. G., R. K. Sinha, F. C. Neuhaus: On the initial stage in peptidoglycan synthesis. Phospho-N-acetylmuramyl-pentapeptide translocase (uridine monophosphate). Biochemistry 5, 82-93 (1966).

Swenson, J. C.: Isolation, characterization, and possible function of a new peptidoglycan precursor [UDP-N-acetylmuramyl-alanyl-γ-D-glutamyl-lysyl-(ε-alanyl)-D-alanyl-D-alanine] from Staphylococcus aureus Copenhagen, Ph.D. thesis, Northwestern University (1974).

Tipper, D. J. and J. L. Strominger: Mechanism of action of penicillins: a proposal based on their structural similarity to acyl D-alanyl-D-alanine. Proc. Nat. Acad. Sci. U.S.A. 54, 1133-1141 (1965).

Wallas, C. H. and J. L. Strominger: Ristocetins, inhibitors of cell wall synthesis in Staphylococcus aureus. J. Biol. Chem. 238, 2264-2266 (1963).

Enzyme Inhibitors as Antimicrobial Agents

J. J. Burchall

The majority of our useful chemotherapeutic agents are not the product of deliberate and rational design. Most new antimicrobial agents discovered during the last 30 years have been isolated from the growth medium of filamentous fungi and *Actinomycetes*. The search for new compounds has been largely empirical with the main effort directed toward further exploitation of the unique synthetic abilities of the organisms in the *Penicillium* and *Streptomyces* group. A major advance in the rational design of antimicrobials was made in 1959 when it was discovered that the growth medium of *Penicillium* could be manipulated so that the organism produced 6-aminopenicillanic acid rather than the entire penicillin molecule (Batchelor *et al.* 1959). This opportunity for partial synthesis of novel penicillins was exploited skillfully by pharmaceutical chemists and compounds appeared with a variety of useful new properties (acid stability, ß-lactamase resistance).

In spite of these early successes, the role of the enzymologist during this period was restricted essentially to drug modification and to studies aimed at elucidating the mechanism of action of the antibiotics at the molecular level. This situation began to change in the early 1950's when Hitchings and his co-workers (1952) began studies which eventually led to synthesis of selective inhibitors of enzymes vital to bacterial growth. These studies led also to an appreciation of the problems that must be solved if an enzyme inhibitor is to be used as an effective antimicrobial agent. Sufficient studies have now been conducted with enzyme inhibitors to allow some generalization of the properties that are most important in this respect. (1) The compound must inhibit a pathway present in the microbe without interference with an apparently identical pathway that may be present in its host. (2) The compound must achieve sufficient intracellular concentrations in relation to its affinity for its target enzyme. (3) It must prevent the synthesis of a vital compound for which no alternative source or substitute is available to the parasite.

The property of selective inhibition is best illustrated by inhibitors of folate biosynthesis and function. The target of these inhibitors, the folate pathway, is shown in Figure 1. Most bacteria are unable to use exogenous sources of folate and must synthesize the vitamin *de novo* from pteridine, pABA, and glutamate. This synthetic capability is lacking in mammals and human needs for folates are satisfied either by folic acid or, more usually, by derivatives (*i.e.* N^5CH_3THFA) found in plant foods which carry a one-carbon adduct and are reduced to the tetrahydro level. The sulfonamide drugs are structural analogs of p-ABA and competitively inhibit dihydropteroate synthetase which condenses a pteridine precursor and p-ABA. Since dihydropteroate synthetase is not present in mammals, the bacteria are inhibited without concomitant toxicity to the host.

FOLATE PATHWAYS IN
BACTERIA AND MAN

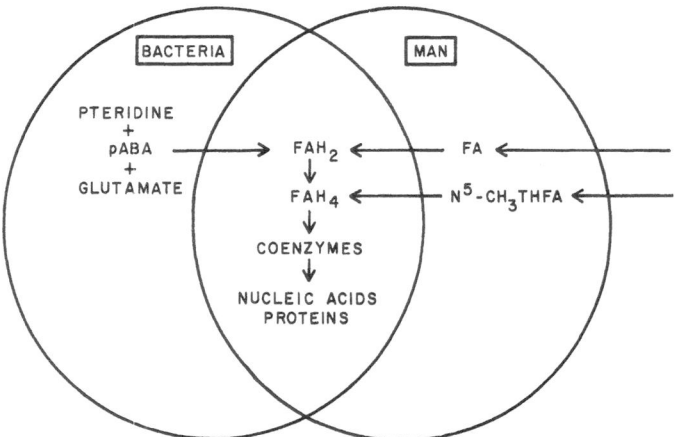

Figure 1.   Folate pathways in bacteria and man.

Sulfonamides are "ideal" drugs in the sense that they inhibit enzymes unique
to bacteria (Woods 1940).   However, as shown in Figure 1, there are a variety of
common reactions that are catalyzed by both bacterial and mammalian enzymes that
are essential to these cells.   For example, dihydrofolate reductase catalyzes the
reduction of dihydrofolate (FAH_2) to tetrahydrofolate (FAH_4) which in turn acts
as a carrier of one-carbon groups for purine, pyrimidine, and amino acid synthesis.   However, during the biosynthesis of thymidylate, tetrahydrofolate also acts
as a reductant and is oxidized back to the dihydro level (Figure 2).   As a result
of this reaction, the function of dihydrofolate reductase becomes critically

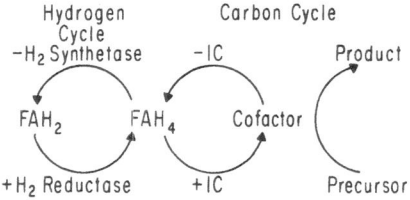

Figure 2.   Hydrogen and carbon cycles within the folate pathway.

important since it must reduce one mole of dihydrofolate for every mole of thymidylate formed.   For this reason, it is clear that inhibition of the reductase
would be injurious to the bacteria cell, but toxicity to the host would also seem
likely.

A number of compounds synthesized by Hitchings *et al*. have been shown to act
as "anti-folic" agents.   The toxicity of these compounds was eliminated by folate
coenzymes (folinic acid) but not by folic acid (FA).   These compounds showed

selective activity against bacteria and protozoa (Hitchings and Burchall, 1965). Although these results suggested a difference in bacteria and mammalian receptors, the possibility remained that differences in permeability or drug metabolism could be responsible for the observed differences among species. In order to document the *locus* of action of these compounds, dihydrofolate reductase was purified from several species of bacteria, from protozoa and human liver. The quantity of each of several potent selective inhibitors required for 50% inhibition of each reductase was determined. The results are shown in Table 1. Methotrexate (MTX), an extremely toxic inhibitor, was shown to bind strongly to all of the enzymes tested. However, the binding of the other three inhibitors was highly selective. Pyrimethamine is an antimalarial compound whose potency appears to be due to its tight binding to the malarial reductase illustrated in this case by the enzyme from *P. berghei*. Trimethoprim (TMP) is a potent antimicrobial agent with very low toxicity for mammalian systems. This selectivity is reflected in the very tight binding of the drug to the bacterial reductase and its poor affinity for the enzyme from human liver (Burchall and Hitchings, 1965). The degree to which selectivity can be manipulated is illustrated by the binding of the dihydrotriazine (DHT). This compound has a very high affinity for the mammalian enzyme but binds poorly to bacterial enzymes. It has been observed that this compound has no antibacterial activity and is highly toxic for rodents.

When more extensive series of compound were examined for the binding to reductases, different groups of bacteria and protozoa could be grouped on this basis alone. In addition, when the antibacterial activity and the affinity for dihydrofolate reductase of a series of compounds were plotted, a linear relation between these values was observed. This is an important relationship since it allows MIC values to be predicted on the basis of enzymatic data. Recently attempts were made to find additional *loci* in the folate pathway which trimethoprim might inhibit (Burchall 1973). Thymidylate synthetase, serine hydroxymethylase, methylene tetrahydrofolate dehydrogenase, and cyclohydrolase were all unaffected by trimethoprim at 1×10^{-4}M.

Table 1. Comparative binding of dihydrofolate reductases from various species.

Species	Concentration ($\times 10^{-8}$M) for 50% inhibition			
	MTX	PYR	TMP	DHT
E. coli	0.1	250	0.5	65,000
S. aureus	0.02	300	1.5	50,000
human liver	0.2	180	30,000	55
P. berghei	0.07	0.05	7.0	0.8

MTX - 2,4-diamino-N^{10}-methylpteroylglutamate (methotrexate)

PYR - 2,4-diamino-5-p-chlorophenyl-6-ethylpyrimidine (pyrimethamine)

TMP - 2,4-diamino-5-(3',4',5'-trimethoxybenzyl)pyrimidine (trimethoprim)

DHT - 1-(p-butylphenyl)-1,2-dihydro-2,2-dimethyl-4,6-diamino-s-triazine

Studies of the spectrum of activity of trimethoprim have shown the importance of determining the ability of the target organism to transport the enzyme inhibitor. Trimethoprim has activity against a wide variety of organisms with the notable exception of *Pseudomonas aeruginosa*. Experiments were conducted to determine the mechanism of resistance of this organism to trimethoprim. The possible explanation of this resistance included the inability of the inhibitor to enter the cell, an alteration in the structure of the Pseudomonal reductase, and metabolism of the compound to an inactive form. A variety of experiments were performed to evaluate these hypotheses, and the relevant data are shown in Table 2.

A series of 2,4-diamino pyridopyrimidines substituted in the 6-position were tested for their ability to inhibit growing cultures of *Pseudomonas aeruginosa* and *E. coli* as well as for their affinity to dihydrofolate reductase purified from these organisms. The first 2 columns show the quantity of each drug required for 50% inhibition of the reductases from each organism. In general, the affinity of the compounds increases for both enzymes to a maximum at 4 carbons in

Table 2. Comparison of enzyme binding and MIC values of various compounds against *Ps. aeruginosa* and *E. coli*.

R	50% I concentration (x 10^{-8}M) [1]		MIC (µg/ml) [2]	
	E. coli	*Ps. aeruginosa*	*E. coli*	*Ps. aeruginosa*
H	270	320	>20	>20
methyl	23	85	2.0	125
propyl	2.0	3	0.5	250
sec-butyl	0.9	0.8	0.3	10
amyl	4.0	1.2	0.6	>20
hexyl	0.9	1.4	0.5	>125
heptyl	0.8	1.8	2.0	>125

[1] Concentration of drug required to inhibit the activity of dihydrofolate reductase to 50% of control value.

[2] Minimum concentration of compound required for inhibition of growth in minimal medium.

the side chain and then gradually decreases. The affinity of each compound is almost identical for the two different enzymes. The activity of the compounds against growing cells (last 2 columns) also increases to a maximum seen with the compound containing the *sec*-butyl substituent. Every compound tested showed greater activity against *E. coli* than against *Ps. aeruginosa*. It should also be noted that as enzyme binding becomes somewhat less favorable with the longer carbon chain substituents, the activity of the compounds against *E. coli* diminishes only slightly whereas a rapid loss of activity against *Ps. aeruginosa* is seen (Hitchings *et al.* 1966 a).

We have interpreted these data in the following manner. The reductase of *Ps. aeruginosa* does not differ from the reductase of *E. coli* in respect to its ability to bind a series of potent inhibitors. However, *Ps. aeruginosa* is less permeable than is *E. coli* to each of these compounds and excludes particularly well compounds that have large hydrophobic side chains. For these reasons we conclude that the "resistance" of *Ps. aeruginosa* to inhibitors of dihydrofolate reductase is not due to an altered enzyme but rather to the failure of these compounds to enter the organism in sufficient quantity.

This conclusion is reinforced by a series of studies on the effect of EDTA and various surface active agents on the MIC of various inhibitors tested on the growth of *Ps. aeruginosa*. EDTA has the ability to alter the permeability barrier of many organisms without interfering with the viability of these cells. In one experiment, EDTA (200 µg/ml) increased the inhibitory effect of trimethoprim (60 µg/ml) 4-fold against *Ps. aeruginosa* without causing inhibition when added alone. Moreover, a number of detergents including Tween 85, sodium lauryl sulfate, Triton X-100, and Brij 30 all increased the activity of trimethoprim against *Ps. aeruginosa* (Hitchings *et al.* 1966 b). All of these experiments suggest that metabolism could not be an important mechanism of drug resistance in *Ps. aeruginosa*. It is interesting to note that a similar increase of the activity of trimethoprim was seen also when *E. coli* was used as the test organism. Although the activity was increased to a much lesser degree than seen with *Ps. aeruginosa*, the results indicate that some permeability barrier to trimethoprim exists even with sensitive, Gram-negative bacilli.

The studies of *Ps. aeruginosa* show clearly that if enzyme inhibitors are to succeed as antimicrobial agents they must be able to achieve intracellular concentrations sufficient to saturate their target enzyme. The minimal concentration required for inhibition can be approximated using the values for the inhibition constants (K_i) obtained from kinetic studies with cell-free extracts of the target enzyme. Thus, for the case where the inhibitor is competitive with a substrate, the relation between the velocity of the reaction, concentration of inhibitor, and the affinity of the inhibitor for the enzyme is given by

$$v = \frac{VS}{K_m(1 + I/K_i) + S} \, .$$

If we assume that the substrate for the enzyme is present in concentrations approximately equal to its Michaelis constant (Cleland 1970), it is possible to calculate the effect of various concentrations of the inhibitor on the activity of the enzyme. When the inhibitor concentration is equal to its inhibition constant (K_i), enzyme velocity is 33% of its maximum velicity and 66% of its normal rate. When the inhibitor concentration is raised to 10 x K_i, the reaction velocity drops to 8% of its maximum velocity and 16% of its normal rate. Although it is difficult to predict *a priori* the degree of inhibition of the enzyme required to produce a specific reduction in cell growth rates, one can safely assume that an inhibitor concentration of ~10 x K_i is highly desirable. It may be useful to determine in preliminary experiments whether a candidate inhibitor will have this essential property. Failure to achieve sufficient intracellular levels

may require re-design of the inhibitor in order to decrease hydrophobic interactions with the cell envelope without concomitant loss of hydrophobic interaction with the target enzyme.

It is important to emphasize again that no conclusion regarding permeability
of the cell to a specific inhibitor should be reached without studies of inhibitor-
enzyme binding. For example, even though yeast and other fungi are highly resistant to reductase inhibition, permeability is not the primary problem. Table 3
shows the quantity of each of a series of drugs required to inhibit 50% reductases
isolated from *E. coli* and *S. cerevisiae*. The reductase from the yeast cells is
5,000-fold less sensitive to trimethoprim than is *E. coli*. A decrease in the affinity of the yeast enzyme is seen to a lesser degree with the phenylpyrimidine
and both pyridopyrimidines. On the other hand, the enzyme is more sensitive to
the dihydrotriazine although this compound is too toxic for use in humans (see
Table 2). Clearly these data show the presence in yeast of an altered enzyme
that does not bind inhibitors sufficiently to inhibit cell growth.

Table 3. Binding of various compounds to reductases
from *E. coli* and *S. cerevisiae*.

	50% I concentration (x 10^{-8}M)	
	E. coli	*S. cerevisiae*
TMP	0.5	2,500
PYR	250	1,200
BPP	50	170

TMP - 2,4-diamino-5-(3',4',5'-trimethoxybenzyl)pyrimidine
(trimethoprim)

PYR - 2,4-diamino-5-p-chlorophenyl-6-ethylpyrimidine
(pyrimethamine)

BPP - 2,4-diamino-5-CH_3-6-butylpyrido(2,3-d)pyrimidine

Altered enzymes may in the future play an even larger role in determining
whether enzyme inhibitors can be used as antimicrobial agents. Investigations
have been reported on the mechanism of action of R-factors that confer on *E. coli*
resistance to trimethoprim. Amyes and Smith (1974) reported that R-factor R388
mediated the synthesis in *E. coli* of a new dihydrofolate reductase which was less
susceptible to trimethoprim by 10,000-fold. Sköld and Widh (1974) reported that
R-factor R483 also was responsible for the introduction of a new, resistant reductase into *E. coli*. R-factor R483 also increases total reductase activity
about 7-fold. The appearance of resistance due to R-factors will require that
detailed studies of these new enzymes be undertaken with a view to the design of
new inhibitors that bind to these enzymes.

The third major property that enzyme inhibitors must possess is the capacity
to prevent the synthesis of a vital compound for which no alternative source or
substitute is available to the parasite. In general there are two ways in which

an organism can overcome a block in the synthesis of a vital metabolite. One possibility is that the organism will take up from its environment the metabolite that ordinarily it must synthesize itself. An alternative possibility is that the organisms may be provided with the end products of a pathway and survive even when a vital cofactor on the pathway is missing.

Inhibitors of folate biosynthesis and functions are interesting since they provide specific examples of the first of these reversal mechanisms. Inhibition of the biosynthesis of folic acid by sulfonamides in E. coli can be reversed by the addition to the growth medium of pABA but not of folic acid. Specific uptake systems for folic acid appear to be lacking in most bacteria except for those that have impaired or missing biosynthesis capacity. pABA, on the other hand, is synthesized by E. coli but is also taken up rapidly. Thus small quantities of pABA in medium can effectively interfere with the activity of several 100-fold greater levels of sulfonamide (Hitchings and Burchall, 1965).

The ability to take up a metabolite or vitamin that is also synthesized is a characteristic of many bacteria. Table 4 shows the capacity of E. coli to synthesize and actively concentrate from the medium several important vitamins. Binding proteins implicated in vitamin uptake have been discovered for thiamine (Griffith et al. 1971), riboflavin (Iwashima et al. 1971), and B_{12} (Taylor et al. 1972). All of these vitamins with the important exception of folate are synthesized and concentrated also by this organism. Thus the growth of E. coli can be effectively inhibited by trimethoprim even when the organism is grown in a medium rich in folates. This is not the case with thiamine where as little as 50 mμg/ml of thiamine restores normal growth to organisms whose synthesis of thiamine has been completely blocked with 2-amino-5-hydroxyethylthiazole (Iwashima 1967). Although not studied in detail as yet, it is clear that there are reciprocal compensatory relationships between the rate of endogenous synthesis and the capacity of the cell to transport the vitamin.

Table 4. The ability of E. coli to synthesize and concentrate various vitamins.

	Synthesis	Active Uptake
Folate	+	−
Riboflavin	+	+
Thiamine	+	+
B_{12}	+	+

An alternative means of reducing or eliminating the activity of an enzyme inhibitor is to supply to the organism end products of the inhibited pathway. Koch and Burchall (1971) showed that the inhibition of the growth of E. coli in minimal medium could be reversed by the addition of thymidine, ribonucleosides, and amino acids. No reversal occurred in the absence of thymidine, and even routine susceptibility testing of trimethoprim was made impossible if thymidine was present in commercial medium used for testing.

Either of the mechanisms of by-pass or reversal of activity discussed above will effectively prevent an enzyme inhibitor from acting as a chemotherapeutic

agent. If blood or urine contained substantial amounts of thymidine or other reversing agents, the inhibitor would fail. In the case of trimethoprim, substantial antibacterial activity is seen in these fluids and direct assay of thymidine shows that it is either absent or barely detectable. In the case of the
vitamins, little is known of the exact tissue levels of each vitamin, and its
distribution into its various cofactor forms and the success of a potential inhibitor is not likely to be known until it has received preliminary testing in
the infected aminal.

The example of trimethoprim has demonstrated that enzyme inhibitors can be
chemotherapeutic agents provided that they are potent, selective, taken up by
the cell in sufficient quantity, and not subject to by-pass or reversal in the
host. It is becoming increasingly clear that useful enzyme inhibitors cannot be
designed in ignorance of bacterial physiology and in the absence of information
concerning the environment in which the drug will be required to act. None of
these requirements encourage the view that the design of antimicrobial enzyme inhibitors will be easy and inexpensive. However, it is useful to note that the
knowledge we need for design is available or obtainable with our present tools
for investigation, and no major conceptual breakthrough seems to be necessary for
success. It is possible that the increasing expense and difficulty of finding
new active compounds by random screening may result eventually in a preference
for rational design solely on economic grounds.

References

Amyes, S.G.B., and J. T. Smith: R-factor trimethoprim resistance mechanism: an
insusceptible target site. Biochem. Biophys. Research Commun 58, 412-418
(1974).

Batchelor, F. R., F. P. Doyle, J.H.C. Nayler, and G. N. Rolinson: Synthesis of
penicillin: 6-aminopenicillanic acid in penicillin fermentations. Nature 183,
257-258 (1959).

Burchall, J., and G. Hitchings: Inhibitor binding analysis of dihydrofolate reductases from various species. Mol. Pharmacol. 1, 126-136 (1965).

Burchall, J.: Mechanism of action of trimethoprim-sulfamethoxazole--II. J. of
Infect. Dis. 128 supplement, S437-S441 (1973).

Cleland, W. W.: Steady state kinetics in "The Enzymes, Kinetics and Mechanism."
Vol. II, 3rd edition, ed. by P. D. Boyer, 1-65 (1970).

Griffith, T. W., C. Carroway, and F. R. Leach: Vitamin transport in *Escherichia
coli*. Fed. Proc. 30, 363 abs. (1971).

Hitchings, G. H., E. A. Falco, H. Vanderwerff, P. B. Russell, and G. B. Elion:
Antagonists of nucleic acid derivatives VII. 2,4-diaminopyrimidines. J. Biol.
Chem. 199, 43-56 (1952).

Hitchings, G. H., and J. Burchall: Inhibition of folate biosynthesis and function
as a basis for chemotherapy. Advances in Enzymology 27, 417-468, Interscience
Publishers, Inc., New York, N. Y. (1965).

Hitchings, G., J. J. Burchall, and R. Ferone: Comparative enzymology of dihydrofolate reductases as a basis for chemotherapy. III Internat. Pharmacol.
Congress, Abstr. 113, Sao Paulo, Brazil, July 24-30 (1966 a).

Hitchings, G. H., J. J. Burchall, and R. Ferone: The comparative enzymology of dihydrofolate reductase and the design of chemotherapeutic agents. Symp. for Gen. Microbiol. 16, 294-300 (1966 b).

Iwashima, A., and Y. Nose: An *Escherichia coli* mutant resistant to 2-amino-hydroxythiazole. J. Biochemistry 62, 537-542 (1967).

Iwashima, A., A. Matsumura, and Y. Nose: Thiamine binding protein of *Escherichia coli*. J. Bact. 108, 1419-1421 (1971).

Koch, A., and J. Burchall: Reversal of the antimicrobial activity of trimetho-prim by thymidine in commercially prepared media. App. Microbiol. 22, 812-817 (1971).

Sköld, O., and A. Widh: A new dihydrofolate reductase with low trimethoprim sensitivity induced by an R factor mediating high resistance to trimethoprim. J. Biol. Chem. 249, 4324-4325 (1974).

Taylor, R. T., S. A. Norell, and M. L. Hanna: Uptake of cyanocobalamin by *Escherichia coli* B: some characteristics and evidence for a binding protein. Arch. Biochem. Biophys. 148, 366-381 (1972).

Woods, D. D.: The relation of p-aminobenzoic acid to the mechanism of action of sulfanilamide. Brit. J. Exptl. Pathol. 21, 74-90 (1940).

Molecular Mechanism of Action of Rifamycins

Guido R. Hartmann

The discussion of the molecular mechanism of action of a drug always involves three central questions: (i) what is the nature of the receptor of the drug; (ii) what is the action of the receptor bound drug; (iii) what is the structural basis of the specificity of action? In this paper more recent findings on the molecular mechanism of action of rifamycins in relation to the three central questions will be discussed. Previous results have been summarized by Wehrli & Staehelin (1971).

MOLECULAR RECEPTOR OF RIFAMYCIN

To discover the receptor of a drug the hypothesis of a particularly tight and specific physical association has proved to be very useful. An excellent example is the classical investigation of Wehrli *et al.* (1968) of the target of the antibiotic rifamycin in bacterial cells. Using gel filtration these authors proved that this inhibitor, even at a low concentration, forms a very stable complex with the DNA directed RNA polymerase core enzyme (EC 2.7.7.6) of rifamycin sensitive bacteria. No stable complex is formed with the enzyme from rifamycin resistant bacterial mutants indicating the RNA polymerase as the target of this antibiotic. However, this physical method for the detection of the molecular receptor of a drug has also some limitations. They become evident in experiments to specify in more detail the receptor area of the target for rifamycin. Bacterial RNA polymerase core enzyme is a very large protein with a molecular mass of about 400 000 daltons. It consists of two large but not identical protein subunits and two copies of a much smaller polypeptide. Considering the much smaller size of rifamycin one is inclined to assume that only one subunit of the enzyme is the molecular receptor of the drug. To answer this question we have studied in some detail the physical binding of rifampicin to the isolated subunits of RNA polymerase. A rather rapid method is coelectrophoresis in polyacrylamide gels of radioactively labelled rifampicin with the isolated polypeptide. If a stable complex is formed both compounds migrate together in the electric field. We found that neither of the isolated RNA polymerase subunits is able to form a tight complex with rifampicin (Lill & Hartmann, 1973). To prove that the subunits used were not altered or degraded during the isolation procedure they were incubated together to reconstitute active enzyme. The reconstituted RNA polymerase was able to bind rifampicin to the extent of the native enzyme (Lill & Hartmann, 1973). We have to conclude from these experiments that none of the isolated subunits fulfil the conformational requirements necessary for the tight binding of rifampicin. If the antibiotic is bound to only one subunit in the enzyme, this polypeptide acquires its proper conformation for binding only in combination with the other subunits. It is also conceivable that the actual binding site is constituted by more than one subunit. This assumption, however, is less likely as will be shown below. These observations are not unique for rifampicin. Similar findings have been reported for the ribosomal protein which is responsible for the binding of streptomycin to the 30S bacterial ribosome. Here, too, the isolated protein itself cannot bind the drug, in contrast to the complete ribosome (Ozaki *et al.*, 1969).

To overcome these limitations, genetic mutants of bacteria have been proved to be most useful. Many mutants have been discovered which possess an RNA polymerase resistant to rifampicin. Heil & Zillig (1970) have prepared subunits from rifampicin sensitive and resistant *E.coli* RNA polymerase. Using our method for the reconstitution of active enzyme (Lill & Hartmann, 1970) these authors formed intrageneric RNA polymerase hybrids by association of subunits from both *E. coli* strains. Upon hybridization of the second largest subunit derived from a rifampicin resistant *E. coli* strain with the other subunits isolated from sensitive *E. coli* they obtained an enzyme which was resistant to the antibiotic. This experiment indicates that the resistance to rifampicin of *E. coli* resides in the second largest subunit of RNA polymerase. Is this conclusion only true for *E. coli* or does it hold also for RNA polymerase from other bacteria? To answer this question we have studied the action of rifampicin on RNA polymerase from *M.luteus*. This gram-positive organism is taxonomically very different from the gram-negative *E. coli* as is evident from its DNA base ratio (A+T)/(G+C) = 0.39 as compared to that of *E. coli* [(A+T)/(G+C) = 0.99]. We have isolated RNA polymerase subunits from rifampicin resistant and sensitive *M. luteus* strains. When the enzyme is reconstituted from the second largest subunit derived from resistant *M. luteus* RNA polymerase and from the other subunits isolated from sensitive *M. luteus* polymerase the resulting hybrid proved to be resistant to the antibiotic. On the other hand formation of a hybrid from the second largest subunit isolated from a sensitive *M. luteus* polymerase and from the other subunits derived from resistant enzyme led to activity which was inhibited to 50 % by just 2×10^{-7} M rifampicin as was the native sensitive enzyme. Obviously in *M. luteus* as in *E. coli* the second largest RNA polymerase subunit plays a decisive role in the action of rifampicin (Lill, U.I., E.M. Behrendt & G.R. Hartmann, submitted for publication). Similarly to *E. coli*, the isolated second largest subunit of *M. luteus* polymerase cannot bind rifampicin in contrast to the intact core enzyme (Behrendt, E.M. & G.R. Hartmann, unpublished). If the property of rifampicin resistance resides completely in the second largest subunit of RNA polymerase it should be possible to confer rifampicin resistance to a sensitive polymerase by intergeneric incorporation of the second largest subunit derived from a resistant polymerase of a different bacterial species. Consequently we have prepared several active intergeneric RNA polymerase hybrids by a new reconstitution technique from isolated subunits derived from rifampicin resistant and sensitive *E. coli* and *M. luteus* strains. These hybrids were tested for activity in presence of rifampicin. The hybrid consisting of the second largest subunit from resistant *E. coli* and of other subunits from sensitive *M. luteus* was resistant to the inhibitor. When the hybrid was formed from the second largest subunit derived from sensitive *E. coli* and from the other subunits isolated from resistant *M. luteus*, the activity was sensitive to rifampicin (Lill, U.I., E.M. Behrend & G.R. Hartmann, submitted for publication). In this context it is interesting to note that the second largest subunit of *M. luteus* has a molecular mass which is approximately 9 000 daltons smaller than the corresponding *E. coli* subunit. In addition, the overall net charge as determined by electrophoresis is distinctly more negative than that of the *E. coli* subunit. These results clearly demonstrate that rifampicin resistance is associated exclusively with one type of subunit in both bacterial species despite of distinct differences in size and overall charge of this type of subunit.

ACTION OF THE POLYMERASE BOUND RIFAMPICIN

The identification of the polypeptide chain responsible for the action of rifampicin does not lead us to an understanding of the inhibition of RNA synthesis by the drug. Therefore, the binding of rifampicin to RNA polymerase in the presence of template and substrate has been studied. It was found that the enzyme involved in active synthesis does not bind the inhibitor. At the same time no inhibition of the enzymatic activity was observed (Lill & Hartmann, 1973; Eilen & Krakow, 1973). These observations suggest that rifampicin acts prior to RNA chain initiation. In order to define more closely the step in RNA synthesis which is blocked by the antibiotic its binding to RNA polymerase in the presence of DNA only was studied. It was found that the binding of the inhibitor to the enzyme is not eliminated by the template (Neuhoff *et al.*, 1969; Eilen & Krakow, 1973). It may be deduced that the antibiotic acts after association of the enzyme with the template but prior to the addition of substrate. However, this deduction is not conclusive. The determination of the binding of the drug to RNA polymerase is too slow to allow a more precise kinetic analysis of the particular step in RNA synthesis which is blocked by the inhibitor. To detect this step we have incubated RNA polymerase containing an excess of sigma factor with a high concentration of T4 DNA to guarantee the association of all enzyme molecules with strong binding sites of the template. Then 2 µg/ml rifampicin together with substrate was added. Usually, rifampicin at this concentration inhibits the initiation of RNA synthesis in less than 5 seconds whereas initiation of RNA synthesis is a rather slow process under our conditions and takes about 45 seconds for completion. Surprisingly, in this experiment no inhibition by rifampicin was observed (Kerrich-Santo & Hartmann, 1974). This result leads to the conclusion that polymerase bound to DNA is completely protected against rifampicin. How can this finding be reconciled with the lack of any protecting effect of DNA on the binding of the inhibitor to the enzyme? The explanation became evident when RNA polymerase was incubated with template at a low temperature such as 5°C. Again all enzyme molecules became attached to strong binding sites of DNA as was shown by competition experiments with poly[d(A-T)]. If now a mixture of rifampicin and substrate is added at 25°C as in the previous experiment only 50 % protection of RNA synthesis is observed (Kerrich-Santo & Hartmann, 1974). We have to conclude that at the low temperature of incubation of enzyme and template a complex of polymerase and DNA is formed which lacks in part the resistance to rifampicin in contrast to the complex which is formed at 25°C. These results suggest the notion that the complex of RNA polymerase and DNA exists in two different states which are interrelated by a temperature dependent equilibrium:

$$(\text{RNA polymerase-DNA})^{\text{rif.sens.}}_{\text{active}} \rightleftharpoons (\text{RNA polymerase-DNA})^{\text{rif.res.}}_{\text{active}}$$

If this hypothesis (Kerrich-Santo & Hartmann, 1974; Mangel & Chamberlin, 1974) is correct it should be possible to change the rifampicin resistance of the enzyme-DNA complex in a reversible way simply by shifting the incubation temperature of the complex. Indeed, this is observed experimentally. When RNA polymerase and DNA are incubated together at 25°C it takes about 2 minutes before full protection against rifampicin is achieved. Cooling the complex to 5°C decreases the protecting effect at 25°C to 50 % within 2 minutes. Upon warming the complex of enzyme and DNA to 25°C again almost full protection is reached within 2 minutes (Kerrich-Santo & Hartmann, 1974). As a further support for the existence of a conformational change in the complex of polymerase and DNA it should be mentioned that this effect depends on the presence of 0.8 mM Mg^{2+} in the incubation mixture (Kerrich-Santo & Hartmann, 1974). This conformational change does not occur in the presence of rifampicin. Therefore we have to conclude that the molecular mechanism of action of rifampicin bound to the second largest subunit of RNA polymerase is the inhibition of a conformational change in the complex of RNA polymerase and DNA (Kerrich-Santo & Hartmann, 1974).

STRUCTURAL BASIS OF SPECIFICITY OF ACTION

The preceding experiments point to an extremely specific action of rifampicin. In contrast to this notion a surprisingly large number of enzymatic activities is inhibited by rifampicin and closely related compounds at higher concentrations. Well known is the inhibition of vaccinia virus multiplication in cell culture by blocking the viral assembly process (Moss & Rosenblum, 1973). Most spectacular was the observation that even cell transformation by RNA tumor viruses is blocked by rifamycin derivatives. Reverse transcriptase and cellular DNA polymerases are inhibited to a different extent (Gurgo *et al.*, 1971; Calvin *et al.*, 1971; Thompson *et al.*, 1974; Bissell *et al.*, 1974). These observations suggest that one single drug may exert its effect by several mechanisms. A first evidence for this notion is the very different dependence of the effects on drug concentration. Whereas for the inhibition of the bacterial DNA directed RNA polymerase a rifamycin concentration as low as 10^{-8} M is sufficient, much higher concentrations up to 10^{-5} M are required for the other inhibitory activities. Comparison of the efficiency of several rifamycin derivatives has clearly shown that for the antiviral effects the hydrophobic nature of the chemically introduced substituents in the 3-position of the naphthohydroquinone residue of the drug is of greater importance than the characteristic ansa-ring structure. Indeed some of the substituents themselves seem to exhibit antiviral activities (Lancini *et al.*, 1971). Careful investigations by Riva *et al.* (1972) have shown that these effects of the hydrophobic substituents are rather unspecific. They act as inhibitors not only on nucleic acid polymerases but also on transaminases and on alkaline phosphatase. Similarly, the association to proteins is rather unspecific at higher concentrations. This is particularly evident upon inspection of the binding of hydrophobic rifamycin derivatives to rifampicin resistant RNA polymerase from *E. coli*. At higher concentrations more than 200 molecules of the drug are bound to the protein. Nevertheless 30 % of the catalytic activity remain unchanged (Riva *et al.*, 1972).

These observations suggest the following rather general conclusions: (i) a drug may exhibit several mechanisms of action at the molecular level; (ii) these different molecular activities may become apparent at different concentrations; (iii) even at a concentration as low as 10 μg/ml unspecific hydrophobic effects may play an important role for the activity of a drug.

Acknowledgments:
Our own investigations have been supported by the Deutsche Forschungsgemeinschaft and by the Fonds der Chemischen Industrie. The generous
gift of rifampicin by Gruppo Lepetit, Milano, is gratefully acknowledged.

REFERENCES

BISSEL, M.J., C. HATIE, A.N. TISCHLER and M. CALVIN: Preferential
    inhibition of the growth of virus-transformed cells in culture by
    rifazone-8_2, a new rifamycin derivative. Proc. Natl. Acad. Sci.
    USA 71, 2520 - 2524 (1974).
CALVIN, M., U.R. JOSS, A.J. HACKETT and R. OWEN: Effect of rifampicin
    and two of its derivatives on cells infected with Moloney sarcoma
    virus. Proc. Natl. Acad. Sci. USA 68, 1441 - 1443 (1971).
EILEN, E. and J.S. KRAKOW: *Azotobacter vinelandii* RNA polymerase
    XI. Effect of transcription on rifampicin binding. Biochem. Biophys.
    Res. Commun. 55, 282 - 290 (1973).
GURGO, C., R.K. RAY, L. THIRY, and M. GREEN: Inhibitors of the RNA
    and DNA dependent polymerase activities of RNA tumor viruses.
    Nat. New Biol. 229, 111 - 114 (1971).
HEIL, A. and W. ZILLIG: Reconstitution of bacterial DNA-dependent RNA
    polymerase from isolated subunits as a tool for the elucidation of
    the role of the subunits in transcription. FEBS Lett. 11, 165 -
    168 (1970).
KERRICH-SANTO, R.E. and G.R. HARTMANN: Influence of temperature on the
    action of rifampicin on RNA polymerase in presence of DNA.
    Eur. J. Biochem. 43, 521 - 532 (1974).
LANCINI, G., R. CRICCHIO and L. THIRY: Antiviral activity of rifamy-
    cins and N-aminopiperazines. J. Antibiotics 24, 64 - 66 (1971).
LILL, U.I. and G.R. HARTMANN: Reactivation of denatured RNA polymer-
    ase from *E. coli*. Biochem. Biophys. Res. Commun. 39, 930 - 935
    (1970).
LILL, U.I. and G.R. HARTMANN: On the binding of rifampicin to the
    DNA-directed RNA polymerase from *Escherichia coli*. Eur. J. Biochem.
    38, 336 - 345 (1973).
MANGEL, W.F. and M.J. CHAMBERLIN: Studies of RNA chain initiation by
    Escherichia coli RNA polymerase bound to T7 deoxyribonucleic acid.
    III. The effect of temperature on ribonucleic acid chain initia-
    tion and on the conformation of binary complexes. J. Biol. Chem.
    249, 3007 - 3013 (1974).
MOSS, B. and E.N. ROSENBLUM: Protein cleavage and poxvirus morpho-
    genesis: Tryptic peptide analysis of core precursors accumulated
    by blocking assembly with rifampicin. J. Biol. 81, 267 - 269 (1973).
NEUHOFF, V., W.B. SCHILL and H. STERNBACH: Mikro-Disk-elektrophore-
    tische Analyse reiner DNA-abhängiger RNA-polymerase aus *E. coli*.
    III. Hoppe Seyler's Z. physiol. Chem. 350, 335 - 340 (1969).
OZAKI, M., S. MIZUSHIMA and M. NOMURA: Identification and functional
    characterization of the protein controlled by the streptomycin-
    resistant locus in *Escherichia coli*. Nature (Lond.) 222, 333 - 339
    (1969).
RIVA, S., A. FIETTA and L.G. SILVESTRI: Mechanism of action of a
    rifamycin derivative (AF/013) which is active on the nucleic acid
    polymerases insensitive to rifampicin. Biochem. Biophys. Res.
    Commun. 49, 1263 - 1271 (1972).
THOMPSON, F.M., A.N. TISCHLER, J. ADAMS and M. CALVIN: Inhibition of
    three nucleotide polymerases by rifamycin derivatives. Proc. Natl.
    Acad. Sci. USA 71, 107 - 109 (1974).

WEHRLI, W., F. KNÜSEL, K. SCHMID and M. STAEHELIN: Interaction of rifamycin with bacterial RNA polymerase. Proc. Natl. Acad. Sci. USA 61, 667 - 673 (1968).

WEHRLI, W. and M. STAEHELIN: Actions of the rifamycins. Bacteriol. Rev. 35, 290 - 309 (1971).

List of Participants

Editors:

Prof.Dr.med. Jürgen Drews
Head, Department of Bacteriology
and Cell Physiology
Sandoz Forschungsinstitut
Gesellschaft m.b.H.
Brunnerstrasse 59
A-1235 Vienna
Austria

Fred E. Hahn, Ph.D.
Professor and Chief of
Department of Molecular Biology
Department of the Army
Walter Reed Army Institute of Research
Walter Reed Army Medical Center
Washington, D.C. 20012
USA

Active Participants:

Ephraim S. Anderson, M.D., F.R.S.
Professor and Director of
Enteric Reference Laboratory
Public Health Laboratory Service
Colindale Avenue
London NW9 5HT
England

Dr. Gregor Högenauer
Department of Bacteriology
and Cell Physiology
Sandoz Forschungsinstitut Ges.m.b.H.
Brunnerstrasse 59
A-1235 Wien
Austria

James J. Burchall, Ph.D.
Head, Department of Microbiology
The Wellcome Research Laboratories
3030 Cornwallis Road
Research Triangle Park, N.C. 27609
USA

Prof.Dr.rer.nat. Helga Kersten
Dozent, Physiol.-Chem. Institut
Universität Erlangen-Nürnberg
Wasserturmstrasse 5
D-8520 Erlangen
Germany

Royston C. Clowes, Ph.D.
Professor and Head of Biology
University of Texas at Dallas
P.O.Box 688
Richardson, Texas 75080
USA

Albert J. Leo, Ph.D.
Director, Medchem. Project
Pomona College
Seaver Laboratory
Claremont, California 91711
USA

Eric Cundliffe, M.A., Ph.D.
Department of Pharmacology
University of Cambridge
Medical School
Hills Road
Cambridge CB2 2QD
England

Francis C. Neuhaus, Ph.D.
Professor of Chemistry and
Biological Sciences
Northwestern University
Department of Biochemistry
and Molecular Biology
Evanston, Illinois 60201 / USA

Fred E. Hahn, Ph.D.
Professor and Chief of
Department of Molecular Biology
Department of the Army
Walter Reed Army Institute of Research
Walter Reed Army Medical Center
Washington, D.C. 20012
USA

Dr.med. Knud Nierhaus
Max-Planck-Institut
für Molekulare Genetik
Abteilung Wittmann
Ihnestrasse 63-73
D-1 Berlin 33 (Dahlem)
Germany

Prof.Dr. Guido R. Hartmann
Institut für Biochemie
der Universität München
Karlstrasse 23
D-8 München 2
Germany

Dr. Olaf Pongs
Max-Planck-Institut
für Molekulare Genetik
Ihnestrasse 63-73
D-1 Berlin 33 (Dahlem)
Germany

William P. Purcell, Ph.D.
Professor and Director
Drug Design Division
University of Tennessee
Center for the Health Sciences
Memphis, Tennessee 38161
USA

Priv.-Doz.Dr.rer.nat. Joachim K. Seydel
Head, Pharmaz.-Chem. Abt.
Forschungsinstitut Borstel
Institut für Experimentelle
Biologie und Medizin
D-2061 Borstel
Germany

Priv.-Doz.Dr.med. Georg Stöffler
Max-Planck-Institut
für Molekulare Genetik
Abt. Wittmann
Ihnestrasse 63-73
D-1 Berlin 33 (Dahlem)
Germany

David Vazquez, DrSc, DrPharm, PhD, DSc.
Director, Instituto de Biologia Celular
Centro de Investigaciones Biologicas
Velazquez, 144
Madrid-6
Spain

Michael J. Waring, Ph.D.
Department of Pharmacology
University of Cambridge
Medical School
Hills Road
Cambridge CB2 2QD
England

Bernard Weisblum, M.D.
Professor of Pharmacology
The University of Wisconsin Med.Center
Department of Pharmacology
426, North Charter Street
383 Med.Sci.Bldg.
Madison, Wisconsin 53706
USA

List of Authors

Subject Index

A

Acceptor site s. Ribosomal A-Site
Acetyl cholinesterase, inhibitors of
   18-20
— — inhibitors, properties of 20
N-Acetylglucosamine 279
Acetyl-leucyl-pentanucleotide
   195, 254, s.a. CACCA-Leu-Ac
N-Acetyl-muramyl-moiety 278
— —, derivatives of 269-283
   s.a. electron spin resonance
N-Acetyl-phenylalanyl-puromycin 131
Acetyl-phenylalanyl tRNA, s. tRNA
Acridine 77, 99, 109
Acridine orange 96, 99, 102, 104, 106,
   107, 110
Acriflavine 99, 100, 103
Actinomycetes 285
Acyl-D-alanyl-D-alanine 274, 275
Adenine-N⁶-dimethylase of 23S rRNA
   146, 147
Adenosine triphosphate (ATP) 279
S-Adenosyl-methionine 158
Adriamycin 79-81
Affinity labeling, principle of
   118, 179
— — with bromoacetylated p-amino-
   phenylhydrazone of streptomycin
   187, 188
— — with N-bromoacetylpuromycin 185
— — with N-iodoacetylpuromycin 183
— — with N-iodo-[2-¹⁴C]acetyl-
   puromycin 183, 184
— — with monoiodoamphenicol
   179, 254
— — with streptomycin-analogs
   123, 130
D-Alanine 274
L-Alanine 276, 281
D-Alanyl-D-Alanine 272
   s.a. Acyl-D-alanyl-D-alanine
Alkaline phosphatase 298
Althiomycin 173, 208
Amicetin 149, 172, 195
Amino acids 291
— —, synthesis of 286
Aminoacridines 109
Aminoacyl-tRNA, s. tRNA
p-Aminobenzoic acid (p-ABA)
   285, 286, 291
Aminoglycosides 12, 123, 130
2-Amino-5-hydroxyethylthiazole 291
6-Aminopenicillanic acid 285
D-AMP-3 208, s.a. Chloramphenicol
   analogs
Ampicillin 60-63, 69-73, 94, 103-110
— resistance determinant 104, 107

Anisomycin 195, 200, 201, 206, 207, 210
— ³H labeled 198, 202, 204, 208, 210
— binding area 203
Ansa-ring 298
Antibiotics 59, 61, 73, 75, 77, 91, 118
   134, 145, 157, 158, 167, 168, 171
—, determination of sensitivity
   against 153
—, self-defence against 171
Antibodies 125-133
— to ribosomal proteins 117, 124
— to 50S subunit proteins 134
Antifolic agents 286
Antimalarial activity 15, 17, 48
Antimetabolite 10
— hypothesis 3
Antipyrine 82
Atropine 46

B

Bacillus megaterium 169-175
— pumilis 172, 173
— stearothermophilus 122, 136, 151
— subtilis 131, 158-161
— —, mutants of 131
Bacitracin 13, 272
Bacteria, enteropathogenic 99
—, gram-negative 99
Bacteriophage P1 60, 65
— P22 60
— PM2 81, 84
— φX174 80
—, DNA of 81, 84
Base-pairs 77, 78
— —, A·T 82
— —, G·C 77
Benzamidine 51
Benzylpenicillin 274, 275, 279
Berberine 104-107
Berenil 9, 79-82
Bioreceptors 3
Blasticidin S 206, 207
Brij 30 289
N-Bromoacetylpuromycin 185
   s.a. affinity labeling
2-Bromo-4-nitro-N¹-phenylsulfanilamide
   33-35
Bryamycin 167, s.a. thiostrepton
1-(p-Butylphenyl)-1,2-dihydro-2,2-dimethyl
   -4,6-diamino-s-triazine 287
Butyramide 53
Butyrylcholinesterase, inhibition of 21